ITI Treatment Guide
Volume 6

ITI Treatment Guide

Editors:
D. Wismeijer, S. Chen, D. Buser

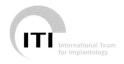

Authors:
J.-G. Wittneben, H. P. Weber

Volume 6

Extended Edentulous Spaces in the Esthetic Zone

Quintessence Publishing Co, Ltd
Berlin, Chicago, London, Tokyo, Barcelona, Beijing,
Istanbul, Milan, Moscow, New Delhi, Paris, Prague,
São Paulo, Seoul, Singapore, Warsaw

German National Library CIP Data

The German National Library has listed this publication in the German National Bibliography. Detailed bibliographical data are available at http://dnb.ddb.de.

© 2012 Quintessence Publishing Co, Ltd
Ifenpfad 2 – 4, 12107 Berlin
www.quintessenz.de

Illustrations: Ute Drewes, CH-Basel,
                    www.drewes.ch
Medical Editing: Dr. Dr. Bernd Stadliner, CH-Zürich
Copyediting: Triacom Dental, D-Barendorf,
                    www.dental.triacom.com
Graphic Concept: Wirz Corporate AG, CH-Zürich
Production: Juliane Richter, D-Berlin
Printing: Bosch-Druck GmbH, D-Landshut,
                    www.bosch-druck.de

Printed in Germany
ISBN: 978-3-86867-141-4

The materials offered in the ITI Treatment Guide are for educational purposes only and intended as a step-by-step guide to treatment of a particular case and patient situation. These recommendations are based on conclusions of the ITI Consensus Conferences and, as such, in line with the ITI treatment philosophy. These recommendations, nevertheless, represent the opinions of the authors. Neither the ITI nor the authors, editors and publishers make any representation or warranty for the completeness or accuracy of the published materials and as a consequence do not accept any liability for damages (including, without limitation, direct, indirect, special, consequential or incidental damages or loss of profits) caused by the use of the information contained in the ITI Treatment Guide. The information contained in the ITI Treatment Guide cannot replace an individual assessment by a clinician, and its use for the treatment of patients is therefore in the sole responsibility of the clinician.

The inclusion of or reference to a particular product, method, technique or material relating to such products, methods, or techniques in the ITI Treatment Guide does not represent a recommendation or an endorsement of the values, features, or claims made by its respective manufacturers.

Some of the manufacturer and product names referred to in this publication may be registered trademarks or proprietary names, even though specific reference to this fact is not made. Therefore, the appearance of a name without designation as proprietary is not to be construed as a representation by the publisher that it is in the public domain.

The tooth identification system used in this ITI Treatment Guide is that of the FDI World Dental Federation.

The ITI Mission is ...

"... to promote and disseminate knowledge on all aspects of implant dentistry and related tissue regeneration through education and research to the benefit of the patient."

Preface

The body of evidence for implant-based dental treatment continues to broaden as more and more clinical research and systematic reviews become available in the peer-reviewed dental literature. Moreover, the widely accepted evidence available for the use of dental implants as the standard of care in numerous clinical situations proves implant therapy to be a safe and efficient treatment option.

However, treatment outcomes depend not only on the level of education, clinical experience, skill, and ability of clinicians but also on their sense of responsibility and ethics. Hence, publications such as the ITI Treatment Guide series are therefore needed to support clinicians in their goal to excel in the field of implant dentistry.

The present Volume 6 of the ITI Treatment Guide series has been compiled to provide clinicians with practice-oriented and evidence-based information about recommended clinical procedures to insert and restore implants in what is possibly the most challenging situation encountered in implant dentistry: extended edentulous spaces in the esthetic zone.

Based in part on the publications that were the results of the Proceedings of the 3rd and 4th ITI Consensus Conferences held in Gstaad (2003) and Stuttgart (2008), this sixth volume in the series of ITI Treatment Guides not only provides an up-to-date analysis of the current literature but also offers an extensive overview of advantages and shortcomings associated with the treatment protocols described. It presents and illustrates eight clinical case studies that follow the guidelines on detailed clinical implant planning as well as prosthetic treatment. The presentations are supplemented by five case reports that focus on the management of complications.

In all respects, the ITI Treatment Guide Volume 6 represents another effort in the mission of the ITI "... to promote and disseminate knowledge on all aspects of implant dentistry to the benefit of the patient."

D. Wismeijer   S. Chen   D. Buser

Acknowledgment

We would like to thank Mr. Thomas Kiss of the ITI Center for his invaluable assistance in the preparation of this volume of the Treatment Guide series. We would also like to express our gratitude to Ms. Juliane Richter (Quintessence Publishing) for typesetting and for coordinating the production workflow, Dr. Dr. Bernd Stadlinger and Mr. Per N. Döhler (Triacom Dental) for their editing support, and Ms. Ute Drewes for her excellent illustrations. We also acknowledge continuing support from Straumann AG, ITI's corporate partner.

Editors and Authors

Editors:

Daniel Wismeijer, DDS, PhD
  Professor and Chairman Department
  of Oral Function and Restorative Dentistry
  Head Section Oral Implantology
  and Prosthetic Dentistry
  Gustav Mahlerlaan 3004
  1081 LA Amsterdam, Netherlands
  E-mail: d.wismeijer@acta.nl

Stephen Chen, MDSc, PhD
  223 Whitehorse Road
  Balwyn VIC 3123, Australia
  E-mail: schen@balwynperio.com.au

Daniel Buser, DDS, Dr med dent
  Professor and Chairman Department
  of Oral Surgery and Stomatology
  University of Bern, School of Dental Medicine
  Freiburgstrasse 7
  3010 Bern, Switzerland
  E-mail: daniel.buser@zmk.unibe.ch

Authors:

Julia-Gabriela Wittneben Matter,
  DMD, Dr med dent, MMSc
  Assistant Professor, Division of Fixed Prosthodontics
  University of Bern, School of Dental Medicine
  Freiburgstrasse 7
  3010 Bern, Switzerland
  E-mail: julia.wittneben@zmk.unibe.ch

Hans-Peter Weber, DMD, Dr med dent
  Professor and Chairman Department
  of Prosthodontics and Operative Dentistry
  Tufts University, School of Dental Medicine
  One Kneeland Street
  Boston, MA 02111, USA
  E-mail: hp.weber@tufts.edu

Contributors

Daniel Buser, DDS, Dr med dent
  Professor and Chairman Department
  of Oral Surgery and Stomatology
  University of Bern, School of Dental Medicine
  Freiburgstrasse 7
  3010 Bern, Switzerland
  E-mail: daniel.buser@zmk.unibe.ch

Stephen Chen, MDSc, PhD
  223 Whitehorse Road
  Balwyn, VIC 3123, Australia
  E-mail: schen@balwynperio.com.au

Urs C. Belser, DMD, Dr med dent
  Professor and Chairman
  Department of Prosthodontics
  University of Geneva, School of Dental Medicine
  Rue Barthélemy-Menn 19
  1205 Genève, Switzerland
  E-mail: urs.belser@unige.ch

William C. Martin, DMD, MS
  Director Center for Implant Dentistry
  Department of Oral and Maxillofacial Surgery
  University of Florida, College of Dentistry
  1600 SW Archer Road, D7-6
  Gainesville, FL 32610, USA
  E-mail: wmartin@dental.ufl.edu

James Ruskin, DMD, MD
  Professor Center for Implant Dentistry
  Department of Oral and Maxillofacial Surgery
  University of Florida, College of Dentistry
  1600 SW Archer Road, D7-6
  Gainesville, FL 32610, USA
  E-mail: jruskin@dental.ufl.edu

Bruno Schmid, DMD
  Bayweg 3
  3123 Belp, Switzerland
  E-mail: brunoschmid@vtxmail.ch

Ronald E. Jung, DMD, PD Dr med dent, PhD
  Vice Chairman
  Clinic for Fixed and Removable Prosthodontics
  Center for Dental and Oral Medicine and
  Cranio-Maxillofacial Surgery
  University of Zurich
  Plattenstrasse 11
  8032 Zurich, Switzerland
  E-mail: ronald.jung@zzm.uzh.ch

Christopher Noel Hart, DMD
  Private Practice
  20 Collins Street, Suite 3/Level 10
  Melbourne VIC 3000, Australia
  E-mail: cnhart@me.com

Hideaki Katsuyama, DDS, PhD
  MM Dental Clinic, Center of Implant Dentistry (CID)
  3F, 3-3-1 Minatomirai
  Nishi-ku, Yokohama 220-0012, Japan
  E-mail: mmdc@cidjp.org

Masaaki Hojo, DDS
   MM Dental Clinic, Center of Implant Dentistry (CID)
   3F, 3-3-1 Minatomirai
   Nishi-ku, Yokohama 220-0012, Japan
   E-mail: mmdc@cidjp.org

Masako Ogawa, DDS
   MM Dental Clinic, Center of Implant Dentistry (CID)
   3F, 3-1-3 Minatomirai
   Nishi-ku, Yokohama 220-8401, Japan
   E-mail: mmdc@cidjp.org

Dejan Dragisic, Dr med dent
   Swiss Smile Dental Centre
   10 Brook Street
   London W1S 1BG, United Kingdom
   E-mail: dejan@dragisic.com

Muizzaddin Mokti, BDS, MMSc
   Division of Regenerative and Implant Sciences
   Department of Restorative Sciences
   and Biomaterial Sciences
   Harvard School of Dental Medicine
   188 Longwood Avenue
   Boston, MA 02115, USA
   E-mail: muizzaddin_mokti@hsdm.harvard.edu

German O. Gallucci, Dr med dent, DMD
   Head Division of Regenerative and Implant Sciences
   Department of Restorative Sciences
   and Biomaterial Sciences
   Harvard School of Dental Medicine
   188 Longwood Avenue
   Boston, MA 02115, USA
   E-mail: german_gallucci@hsdm.harvard.edu

Urs Brägger, Dr med dent
   Professor Division of Fixed Prosthodontics
   University of Bern, School of Dental Medicine
   Freiburgstrasse 7
   3010 Bern, Switzerland
   E-mail: urs.braegger@zmk.unibe.ch

Sybille Scheuber, Dr med dent
   Clinical Instructor Division of Fixed Prosthodontics
   University of Bern, School of Dental Medicine
   Freiburgstrasse 7
   3010 Bern, Switzerland
   E-mail: sybille.scheuber@zmk.unibe.ch

Lisa Heitz-Mayfield, BDS, MDSc, Dr Odont
   Professor University of Sydney
   University of Western Australia
   West Perth Periodontics
   21 Rheola Street
   West Perth, WA 6005, Australia
   E-mail: heitz.mayfield@iinet.net.au

Scott E. Keith, DDS, MS, FACP
   Dental Implant Center Walnut Creek
   1111 Civic Drive, Suite 320
   Walnut Creek, CA 94596, USA
   E-mail: drkeith@implantcenterwc.com

Gregory J. Conte, DMD, MS
   The Practice SF
   345 West Portal Avenue
   San Francisco, CA 94127, USA
   E-mail: gregory@thepracticesf.com

Table of Contents

1   Introduction

J.-G. Wittneben, H. P. Weber

The use of dental implants in the esthetic zone is well documented in the literature. Numerous controlled clinical trials have shown that the overall implant survival and success rates involved are similar to those reported for other indications. However, few studies have been published in which the actual success of the treatment was measured. This would have to include a critical and systematic assessment of short-term and long-term outcomes with implant-supported prostheses in the esthetic zone, including esthetic parameters.

Implant therapy in the esthetic zone is considered an advanced or complex procedure that requires comprehensive preoperative planning and precise surgical execution based on a restoration-driven approach. The esthetic zone is generally defined as any dentoalveolar segment that is visible in full smile. For the purposes of this text, the esthetic zone has been defined as the portion of the dentition that is predominantly visible when facing an individual, encompassing the maxillary anterior teeth from the right to the left canine.

There is convincing evidence that replacement of single teeth with implant-supported restorations in the esthetic zone will yield esthetically and functionally successful treatment outcomes if the hard and soft tissues surrounding the adjacent natural teeth are intact and if guidelines for correct three-dimensional implant placement and restoration, as appropriate for the respective indications, are properly followed.

By contrast, esthetically ideal outcomes are less predictably achieved when replacing multiple adjacent missing teeth in the anterior maxilla with fixed implant-supported restorations, the main problem being that the bone and soft-tissue volume is often deficient both vertically and horizontally in multi-tooth edentulous areas. Deficiencies of this type will require appropriate procedures to augment the hard or soft tissues affected. But the efficacy and predictability of these procedures are limited when it comes to vertical augmentation and, for that matter, biologic ways of replacing any missing soft tissue between implants.

The present volume within the ITI Treatment Guide series summarizes the results and consensus statements of the 3rd and 4th ITI Consensus Conferences. It also contains a review of current evidence regarding the treatment of extended edentulous spaces in the esthetic zone with implant-supported restorations. Clinical recommendations for treatment alternatives and procedures are based, as much as possible, on existing scientific and clinical evidence, including the experiences and suggestions of many seasoned clinicians within the ITI and outside. Special emphasis is given to the preoperative evaluation, treatment planning, and assessment of risk factors for these—often complex—indications. Surgical and prosthodontic procedures are presented with detailed descriptions and illustrations followed by a number of step-by-step clinical case presentations. Complications of various etiologies are highlighted and suggestions are made on how to avoid them. A number of clinical cases documenting various complications and their treatment complete this volume of the ITI Treatment Guide.

In summary, the purpose of this sixth volume of the ITI Treatment Guide series is to provide clinical recommendations for implant-supported prosthodontic treatments in patients with multiple missing adjacent teeth in the esthetic zone. The authors hope that they have created a valuable resource for clinicians who perform implant treatment on patients with indications of this type and that they can enhance the ability of clinicians to achieve successful long-term outcomes in these situations despite their often complex esthetic nature.

2 <u>Proceedings of the 3rd and 4th
ITI Consensus Conferences
and Literature Review:
Extended Edentulous Spaces
in the Esthetic Zone</u>

The International Team for Implantology (ITI) is an independent academic organization that brings together professionals from various fields in implant dentistry and tissue regeneration. The ITI regularly publishes treatment guidelines based on evidence from systematic reviews or clinical studies with long-term clinical results. Information of this type is also included in the ITI Treatment Guides, which have become a valuable resource for clinicians engaging in patient care involving implant dentistry of various degrees of difficulty.

The ITI regularly organizes Consensus Conferences to review the current literature in the field with the aim of evaluating and updating the scientific evidence supporting the entire variety of clinical materials and techniques. The resulting consensus statements and clinical recommendations are agreed upon by invited panels of experts, and the results are published in peer-reviewed journals.

In keeping with the topic of Volume 6 of the ITI Treatment Guide, "Extended Edentulous Spaces in the Esthetic Zone," Consensus Statements and Clinical Recommendations from the 3rd ITI Consensus Conference in 2003 in Gstaad, Switzerland and the 4th ITI Consensus Conference in 2008 in Stuttgart, Germany have been extracted from the original Consensus Proceedings. The following paragraphs will list the Consensus Statements with direct relevance to the main objectives of this text, namely considerations of treatment planning, risk assessment, and prosthodontic concepts to successfully replace multiple missing teeth in the maxillary anterior region with implant-supported restorations.

2.1 Consensus Statements

2.1.1 Proceedings of the 3rd ITI Consensus Conference 2003

International Journal of Oral and Maxillofacial Implants 2004, Vol. 19 (Supplement)
Consensus Statements and Recommended Clinical Procedures Regarding Esthetics in Implant Dentistry (Belser and coworkers 2004)

Long-term results
- The use of dental implants in the esthetic zone is well documented in the literature. Numerous controlled clinical trials show that the respective overall implant survival and success rates are similar to those reported for other segments of the jaws. However, most of these studies do not include well-defined esthetic parameters or criteria of patient satisfaction.
- The replacement of multiple adjacent missing teeth in the anterior maxilla with fixed implant restorations is poorly documented. Esthetic reconstructions, particularly regarding the contours of the interimplant soft tissue, are not predictable in this situation.

Surgical considerations
- *Planning and execution.* Implant therapy in the anterior maxilla is considered an advanced or complex procedure that requires comprehensive preoperative planning and precise surgical execution based on a prosthetically driven approach.
- *Patient selection.* Appropriate patient selection is essential to achieving esthetic treatment outcomes. Treatment of high-risk patients identified through site analysis and a general risk assessment (medical status, periodontal susceptibility, smoking, and other risks) should be undertaken with caution, since esthetic results are less consistent in these cases.

- *Implant selection.* Implant type and dimensions should be selected based on site anatomy and on the planned restoration. Inappropriate dimensions of the implant body and shoulder may result in hard- or soft-tissue complications.
- *Implant positioning.* Correct three-dimensional implant placement is essential to an esthetic outcome of treatment. If the comfort zones are respected in all three dimensions, the implant shoulder will be located in an ideal position, allowing for an esthetic implant restoration with long-term stability of the peri-implant tissue support.
- *Soft-tissue stability.* For long-term stability of esthetic soft tissue, an adequate horizontal and vertical bone volume is essential. Where deficiencies exist, appropriate grafting or procedures to augment hard or soft tissue are required. Correcting deficiencies in bone height remains a challenge, often resulting in esthetic shortcomings.

Prosthodontic considerations
- *Esthetic fixed implant-supported restorations.* An esthetic implant-supported restoration was defined as one that is in harmony with the perioral facial structures of the patient. The esthetic peri-implant tissues must be in harmony with the healthy surrounding dentition—including health, height, volume, color, and contours. The restoration should imitate the natural appearance of the missing dental unit(s) in color, form, texture, size, and optical properties.
- *Esthetic zone.* Objectively, the esthetic zone can be defined as any dentoalveolar segment that is visible in full smile. Subjectively, the esthetic zone can be defined as any dentoalveolar area of esthetic importance to the patient. (Note: For purposes of the present volume, the esthetic zone is defined as being limited to the anterior maxilla, from right to left canine.)

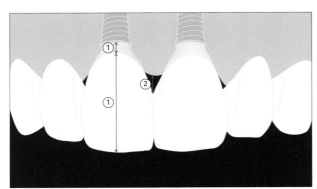

Fig 1   Illustration of esthetic soft-tissue parameters: (1) location of the mid-facial soft-tissue margin adjacent to an implant-supported restoration in relation to the incisal edge or implant shoulder; (2) distance between the tip of the papilla and the most apical interproximal contact.

2.1.2   Proceedings of the 4th ITI Consensus Conference 2008

International Journal of Oral and Maxillofacial Implants 2009, Vol. 24 (Supplement)
Consensus Statements and Recommended Clinical Procedures Regarding Loading Protocols (Weber and coworkers 2009)

Principal consensus
In agreement with the 2007 Cochrane Report (Esposito and coworkers 2007), the ITI proposes the following definitions for the loading of dental implants (Weber and coworkers 2009):

- Conventional loading of dental implants is defined as later than 2 months following implant placement.
- Early loading of dental implants is defined as between 1 week and 2 months following implant placement.
- Immediate loading of dental implants is defined as earlier than 1 week following implant placement.
- A separate definition for delayed loading is no longer required.

Consensus statements relative to loading protocols for the esthetic zone (Grütter and Belser 2009)
While implant survival in partially edentulous areas of the esthetic zone does not appear to be affected by loading protocols, success criteria and patient-centered outcomes may be. As no data evaluating these aspects are available, clinical trials are recommended.

- *Early loading* of microrough implants between 6 and 8 weeks following implant placement can be considered routine in partially edentulous areas of the esthetic zone.
- *Immediate loading* of microrough dental implants can be considered a viable treatment option for partially edentulous areas in the esthetic zone. Treatment within this time frame is, however, complex and can be considered a valid treatment option for clinicians with an appropriate level of education, experience, and skills.
- *Conventional loading* (later than 2 months following implant placement) remains the procedure of choice in partially edentulous areas of the esthetic zone in the following situations:
  - Stability is considered inadequate for early or immediate loading
  - Specific clinical conditions such as compromised host or implant site
  - Presence of parafunction or other dental complications
  - Need for extensive or simultaneous augmentation procedures or sinus floor elevation

- *Esthetic outcomes.* The following soft-tissue parameters were considered esthetically relevant and proposed for use in clinical studies:
  - Location of the mid-facial soft-tissue margin adjacent to an implant-supported restoration in relation to the incisal edge or implant shoulder (Fig 1).
  - Distance between the tip of the papilla and the most apical interproximal contact (Fig 1).
  - Width of the facial keratinized mucosa.
  - Assessment of mucosal conditions (modified gingival index, bleeding on probing).
  - Subjective (patient-centered) measures of esthetic outcomes, such as visual analog scales.
- *Provisional restorations.* To optimize esthetic treatment outcomes, the use of provisional restorations with adequate emergence profiles is recommended to guide and shape the peri-implant tissue prior to definitive restoration.
- *Implant shoulder.* In most esthetic areas, the implant shoulder is located subgingivally, resulting in a deep interproximal margin. This shoulder location makes it difficult to seat the restoration and to remove cement. A screw-retained restoration (or a cemented restoration over a screw-retained custom abutment) is recommended to minimize these potential problems resulting from cementation errors.

2.2 Literature Review

H. P. Weber, J.-G. Wittneben

2.2.1 General Aspects and Biological Considerations

The use of dental implants in the esthetic zone is well documented in the literature. Numerous controlled clinical trials have shown that the overall implant survival and success rates are similar to those reported for other indications. However, most of these studies did not include well-defined esthetic parameters (Belser and co-workers 2004a; Belser and coworkers 2004b; Grütter and Belser 2009).

Implant therapy in the esthetic zone is considered an advanced or complex procedure that requires comprehensive preoperative planning and precise surgical execution based on a prosthetically driven approach (Buser and coworkers 2004). In general, the esthetic zone is defined as any dentoalveolar segment that is visible in full smile. Subjectively, the esthetic zone can be defined as any dentoalveolar area of esthetic importance to the patient (Higginbottom and coworkers 2004). (Note: For the purpose of this text, the esthetic zone has been defined as the portion of the dentition that is predominantly visible when facing an individual, encompassing the maxillary anterior teeth from right to left canine.)

There is convincing evidence that the replacement of single teeth with implant-supported restorations in the esthetic zone will be successful both esthetically and functionally if the hard and soft tissues at the adjacent natural teeth are intact and if the guidelines for correct three-dimensional implant placement for the respective indication are properly followed (Garber and Belser 1995; Buser and coworkers 2004).

Conversely, the esthetic result when replacing multiple adjacent missing teeth in the anterior maxilla with fixed implant-supported restorations is not as predictable (Kan and Rungcharassaeng 2003; Mitrani and coworkers 2005). The main problem is that vertical as well as horizontal bone and soft-tissue volumes in the affected area

are often deficient in these cases. When deficiencies are present, appropriate grafting procedures are required (Buser and coworkers 2004).

A major concern in the presence of multiple adjacent missing teeth in the esthetic zone is the lack of interimplant soft tissue. The height of a papilla between two implant crowns is dictated by the interimplant bone level (Tarnow and coworkers 2000, 2003; Kourkouta and coworkers 2009). Frequently, the interimplant crestal bone presents at a lower level than next to a tooth with intact periodontal bone height. This can be due to a preexisting condition (i.e. reduction of or flattening of the alveolar ridge after a previous extraction) or to inadequate interimplant distance. If two implants are placed extremely close (3 mm or more, according to Tarnow and coworkers 2000), a loss of interimplant crestal bone height must be expected. This is caused by the configuration of the biologic width around dental implants (Cochran and coworkers 1997), which will lead to a circumferential vertical bone loss of approximately 2 mm from the level of the implant-abutment or implant-restoration interface. The width of this peri-implant "bone defect" is up to 1.5 mm circumferentially (Hermann and coworkers 1997, 2000; Tarnow and coworkers 2000; Cardaropoli and coworkers 2006). If two implants are too close, the adjacent interproximal resorption defects will overlap, resulting in a reduction in interimplant bone height and, consequently, in a shortened papilla (Hermann and coworkers 1997; Tarnow and coworkers 2000, 2003; Kourkouta and coworkers 2009). The result will be a black triangle (or several), which can only be managed by accepting a prosthodontic compromise—square teeth with long proximal contacts or prosthetic papillae in pink ceramic (Mitrani and coworkers 2005).

Due to the biologic changes in crestal bone, one of the main rehabilitative goals in the esthetic zone must be to preserve the peri-implant bone at the optimal vertical height as much and as diligently as possible. For adjacent implants, this means that an interimplant distance of at least 3 mm at the level of the alveolar crest needs to be respected. This can be difficult if the missing adjacent teeth in the maxillary anterior segment are a canine and a lateral incisor or a lateral and a central incisor, since the interdental space is often too narrow to meet this requirement even when implants with reduced diameters or restorative platforms are used (Tymstra and coworkers 2011).

More recently, it has been suggested that implant-abutment interfaces with a horizontal offset (platform switching) will minimize crestal bone resorption and improve the chances of achieving more favorable interimplant bone levels (Rodriquez-Ciurana and coworkers 2009). Clinical reports have been promising, so this may be a valid recommendation. However, conclusive evidence from comparative outcome studies is still unavailable at this time (Bateli and coworkers 2011).

Attempts have also been made to use implants with a scalloped top for better preservation of the proximal peri-implant bone height. Clinical outcomes with this design have not found to have any advantages over flat-top implants; instead, more extensive bone loss has been reported than for conventional implant designs (den Hartog and coworkers 2011).

Consideration has to be given to alternate implant-supported restorative units with pontics or cantilevers if the interimplant distance is limited. A prosthodontic mock-up helps evaluate implant locations and interimplant distances. Today, with the help of cone-beam computed tomography and three-dimensional modeling of implant positions via treatment planning software, these parameters can be previsualized even more accurately at the planning stage. In contrast to the potential consequences of implants, pontics or cantilevers will not adversely affect the crestal bone height. In a recent prospective comparative pilot study, Tymstra and coworkers (2011) evaluated peri-implant tissue levels in patients with both a central and a lateral maxillary incisor missing, treated either with one implant supporting a cantilever restoration or with two implants supporting solitary restorations. Implant survival, pocket probing depths, papilla index, marginal bone levels, and patient satisfaction were assessed during the 1-year follow-up. No implants were lost; the mean peri-implant probing values were comparable in both groups. Papillary index scores were relatively low in both groups, pointing toward a compromised papilla. Marginal bone loss was minimal and comparable in both groups. Patient satisfaction was very high in both groups. The authors concluded that, based on this 1-year prospective comparative study, no substantial differences in hard- and soft-tissue levels were demonstrable in patients with a central and a lateral maxillary incisor

missing, who were treated either with one implant supporting a crown with a cantilever or with two implants supporting solitary crowns.

Biologically interesting but clinically not well documented (not by any comparative outcome studies) is the "root submergence technique" (Salama and coworkers 2007). By preserving a natural dental root below the local keratinized mucosa in areas where adjacent teeth need to be replaced, the surrounding tissues can be predictably maintained, as the periodontal attachment apparatus will preserve the surrounding alveolar bone. In situations of periodontal bone loss, orthodontic extrusion will need to be performed before submerging the roots to bring the local tissues back to a desirable level (Zuccati and Bocchieri 2003).

2.2.2   Treatment Planning and Risk Assessment

As stated earlier, implant therapy in the esthetic zone is considered an advanced or complex procedure that requires comprehensive preoperative planning and precise surgical execution based on a prosthetically driven approach (Buser and coworkers 2004). Appropriate patient selection and information is essential in achieving esthetic treatment outcomes that are acceptable to both the patient and the dentist. The patient's expectations, attitude, and smile line are important determinants in predicting treatment success subjectively (in the patient's view) or objectively (in the dentist's view). Similarly, there is a need to identify patients with significant systemic risks (compromised medical status, periodontal susceptibility, smoking, lack of compliance) because esthetic outcomes are less consistent here (Weber and coworkers 2009). The SAC Assessment Tool, freely available at no cost on the ITI website (iti.org), is helpful in determining the complexity (SAC = Straightforward, Advanced, Complex) of specific treatment cases (Dawson and Chen 2009).

2.2.3   Surgical Procedures

Correct three-dimensional implant placement is essential to esthetic treatment outcomes. If the comfort zones in all three dimensions are respected, the implant shoulder will be located in an ideal position, allowing for an esthetic implant-supported restoration with stable, long-term peri-implant tissue support (Buser and coworkers 2004). Implant type and dimensions should be selected based on site anatomy and on the planned restoration. An inappropriate implant body or restorative platform may result in tissue complications.

As mentioned above, an adequate horizontal and vertical bone volume is essential to the long-term stability of esthetic soft tissue. Where deficiencies exist, appropriate augmentation procedures are required (Buser and coworkers 2004). A number of effective surgical approaches are available for the augmentation of deficient edentulous ridges to allow placement of implants. However, most relevant studies in the literature have been retrospective in nature, with small sample sizes and short follow-up periods. No direct comparisons should therefore be made between those studies, and caution must be exercised in drawing any definitive conclusions (Chiapasco and coworkers 2009).

A variety of techniques and grafting materials are available to increase the width of the alveolar ridge effectively and predictably. Autologous bone blocks for grafting, used with or without membranes, achieve greater horizontal bone gains and involve lower complication rates than particulate materials used with or without a membrane (Jensen and Terheyden 2009).

Different techniques to increase the height of the alveolar ridge have been described. Overall, they are much less predictable and involve a substantially higher complication rate than procedures for horizontal ridge augmentation. Generally, autologous bone blocks, used with or without membranes, result in greater vertical bone gains than particulate materials used with or without a membrane (Jensen and Terheyden 2009).

Given the limited predictability of vertical augmentation, it is important to consider orthodontic extrusion of prognostically unfavorable teeth with periodontal bone loss prior to their extraction. This will allow the regeneration of deficient hard and soft tissues in the vertical dimension before the teeth are removed (Zuccati and Bocchieri 2003; Brindis and Block 2009).

Some clinicians use alveolar distraction osteogenesis to augment vertically deficient alveolar ridges in selected cases. But this procedure has a high complication rate, including changes of the distracting vector, incomplete distraction, fracture of the distracting device, and partial relapse of the initial bone gain, and must therefore be considered a complex procedure that is highly technique-sensitive and has limited applicability and predictability (Chiapasco and coworkers 2009).

In summary, vertical bone deficiencies continue to be a challenge and often lead to esthetic shortcomings. The use of pink ceramic or resin materials to replace missing soft tissues will often be necessary in these indications (Salama and coworkers 2009; Coachman and coworkers 2009). In the phase of treatment planning, it is impor-

tant to discuss with the patient the option or need for "artificial gingiva" as a non-invasive alternative to overcome the problem (Mitrani and coworkers 2005).

Regarding the actual surgical placement of dental implants, techniques and biomaterials continue to develop and have facilitated the expansion of clinical indications for implant therapy (Chen and coworkers 2009c). The variety of procedures and biomaterials available may offer a confusing picture for the implant surgeon, who is responsible for recommending the best surgical approach with the lowest risk of complications and morbidity to the patient (Chen and coworkers 2009c). Some of the important aspects relevant to the objectives of this treatment guide are summarized in the paragraphs that follow.

Timing of implant placement after tooth extraction

At the 3rd ITI Consensus Conference in 2003, a classification system for the timing of implant placement after tooth extraction was proposed (Hämmerle and coworkers 2004). This system is based on desired levels of healing following tooth extraction rather than on descriptive terms or rigid time frames. Type 1 refers to placement of an implant into a tooth socket at the time of extraction ("immediate implant placement"); type 2 refers to the placement of an implant after completion of soft-tissue healing but before clinically significant bone fill within the socket has occurred; type 3 refers to placement of an implant following significant clinical or radiographic socket bone fill (types 2 and 3 fall in the category of "early implant placement"); and type 4 refers to placement of an implant into fully healed alveolar bone ("late implant placement").

Advantages and disadvantages of implant-placement times

The survival rates of implants placed immediately or early after extraction are high and comparable to those of implants placed in healed sites (Grütter and Belser 2009; Chen and coworkers 2009c). All of these approaches have specific advantages and disadvantages, which should be carefully considered at the time of treatment planning (Chen and coworkers 2004; Chen and Buser 2008). As for immediate implant placement (type 1), the combined approach to extracting the tooth and inserting the implant reduces the number of surgical procedures that the patient needs to undergo. Extraction socket defects will normally feature two or three walls, and this renders simultaneous bone augmentation highly predictable. Also, this protocol offers an opportunity to attach a provisional restoration to the implant immediately or soon after implant placement. This may prevent the patient from having to wear an interim removable prosthesis. However, these advantages are counteracted by the technical challenges inherent in preparing intra-socket implant sites such that the implant exhibits good primary stability in the desirable prosthodontic position.

An increased risk of mucosal recession is also associated with immediate implant placement (Chen and coworkers 2007; Evans and Chen 2008), which can compromise the esthetic outcome. Mucosal recession is mostly associated with the resorption of labial bone after extraction (Araújo and coworkers 2006a; Araújo and coworkers 2006b; Chen and coworkers 2007; Evans and Chen 2008). This may even be more pronounced when multiple adjacent teeth are extracted (Al-Askar and coworkers 2011). Additional tissue augmentation procedures are usually required to overcome this risk, further increasing the technical complexity of the procedure. While the grafting of peri-implant defects with particulate bone or bone substitutes is readily achieved, grafting of the external surfaces of the facial bone is more demanding due to the convexity of the bone wall. If primary soft-tissue closure is required, the lack of soft tissue increases the difficulty of attaining tension-free closure, and flap advancement may alter the mucogingival line (Chen and coworkers 2009c).

Bone modeling following tooth extraction is unpredictable and may lead to suboptimal bone-regenerative outcomes and seemingly random dimensional changes. With early implant placement (type 2), healing of the soft tissues increases the volume of mucosa at the site. This facilitates manipulation of the surgical flaps, and flap advancement for partial implant submersion or primary closure can be more readily achieved. In areas of high esthetic importance, the increased soft-tissue volume of may enhance soft-tissue esthetic outcomes.

In the 4- to 8-week period following tooth extraction, a slight flattening of the facial bone wall is commonly observed. This facilitates grafting of the facial surface of the bone with bone substitutes possessing low rates of substitution. These grafts may limit long-term dimensional changes of the ridge (Buser and coworkers 2009). As there is minimal bone regeneration within the socket at this point, peri-implant defects are usually still present. However, the defects usually present with two or three intact walls amenable to simultaneous bone augmentation techniques. The lack of bone regeneration within the socket may increase the difficulty of attaining initial stability of the implant. Implant placement 4 to 8 weeks after tooth extraction also allows pathology associated with the extracted tooth to resolve prior to implant placement.

For type 3 implant placement (approximately 12 weeks after extraction), soft tissues are fully healed and will also facilitate a tension-free closure of the site after implant placement and contour augmentation. Since partial bone healing in the socket has been achieved, implant stability can be more readily attained compared to type 1 and type 2 placement. However, it should be noted that the modeling of the bone is more advanced than with type 2 implant placement (Chen and coworkers 2009).

In late implant placement (type 4), the socket walls exhibit the greatest amount of resorption. Although the soft tissues are fully healed and manipulation of the surgical flaps is facilitated, ongoing modeling/remodeling and horizontal resorption will increase the chances of having insufficient bone width to place the implants so that horizontal ridge augmentation prior to implant placement will become necessary.

Effectiveness of ridge-preservation techniques
The effectiveness of post-extraction ridge preservation has been reviewed by Darby and coworkers (2009). Those authors found that ridge-preservation procedures ("socket preservation") following tooth extraction are effective in limiting horizontal and vertical ridge alterations. There was no evidence for one published procedure being superior to another. There was also no conclusive evidence that such procedures improved the ability to place implants at a later point in time, although intuitively this would seem to be the case.

Computer technology in surgical implant dentistry
According to the Glossary of Oral and Maxillofacial Implants (Laney 2007), one has to differentiate between different terms. Two of them appear relevant to this review:

- Computer-guided (static) surgery: The use of a static surgical template that reproduces the virtual implant position directly from computed tomographic data and does not allow for intraoperative modification of the implant position.
- Computer-navigated (dynamic) surgery: The use of a surgical navigation system that reproduces the virtual implant position directly from computed tomographic data and allows for intraoperative changes in implant position.

Computer-aided planning offers potential advantages and may result in less complex surgery (Jung and coworkers 2009). By visualizing bone volume preoperatively, it may be possible to place implants more precisely within the existing bone structure, consequently reducing any grafting requirements. Computer-aided planning also helps to avoid anatomical complications, and it can be used with flapless surgery, possibly leading to reduced morbidity. It might even allow for the provision of implant therapy where complex anatomical limitations had previously precluded treatment. The improved accuracy of implant placement should improve the prosthetic outcome and could facilitate prefabrication of the prosthesis. Finally, increased surgical precision may improve implant survival rates. These systems may also soon demonstrate their potential as teaching tools.

But there is a learning curve for this technique-sensitive procedure, and it can be quite steep. Caution should be exercised in the early stages of acquiring these skills. The current literature fails to provide any long-term data to support the assumption that implant and prosthetic survival and success with computer-assisted surgical techniques are similar or superior to traditional procedures of implant placement. Unfortunately, the rapid development of this poorly documented technology in a commercially driven marketplace has led to unrealistic clinical expectations with regard to its efficacy and ease of use. Clinicians are advised to exercise caution in interpreting the claims made by companies promoting this computer technology for implant surgery as easy and unproblematic.

Flapless surgery
The data on implant survival suggest that flapless implant surgery is efficacious and clinically effective in patients (Brodala 2009). However, this information has been derived from relatively short-term studies (mean observation time 19 months) and is based on a systematic review by Brodala (2009) that found no comparative evidence regarding soft-tissue response. The reported incidence of intraoperative complications (3.2%) may be clinically relevant. According to Brodala, the literature does not offer any information on bone perforations rates associated with flapless surgery, as the majority of articles did not report the presence or absence of this complication. It is also unclear whether such bony perforations will have long-term adverse effects on implants. Reported data demonstrated statistically significant improvements in patient comfort for flapless versus conventional implant surgery—based on evidence from two high-level studies. But again, the same systematic review did not identify any comparative evidence regarding soft-tissue responses or esthetic outcomes.

2.2.4 Restorative Procedures

Today a multiplicity of procedures and materials exist to produce esthetic implant-supported restorations as required especially for the indications discussed in this Treatment Guide. Materials and techniques will be discussed in detail in Chapter 5 along with the relevant evidence from the literature. In this section, therefore, only a few key principles relative to implant prosthodontics and esthetic outcomes are reviewed.

Esthetic implant-supported restorations
An esthetic implant-supported restoration is defined as one that is in harmony with the perioral facial structures of the patient (Higginbottom and coworkers 2004). Height, volume, color, and contours of healthy peri-implant tissues must be in harmony with an intact surrounding dentition. The restoration(s) should imitate the natural appearance of the missing tooth (teeth) in color, form, texture, size, translucency, and other visual characteristics.

Unfortunately, much of the existing literature pertaining to implant prosthodontics falls short of using evaluation criteria more specific than implant or prosthodontic survival or success. Despite relatively recent efforts by a number of authors assessing prosthodontic or esthetic outcomes (Higginbottom and coworkers 2004; Fürhauser and coworkers 2005: Belser and coworkers 2009; Buser and coworkers 2011), similar data about treatment success in the context of multiple missing adjacent teeth in the esthetic zone continues to be lacking.

As discussed earlier, prosthodontically correct implant placement in all three (apicocoronal, buccolingual, mesiodistal) dimensions is a prerequisite for ultimate prosthodontic success. It is exponentially more difficult to achieve such three-dimensional placement in situations of multiple missing teeth, as numerous landmarks are missing that may otherwise be offered by contralateral teeth. Proper planning via diagnostic and surgical guides produced from prosthodontic mock-ups that have been tried in the patient's mouth is instrumental.

It has also been demonstrated that provisional restorations are essential to optimizing esthetic treatment outcomes. The use of provisional restorations with adequate emergence profiles is necessary to develop the peri-implant tissue frame prior to the definitive restoration (Garber and Belser 1995; Higginbottom and coworkers 2004).

CAD/CAM manufacturing
in prosthetic implant dentistry

A systematic review by Kapos and coworkers (2009) suggested that while preliminary evidence for CAD/CAM in implant dentistry appears promising, the literature concerning its use for the fabrication of frameworks and abutments fails to provide meaningful clinical evidence of safety and effectiveness associated with the routine application of this technology. The current body of information provides insufficient data for long-term documentation. As technological developments outpace clinical research into CAD/CAM implant abutments and frameworks, users of this technology should acknowledge this limitation when interpreting clinical research data. Clinicians and technicians should also be aware that new materials and techniques are now being combined in previously undocumented ways (Hämmerle and coworkers 2009).

Implant loading protocols

The literature associated with loading protocols for dental implants remains limited, particularly with regard to studies of high scientific quality such as randomized controlled trials (RCTs) or systematic reviews (Weber and coworkers 2009). In agreement with the 2007 Cochrane Review (Esposito and coworkers 2007), consensus was obtained at the 4th ITI Consensus Conference in 2008 that, for future evaluations, the ITI definitions for dental implant loading should be modified from the 2004 ITI Consensus Report such that "conventional loading" refers to the loading of implants later than 2 months following their placement; early loading to the time frame between 1 week and 2 months following placement; and immediate loading to the period of less than 1 week following placement. It was proposed that a separate definition for delayed loading was no longer required.

Specifically referring to implant loading protocols in the esthetic zone, a systematic review by Grütter and Belser (2009) revealed that while implant survival at partially edentulous sites in the esthetic zone does not appear to be affected by loading protocols, success criteria and patient-centered outcomes might be. As insufficient pertinent data is available in the literature, clinical trials are recommended to address this kind of questions (Weber and coworkers 2009).

The review by Grütter and Belser (2009) also concluded that early loading of microrough implants between 6 and 8 weeks after implant placement in partially edentulous areas of the esthetic zone can be considered routine. While immediate loading of microrough dental implants may be a viable treatment option to deal with partially edentulous areas of the esthetic zone, this approach must be considered complex and should be performed by clinicians with a high level of experience and skills. Conventional loading (later than 2 months after implant placement) remains the procedure of choice for partial edentulism in the esthetic zone whenever primary implant stability is considered inadequate for early or immediate loading or in the presence of specific clinical conditions such as compromised host or implant sites, the presence of parafunction or other dental complications, or a need for extensive or simultaneous augmentation procedures including sinus floor elevation.

2.2.5 Complications

Risk factors for complications in the treatment of extended edentulous spaces in the esthetic zone with implant-supported restorations are manifold and need to be taken into consideration. They include early or late complications or failures caused by systemic or local biologic (Martin and coworkers 2009; Cochran and coworkers 2009; Heitz-Mayfield and Huynh-Ba 2009), technical or mechanical factors (Goodacre and coworkers 2003; Cochran and coworkers 2009; Salvi and Brägger 2009). An extensive review of these generally recognized complications would be beyond the scope of this chapter. It is important to understand that any risk for complications can be substantially reduced with proper diagnosis, treatment planning and risk assessment, followed by a state-of-the-art execution of the various treatment steps involved.

The most prominent complications in the treatment of multiple missing teeth in the maxillary anterior segment are related to esthetics. Chapter 7 will discuss the nature of these complications in more detail and examine how they can be avoided or resolved.

3 <u>Preoperative Evaluation and Treatment Planning</u>

H. P. Weber, J.-G. Wittneben

3.1 Introduction

Any effort to provide comprehensive dental care in situations with missing teeth or teeth with an unfavorable prognosis has to consider the dental implant option. Ever since the first reports on osseointegration were published (Brånemark and coworkers 1969, 1985; Schroeder and coworkers 1976, 1981), clinical studies have established scientific evidence that dental implants can serve as long-term predictable anchors for fixed or removable prostheses in completely and partially edentulous patients and that patient satisfaction with dental implant therapy is high (Adell and coworkers 1990; Fritz 1996; Buser and coworkers 1997; Lindh and coworkers 1998; Moy and coworkers 2005; Pjetursson and coworkers 2005). Furthermore, substantial scientific and clinical evidence has improved our understanding of factors that enhance or compromise the treatment outcome in esthetic terms (Belser and coworkers 2004a; Belser and coworkers 2004b; Buser and coworkers 2004; Higginbottom and coworkers 2004; Buser and coworkers 2007a; Grütter and Belser 2009; Weber and coworkers 2009). The overall body of information on success factors continues to grow; and despite its diversity and scientific inconsistencies, it is becoming more valuable. This was made possible, to a large extent, by systematic reviews offering focused interpretations of the published data.

The generally supportive evidence for most implant indications—including the esthetically demanding maxillary anterior region—has to be weighed against the long-term performance of dental implants in patients with (a history of) systemic disease, including periodontal disease, which has attracted increasing attention in the more recent peer-reviewed literature (Ellegaard and coworkers 1997; Baelum and Ellegaard 2004; Ellegaard and coworkers 2006). While no difference was observed between patients with and without periodontal disease after 5 years of function, a slightly increased risk for peri-implantitis with bone loss and subsequent implant failure was found for certain implants after 10 years. Nevertheless, the authors concluded that dental implants remained a good treatment alternative for patients with periodontal disease.

In patients with residual teeth in the maxillary anterior segment, the decision whether residual natural teeth should be used as abutments for conventional fixed prostheses or whether dental implants should be added to replace compromised natural teeth is influenced by factors such as the location, strategic value, and treatment prognosis of the teeth in question, the subjective and objective need for tooth replacement, the dimensions of the alveolar process, and esthetic considerations. Especially in tooth loss due to periodontal disease, the alveolar process may be substantially reduced (Fig 1).

This introduces a number of concerns related to function and esthetics. In the anterior segment, any loss of periodontal hard and soft tissues and the consequent "lengthening" of teeth raise esthetic concerns that may complicate matters, especially in patients with high expectations or in the presence of a high smile line (Fig 1). It is important to anticipate problems of this type and to analyze local conditions carefully so that expected outcomes can be appropriately discussed with the patient before any treatment steps are taken.

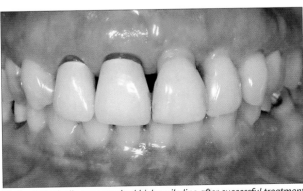

Fig 1 Esthetically compromised high smile line after successful treatment of periodontal disease. In situations such as these, treatment options become complex. (Image courtesy of Prof. Urs Belser.)

3.2 Patient History

Implant therapy is part of a comprehensive treatment plan. For the treatment to be successful, an understanding of patient-related factors such as individual needs, social and economic background, or general medical condition is required. In order to expedite history taking, the patient should fill out a health questionnaire prior to the initial examination. Questionnaires of this type should ideally be designed such that they immediately reveal any compromising factors that may modify the treatment plan. These factors need to be discussed in detail with the patient during the initial visit or may require consultation with medical colleagues to allow for proper treatment planning. Assessment of the patient's history should include (1) chief complaint and expectations; (2) social and family history; (3) dental history; (4) motivation and compliance, including oral hygiene; (5) relevant habits such as smoking or recreational drug use or bruxism; and (6) medical history and medications.

3.2.1. Main Complaints and Expectations

To get a successful treatment outcome, it is essential to identify and understand the patient's therapeutic needs and desires. Most patients have specific desires and expectations regarding the treatment and its results, even though these are not always consistent with the attainable outcome projected by the clinician after assessing the specific clinical situation. Ideal outcomes can only be achieved if the patient's demands are in line with objective clinical findings and projected treatment outcomes. Patient expectations must be taken seriously and included in the evaluation. A clear understanding of patient views is essential for dentofacial esthetics. For implant restorations in periodontally compromised dentitions, it is often necessary to accept the esthetic compromises mandated by tissue loss. If a patient has been referred for a specific kind of treatment, the extent of the desired treatment has to be defined, and the referring dentist has to be informed of the intended treatment steps and expected outcomes.

3.2.2 Social and Family History

Before assessing the clinical situation in detail, it is helpful to interview patients about their occupational and social environment and about their priorities in life. An understanding of these factors is particularly important when extensive, time-consuming, and costly treatment steps are anticipated envisioned, which is often the case in implant therapy. Likewise, family histories may offer important clues as to when and why tooth loss occurred, about systemic or local diseases such as aggressive forms of periodontitis, or about any other genetic dispositions, habits, levels of compliance, and other behavioral aspects.

3.2.3 Dental History

Unless already reported by the referring dentist, any previous dental care, including prophylaxis and maintenance, must be explored with the patient. Information regarding the causes of tooth loss, tooth migration and progressive mobility, gingival bleeding, food impaction, and chewing difficulties needs to be explored. Other points that should be assessed at this time include the patient's esthetics and functional comfort and the perceived need for tooth replacement.

3.2.4 Motivation and Compliance

This part of the dentist-patient communication is about assessing the patient's interest in and motivation for extended and potentially expensive treatment. Helpful information include the patient's views on oral health, his or her last visit to a dentist or hygienist, frequency and regularity of dental visits, and details about routine oral hygiene.

3.2.5 Habits

Cigarette smoking has been known to be a risk factor for implant therapy for some time now (Bain and Moy 1993; Chuang and coworkers 2002; McDermott and coworkers 2003; Heitz-Mayfield and Huynh-Ba 2009). The importance of counseling patients with regard to this issue cannot be overestimated. Assessment of the smoking status should include details on exposure time and quantity. Patients should be encouraged to enter a cessation program.

Bruxism has not been shown to be a risk factor for implant survival, but an increased risk for mechanical and technical complications related to the superstructures and associated components—including implant abutments and screws—has been identified (Salvi and Brägger 2009). Reports in the literature attest to the usefulness of precautionary measures in terms of selecting implants of sufficient length and diameter, splinting multiple implants, and using retrievable restorations and occlusal jigs. Early identification of bruxism or clenching is conducive to successful treatment planning (Lobbezoo and coworkers 2006), but these conditions often simply cannot be diagnosed and assessed at the outset.

3.2.6 Medical History and Medications

A thorough review of the patient's medical history is essential. Specific medical conditions may constitute contraindications to dental implant therapy (Bornstein and coworkers 2009). Any factors that could affect wound healing should at least be regarded as a conditional contraindication. Factors of this type include chemotherapy and radiation therapy for cancer treatment, bisphosphonate therapy, anti-metabolic therapy for the treatment of arthritis, uncontrolled diabetes, seriously impaired cardiovascular function, bleeding disorders including medication-induced anticoagulation, and active drug addiction, including alcohol and heavy smoking. Patients with mental health conditions may not be good candidates for implant therapy, either. Conditions of this type are often difficult to identify during a first examination. If noticed, care should be taken that the patients are thoroughly examined by medical specialists before they are accepted for implant treatment.

Given the increasing need for medications in an aging population, an accurate assessment has to be made of each patient's prescribed and over-the-counter drugs, including potential interactions and effects on therapeutic procedures. Of particular relevance is the use of anticoagulants such as coumarin derivatives and aspirin. Clinicians should also recognize the need for antibiotic prophylaxis during dental surgical procedures. Recently, osteonecrosis of the jaw has been reported in patients who were undergoing, or had previously undergone, long-term therapy with bisphosphonates. Cases of osteonecrosis have been observed mainly after oral surgical procedures in patients on long-term intravenous bisphosphonate therapy as used in the treatment of cancers, although some cases were also observed in connection with oral intake of these drugs (Marx and coworkers 2005). According to online member information offered by the American Dental Association, the risk for osteonecrosis translates into about 7 cases per year for every million people taking oral bisphosphonates. Addressing this issue, Mortensen and coworkers (2007) concluded that the increasing number of reports about bisphosphonate-associated osteomyelitis and the difficulties encountered in treating these patients require further investigation to identify risk patients. Furthermore, the maximum effective and safe duration of bisphosphonate treatment remains to be determined. A systematic review examining the impact of systemic bisphosphonates on oral implant therapy (Madrid and Sanz 2009) arrived at the following conclusions and clinical recommendations with regard to implant surgery in patients on oral or systemic bisphosphonates: There is consensus in the literature that (1) dental implants are contraindicated in cancer patients on intravenous bisphosphonates; and that (2) the placement of dental implants may be considered safe in patients who have taken oral bisphosphonates to manage osteoporosis for under 5 years. Moreover, the intake of oral bisphosphonates did not adversely affect short-term implant survival rates (1–4 years) in the surveyed literature. Because of these uncertainties, patients on bisphosphonates need to be identified, communication with the treating physician(s) established, and a risk/benefit assessment made whenever implant therapy is being considered.

In summary, while most of this medical information can be extracted from the health questionnaire mentioned earlier, it is important for the clinician to ask specific questions relating to the patient's replies to that questionnaire in order to clarify the potential impact these points might have on dental implant treatment. In many cases, it will be necessary to contact the patient's physician for detailed information relevant to the planned treatment.

3.3   Local Examination

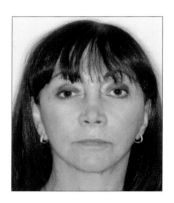

Fig 2a   Portrait view during passive lip closure.*

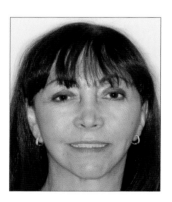

Figs 2b   Portrait view during partial smile.

3.3.1   Extraoral

Extraoral parameters should be a part of any initial patient examination. The clinician should look for asymmetries, lesions, or swelling in the head and neck area. In addition to a visual functional evaluation, the head and neck muscles and the temporomandibular joints should be palpated. Although the upper anterior segment in the oral cavity can usually be accessed without problems, evaluating the opening amplitude of the mandible is still useful to ensure that mouth opening is sufficient to accommodate the instruments used in dental implant therapy. This is also the perfect time to verify the accuracy of the patient's vertical dimension of occlusion as well as esthetic characteristics such as the smile, lip, and gingival lines or the facial and dental midline (Figs 2a-d).

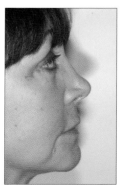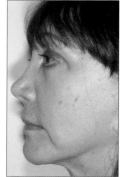

Fig 2c   Profile views with the teeth in contact. The vertical dimension of occlusion appears to be accurate.

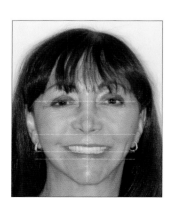

Fig 2d   Portrait view during full smile. Facial and dental landmarks are identified.

* The patient consented to her full portrait being shown.

3.3.2 Intraoral General Examination

The intraoral general examination includes an assessment of tissue conditions, including a careful screening for cancer or other tumor activity. Any tissue lesions will most likely require treatment before dental implants can be placed. Soft-tissue pathologies may include herpetic stomatitis, candidiasis, prosthesis-induced stomatitis, tumors, or hyperplasia. Hard-tissue pathologies that normally require pretreatment may include any impacted teeth, bone cysts, root fragments, residual infections in the alveolar bone (e.g. those caused by failed endodontic treatment), or tumors.

Periodontal tissues and dental hard tissues are examined with equal care to determine the need for periodontal, endodontic, and prosthetic treatment of the remaining dentition, most importantly for teeth directly adjacent to the edentulous space. The need for treating the latter may influence the treatment plan in terms of selecting a conventional fixed partial denture instead of an implant-supported restoration to replace a missing tooth. Note is taken of any pathologies such as gingival recession, bleeding on probing, increased periodontal probing depths, carious lesions, fractures, attrition, abrasion, abfraction, tooth mobility, or tooth misalignment. Existing restorations are recorded and deficiencies such as open margins, open contacts, or fractures identified (Figs 3a-c). Vitality tests, especially of teeth adjacent to potential implant sites, will point to possible endodontic pathologies. It should be understood that the treatment plan addresses all of these pathologies and that carious lesions and periodontal or endodontic problems are appropriately resolved prior to placing implants. It is also important that any treatment plan including orthodontics needs to sequence the active orthodontic phase with the timing of implant placement.

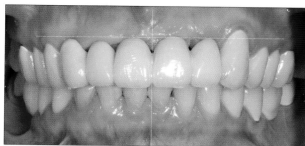

Fig 3a   Intraoral examination revealing the presence of an extended maxillary anterior fixed prosthesis. The patient's dissatisfaction with her teeth was due to the open embrasure spaces at the cervical level. Inflamed marginal tissues at tooth 13, the difference in cervical length between the two canines, and the repaired ceramic fracture on the mesiobuccal side of tooth 13.

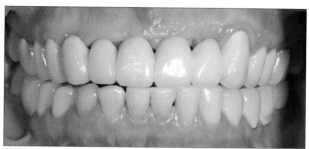

Fig 3b   Close to unilateral guidance in anterior excursive movements.

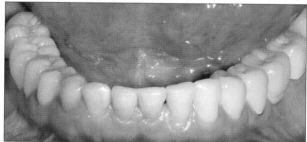

Fig 3c   View of mandibular arch with extended posterior fixed metal-ceramic prostheses, wear signs of the anterior teeth and generalized mild to moderate gingivitis with various degrees of gingival recession.

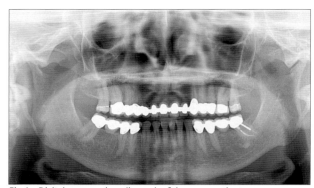

Fig 4   Digital panoramic radiograph of the same patient.

3.3.3   Initial Radiographic Examination

The initial patient assessment will include a radiographic survey. A full-mouth set of periapical radiographs or a high-quality panoramic radiograph is required to supplement the intraoral examination (Fig 4).

Minimum requirements for implant placement in terms of bone height depend on a number of factors, including the recommended implant length for a single-implant restoration, single versus multiple adjacent implants, jaw location, and the ease and predictability of ridge augmentation at the site in question. Additional radiographs such as occlusal views, cephalometric images, conventional radiographs, or CT scans may be indicated for detailed planning of implant placement (see Section 3.5).

3.3.4 Mounted Diagnostic Casts

The static and dynamic aspects of the patient's occlusion also need to be determined. This is especially important when multiple anterior teeth have to be replaced to reestablish a mutually protected occlusion with an anterior guidance that is consistent with the path of movement of the temporomandibular joints. Diagnostic casts mounted in a semi-adjustable articulator by way of a facebow transfer and a wax or silicone bite record are essential. It is frequently easier to assess parameters such as maxillomandibular relations (Angle class), overbite, overjet, stability in habitual occlusion, centric relation, slide in centric, or lateral and anterior excursive contacts (canine guidance, group function, anterior guidance) in this way than intraorally (Figs 5a-e). No less important is a detailed three-dimensional assessment of the available space.

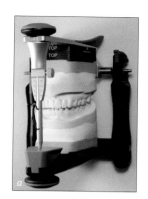

Figs 5a-b Semi-adjustable articulator and mounted casts (same patient).

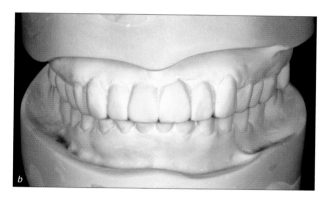

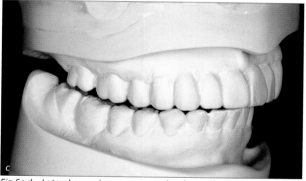
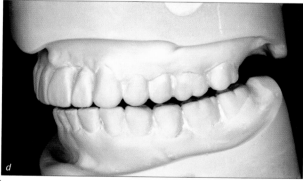

Fig 5c-d Lateral excursive movements showing canine guidance on both sides.

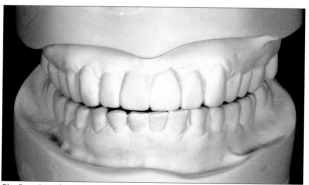

Fig 5e Anterior excursive movements supported exclusively by teeth to the left of the patient's midline.

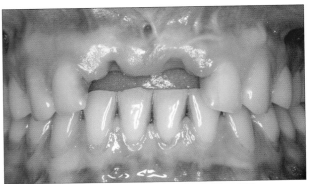

Fig 6a   Soft-tissue defects after extraction of teeth 11 and 21.

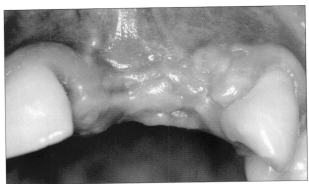

Fig 6b   Pathology and deficiency of the local alveolar ridge at sites 21 and 22 after traumatic loss of both teeth.

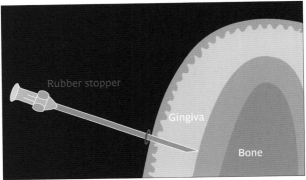

Fig 7a   Bone mapping, schematically.

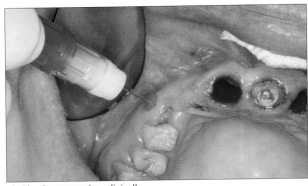

Fig 7b   Bone mapping, clinically.

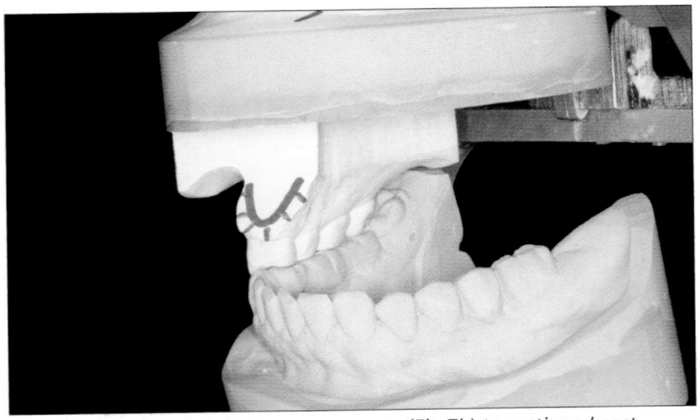

3.3.5   Intraoral Implant-Specific Examination

An implant-specific intraoral examination emphasizing the local characteristics of potential implant sites is important. Due to the esthetic impact of implant treatment, anterior locations in the oral cavity require special attention. Evaluating the condition of the local mucosa must be part of the examination. Note is taken of any soft-tissue defects or pathological changes, and an assessment is made as to whether these factors necessitate modifications to the treatment plan or risk compromising the treatment outcome (Figs 6a-b).

To give the patient realistic information on the feasibility of treatment with dental implants, probing of the local tissues may be indicated to assess tissue thickness and to confirm that sufficient alveolar bone is present. This can be accomplished in a bone mapping procedure using a fine needle or explorer after a small amount of local anesthetic has been applied to the area of interest (Figs 7a-c).

Fig 7c   Transfer of clinical measurements (Fig 7b) to sectioned cast.

3.3.6 Summary

In the specific context of implant prosthetic therapy to be performed in the maxillary anterior segment, the local implant-related examination has to focus particularly on the esthetic consequences of treatment (Table 1).

Depending on the patient's smile line, the most common visible compromises that have a direct bearing on esthetic appearance would include (excessively) long clinical crowns and flattening of the originally scalloped course of the gingival line, as well as loss of papillary tissue leading to unsightly "black triangles" in the interproximal areas (Fig 8).

These factors are particularly pronounced in patients exhibiting an originally "scalloped-thin" gingival biotype instead of a "flat-thick" one (Olsson and Lindhe 1991). Not infrequently, the situation may be compounded by vertical or lateral migration of teeth, which is capable of significantly affecting esthetic parameters in their own turn. Furthermore, in situations of more localized periodontal disease and attachment loss, abrupt changes in vertical tissue levels may be present between neighboring teeth.

The resultant major esthetic shortcomings mainly consist of an altered length-to-width ratio of the clinical crowns ("long-tooth syndrome") and of interproximal spaces that are incompletely filled by gingival tissue. The latter may not only affect esthetics but may also give rise to food retention and phonetic problems. As a consequence, reconstructive measures in general and implant therapy in particular need to be performed not only with a predictable and long-lasting functional rehabilitation in mind, but also with the goal of reestablishing harmony from an esthetic and phonetic viewpoint. The potential of fixed prosthodontics is somewhat limited when it comes to correcting length-to-width discrepancies of clinical crowns and to reducing any open interproximal embrasures. Furthermore, clinicians should be aware of the additional specific limitations associated with implant therapy, notably in connection with esthetic parameters, and use this awareness in conducting the local examination. Once again, the importance of assessing the height of each patient's smile line, as well as their individual therapeutic expectations, must be emphasized (Fig 9).

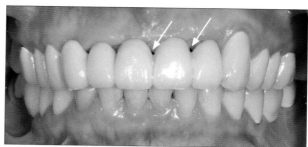

Fig 8 "Black triangles" in the anterior dentition.

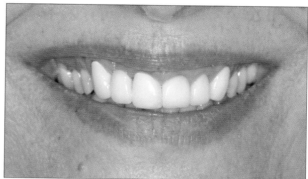

Fig 9 Failing dental restoration with disharmonious marginal gingival contour in a patient with a high smile line.

Table 1 Elements of the implant-specific local examination of the anterior maxilla.

Patient's smile line
Periodontal examination (gingival index, plaque index, probing pocket depths, clinical attachment level, bleeding on probing, width of keratinized mucosa, recessions, tooth mobility, etc.)
Gingival phenotype ("scalloped-thin" or "flat-thick")
Anatomy of the soft tissue and the bone
Interproximal bone level (as assessed on radiographs)
Shape of tooth crowns
Length of clinical crown
Overbite, overjet, malpositioned teeth
Restorative status of teeth
Width of existing or prospective edentulous spaces

Any tooth extraction or surgical removal results in horizontal and vertical tissue loss of varying magnitudes, including both the soft tissue and the underlying bone. This loss has been reported to vary between 2 and 3 mm vertically (Kois 1996; Cardaropoli and coworkers 2003; Araújo and coworkers 2005). For teeth still present but considered irrational to treat, further aggravation of the esthetic outcome should be expected. A slow orthodontic forced-eruption procedure may be beneficial prior to extracting the tooth (Salama and Salama 1993). One should also keep in mind that the esthetic outcomes of multiple adjacent implant restorations are significantly less predictable than the esthetic outcomes of single-tooth restorations in the anterior maxilla (Belser and coworkers 2004a; Buser and coworkers 2004; Higginbottom and coworkers 2004; Buser and coworkers 2007). Implant-supported single-tooth restorations clearly benefit from the tissue support offered by the adjacent natural teeth. As a consequence, the currently recommended extraction strategy is to avoid two adjacent gaps in this jaw segment (Martin and coworkers 2007). In other words, one should aim either for single-tooth gaps or, unless this is not possible, for extended edentulous areas

that span the sites of 3 or more adjacent missing teeth. The latter concept allows taking advantage of the superior inherent esthetics of pontics as replacement of some of the missing teeth (with or without enhancement by connective tissue grafting) and of the fact that adjacent implant restorations can be avoided in this way. This concept and its applications will be explained in detail in Section 3.5 (Prosthodontic Planning Considerations).

3.3.7 Implant-Specific Radiographic Evaluation

To determine the feasibility of implant-supported replacements of multiple missing teeth in the anterior maxilla, it is usually indicated to obtain additional radiographic information in the form of cone-beam computed tomography (CBCT) scans. These should be taken with a diagnostic (radiographic) template in place that accurately reflects the position and axis of the planned restoration. Consequently, these templates need to be based on a mock-up and a prosthodontic plan (Figs 10a-d), which will be further discussed in Section 3.5.

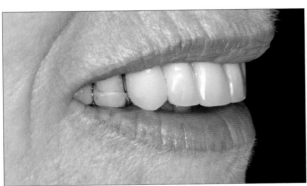

Fig 10a   Intraoral mock-up stage.

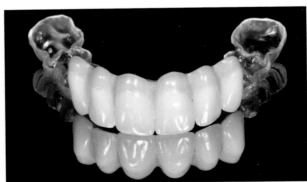

Fig 10b   Tooth-supported diagnostic template (Essex type).

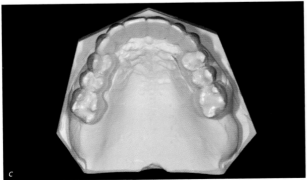

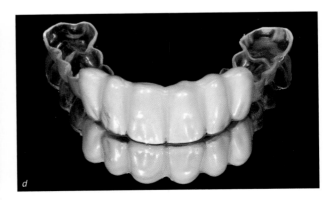

Figs 10c-d   Duplication of mock-up into a template with radiopaque teeth.

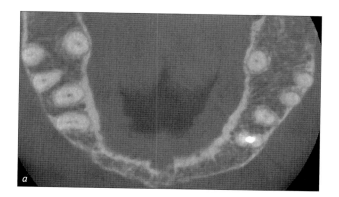

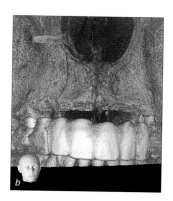

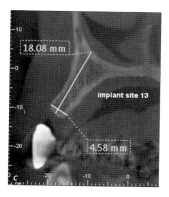

18.08 mm

implant site 13

4.58 mm

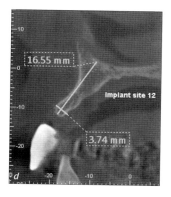

16.55 mm

implant site 12

3.74 mm

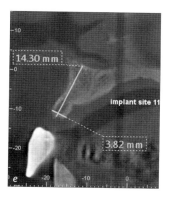

14.30 mm

implant site 11

3.82 mm

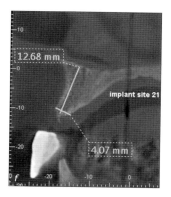

12.68 mm

implant site 21

4.07 mm

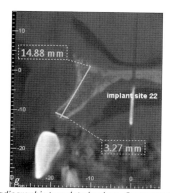

14.88 mm

implant site 22

3.27 mm

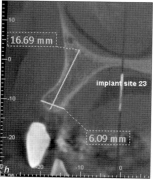

16.69 mm

implant site 23

6.09 mm

Figs 11a-h   CBCT scans with the radiographic template in place. Contours of individual teeth to be replaced are visualized by the use of radiopaque teeth in the template.

3.4   Risk Assessment

To summarize the aforementioned elements of a comprehensive preoperative examination, an individual risk profile is compiled for each potential implant patient, and this assessment needs to be especially detailed in the anterior maxilla where esthetic considerations are paramount (Table 2).

Any risk assessment for anterior implant sites of high esthetic impact is a detailed and complex task. General/systemic and esthetic/restorative criteria that are relevant to predicting the chances of an esthetically acceptable treatment outcome need to be included. These parameters were outlined in detail by Martin and coworkers (2006) in the first ITI Treatment Guide and have since been further refined through the SAC classification of surgical procedures as Straightforward, Advanced, or Complex (Dawson and Chen 2009). The SAC assessment tool is available to the clinical community as an interactive online tool at www.iti.org. It allows clinicians to categorize clinical scenarios and to determine the complexity of a given patient treatment based on a number of variables that may decrease or increase the risk for a desirable outcome. The replacement of multiple missing teeth in the maxillary anterior segment, whether short or extended, usually involves complex surgical and prosthodontic treatment protocols with a high esthetic risk (Table 3a-e). As mentioned previously, this is compounded by the fact that vertical tissue deficiencies due to tooth loss, periodontal disease, or trauma are relatively common in these situations (Fig 12). As a result, only clinicians with well-developed knowledge and expertise should be in charge of these treatments to attain successful outcomes as predictably as possible.

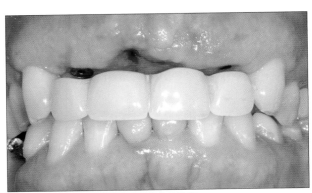

Fig 12   Vertical tissue deficiency at sites 11-21.

Table 2   Esthetic Risk Assessment (ERA).

Esthetic Risk Factor	Level of Risk		
	Low	Moderate	High
Medical status	Healthy, cooperative patient with an intact immune system.		Reduced immune system
Smoking habit	Non-smoker	Light smoker (< 10 cigs/day)	Heavy smoker (≥ 10 cigs/day)
Patient's esthetic expectations	Low	Medium	High
Lip line	Low	Medium	High
Gingival biotype	Low-scalloped, thick	Medium-scalloped, medium thick	High-scalloped, thin
Shape of tooth crowns	Rectangular		Triangular
Infection at implant site	None	Chronic	Acute
Bone level at adjacent teeth	≤ 5 mm to contact point	5.5 to 6.5 mm to contact point	≥ 7 mm to contact point
Restorative status of neighboring teeth	Virgin		Restored
Width of edentulous span	1 tooth (≥ 7 mm)	1 tooth (≤ 7 mm)	2 teeth or more
Soft-tissue anatomy	Intact soft tissue		Soft-tissue defects
Bone anatomy of alveolar crest	Alveolar crest without bone deficiency	Horizontal bone deficiency	Vertical bone deficiency

Table 3a   Surgical modifying factors.

Site Factors	Risk or Degree of Difficulty		
	Low	**Moderate**	**High**
Bone Volume			
Horizontal	Adequate	Deficient, but allowing simultaneous augmentation	Deficient, requiring prior augmentation
Vertical	Adequate	Small deficiency crestally, requiring slightly deeper corono-apical implant position. Small deficiency apically due to proximity to anatomical structures, requiring shorter than standard implant lengths.	Deficient, requiring prior augmentation
Anatomic Risk			
Proximity to vital anatomic structures	Minimal risk of involvement	Moderate risk of involvement	High risk of involvement
Esthetic Risk			
Esthetic zone	No		Yes
Biotype	Thick		Thin
Thickness of facial bone wall	Sufficient ≥ 1 mm		Insufficient < 1 mm
Complexity			
Number of prior or simultaneous procedures	Implant placement without adjunctive procedures	Implant placement with simultaneous procedures	Implant placement with staged procedures
Complications			
Risk of surgical complications	Minimal	Moderate	High
Consequences of complications	No adverse effect	Suboptimal outcome	Severely compromised outcome

Table 3b   Surgical risk assessment and SAC classification for short edentulous spaces in areas of high esthetic risk.

Areas of High Esthetic Risk	Case Type: Short Edentulous Space					
Risk Assessment					Normative Classification	Notes/Adjunctive procedures that may be required
Bone Volume	Anatomic Risk	Esthetic Risk	Complexity	Risk of Complications		
Defining Characteristics: Two implants and up to 4 teeth replaced						
Sufficient	Low	High	Moderate	Moderate	Advanced	Adjunctive soft-tissue graft
Deficient horizontally, allowing simultaneous grafting	Low	High	Moderate	Moderate	Advanced	Adjunctive soft-tissue graft Procedures for simultaneous horizontal bone augmentation In the anterior maxilla, the nasopalatine canal may increase the anatomic risk and influence implant position
Deficient horizontally, requiring prior grafting	Low	High	Moderate	Moderate	Complex	Adjunctive soft-tissue graft Procedures for horizontal bone augmentation In the anterior maxilla, the nasopalatine canal may increase the anatomic risk and influence implant position
Deficient vertically and/or horizontally	High	High	High	High	Complex	Adjunctive soft-tissue graft Risk to adjacent teeth Procedures for vertical and/or horizontal bone augmentation In the anterior maxilla, the nasopalatine canal may increase the anatomic risk and influence implant position

Table 3c   Surgical classification of cases in long edentulous spaces in areas of high esthetic risk.

Areas of High Esthetic Risk					Case Type: Long Span	
Risk Assessment					Normative Classification	Notes/Adjunctive procedures that may be required
Bone Volume	Anatomic Risk	Esthetic Risk	Complexity	Risk of Complications		
Defining Characteristics: More than 2 implants, span of more than 3 teeth						
Sufficient	Low	High	Moderate	Moderate	Advanced	Adjunctive soft-tissue graft Adjacent implants increase the complexity and risk of complications
Deficient horizontally, allowing simultaneous grafting	Low	High	Moderate	Moderate	Advanced	Adjunctive soft-tissue graft Procedures for simultaneous horizontal bone augmentation The nasopalatine canal may increase the anatomic risk and influence implant position Adjacent implants increase the complexity and risk of complications
Deficient horizontally, requiring prior grafting	Moderate	High	Moderate	Moderate	Complex	Adjunctive soft-tissue graft Procedures for horizontal bone augmentation The nasopalatine canal may increase the anatomic risk and influence implant position Adjacent implants increase the complexity and risk of complications
Deficient vertically and/or horizontally	High	High	High	High	Complex	Adjunctive soft-tissue graft Risk to adjacent teeth Procedures for vertical and/or horizontal bone augmentation The nasopalatine canal may increase the anatomic risk and influence implant position Adjacent implants increase the complexity and risk of complications

Table 3d   Prosthetic risk assessment and SAC classification for anterior extended spaces in areas with different levels of esthetic risk. Note that prosthetic treatment is considered complex if the esthetic risk is high.

Anterior Extended Edentulous Spaces	Notes	Straightforward	Advanced	Complex
Esthetic risk	Refer for ERA (Treatment Guide 1)	Low	Moderate	High
Intermaxillary relationship	Refers to horizontal and vertical overlap and the effect on restorability and esthetic outcome	Class I and III	Class II Div 1 and 2	Non-restorable without adjunctive preparatory therapy due to severe malocclusion
Mesiodistal space		Adequate for required tooth replacement	Insufficient space available for replacement of all missing teeth	Adjunctive therapy necessary to replace all missing teeth
Occlusion/ articulation		Harmonious	Irregular, with no need for correction	Changes of existing occlusion necessary
Interim restorations during healing		RDP	Fixed	
Provisional implant-supported restorations	Provisional restorations are recommended		Restorative margin < 3 mm apical to mucosal crest	Restorative margin ≥ 3 mm apical to mucosal crest
Occlusal parafunction	Risk of complication is to the restoration, not to implant survival	Absent		Present
Loading protocol	To date, immediate restoration and loading procedures are lacking scientific documentation	Conventional or early		Immediate

Table 3e *Restorative modifying factors that may influence the SAC classification of an individual case.*

Issue	Notes	Degree of Difficulty		
		Low	Moderate	High
Oral Environment				
General oral health		No active disease		Active disease
Condition of adjacent teeth		Restored teeth		Virgin teeth
Reason for tooth loss		Caries/Trauma		Periodontal disease or occlusal parafunction
Restorative Volume				
Inter-arch distance	Refers to the distance from the proposed implant restorative margin to the opposing occlusion	Adequate for planned restoration	Restricted space, but can be managed	Adjunctive therapy will be necessary to gain sufficient space for the planned restoration
Mesiodistal space	The arch length available to fit tooth replacements	Sufficient to fit replacements for missing teeth	Some reduction in size or number of teeth will be necessary	Adjunctive therapy will be needed to achieve a satisfactory result
Span of restoration		Single tooth	Extended edentulous space	Full arch
Volume and characteristics of the edentulous saddle	Refers to whether there is sufficient tissue volume to support the final restoration, or some prosthetic replacement of soft tissues will be necessary.	No prosthetic soft-tissue replacement will be necessary		Prosthetic replacement of soft tissue will be needed for esthetics or phonetics

Table 3e (continued)

Issue	Notes	Degree of Difficulty		
		Low	Moderate	High
Occlusion				
Occlusal scheme		Anterior guidance		No guidance
Involvement in occlusion	The degree to which the implant prosthesis is involved in the patient's occlusal scheme	Minimal involvement		Implant restoration is involved in guidance
Occlusal parafunction	Risk of complication to the restoration, but not to implant survival	Absent		Present
Provisional Restorations				
During implant healing		None required	Removable	Fixed
Implant-supported provisionals needed	Provisional restorations will be needed to develop esthetics and soft tissue transition zones	Not required	Restorative margin < 3 mm apical to mucosal crest	Restorative margin ≥ 3 mm apical to mucosal crest
Loading protocol	To date immediate restoration and loading procedures are lacking scientific documentation	Conventional or early loading		Immediate loading
Materials/manufacture	Materials and techniques used in the manufacture of definitive prostheses	Resin-based materials ± metal reinforcement	Porcelain fused to metal	
Maintenance needs	Anticipated maintenance needs based on patient presentation and the planned prosthesis	Low	Moderate	High

3.5   Prosthodontic Planning Considerations

3.5.1   Introduction

Considering that treatment of multiple adjacent missing teeth in the maxillary anterior zone is considered complex or, in other words, involves a high risk of dissatisfying esthetic outcomes, careful planning is of utmost importance. As concluded in the consensus statements of the 3rd ITI Conference with regard to esthetics in implant dentistry, long-term esthetic outcomes can be predictably achieved with single-tooth replacement in

the absence of tissue deficiencies because of the tissue support provided by the adjacent teeth (Belser and co-workers 2004a). Replacement of multiple adjacent teeth with fixed restorations in the anterior maxilla was, by contrast, found to be poorly documented and its esthetic outcomes to be unpredictable, specifically with regard to the contours of the interimplant soft tissue (Belser and coworkers 2004a; Belser and coworkers 2004b; Martin and coworkers 2007) (Figs 13a-d).

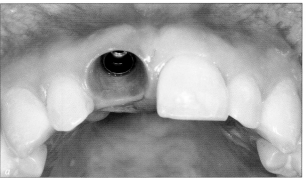
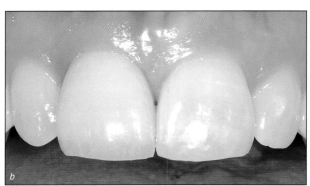

Figs 13a-b   Esthetic single-tooth replacement at a site delimited by neighboring teeth with intact tissue.

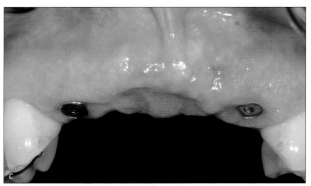
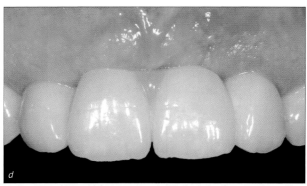

Figs 13c-d   Multiple adjacent missing teeth with a deficient ridge morphology at sites 11 and 21, which was restored with the help of a ceramic papilla.

Interimplant support by soft and hard tissues is largely unpredictable because implant and abutment design characteristics in conjunction with an overly small inter-implant distance will cause the peri-implant crestal bone adjacent to the two implants to decrease (Tarnow and coworkers 2003; Buser and coworkers 2004; Martin and coworkers 2007). This, in turn, will lead to an insufficient height of the bony support for the papilla between the two implant restorations and, consequently, to a short papilla opening an unsightly black triangle, especially in patients with triangular tooth forms in the anterior segment (Fig 14).

Particular caution is needed when replacing adjacent central and lateral incisors or adjacent canines and lateral incisors. The available space may be too narrow to place two implants next to each other while still allowing esthetically pleasing restorative and soft-tissue contours to be created. As stated in Volume 1 of the ITI Treatment Guide, treatment options should be explored in situations of this type that will not require placement of adjacent implants whenever possible (Martin and coworkers 2007). Various options to achieve this goal are illustrated in the following schematics (Figs 15a-e).

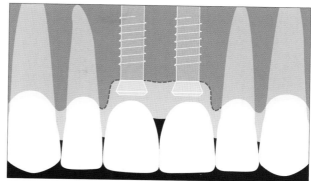

Fig 14   Proximal bone loss and insufficient papilla height.

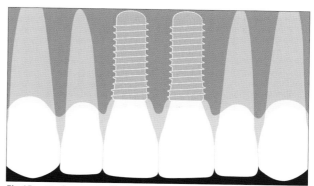

Fig 15a   Replacement of both central incisors with non-splinted implant crowns.

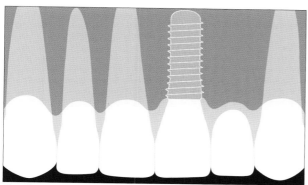

Fig 15b   Replacement of a central incisor with an implant and of the lateral incisor next to it with a cantilever.

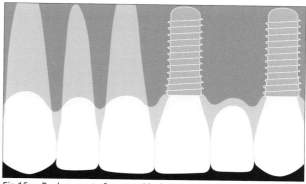

Fig 15c   Replacement of a central incisor, lateral incisor and canine with two implants and a pontic in between.

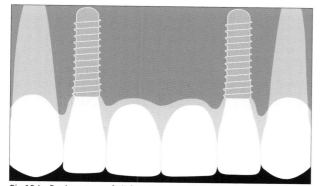

Fig 15d   Replacement of all four incisors with two implants and two pontics in between.

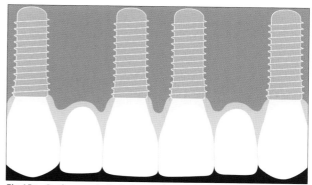

Fig 15e   Replacement of all six anterior teeth with implants in positions 13, 11, 21, 23 and pontics in positions 12, 22.

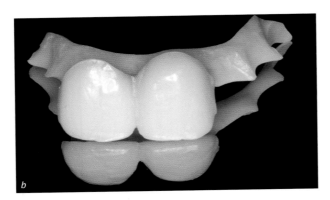

Figs 16a-b   Removable diagnostic setup (either in wax or in resin).

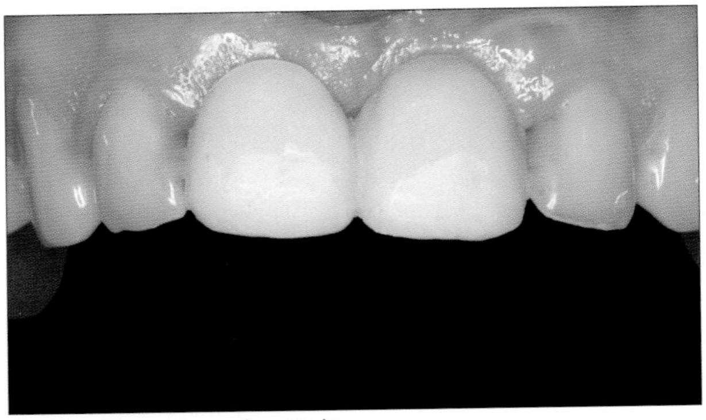

3.5.2 Diagnostic Wax-up

A top-down approach (i.e. prosthodontically driven) needs to be taken for esthetic implant placement. A diagnostic wax-up, setup or mock-up becomes especially important when both multiple adjacent teeth and contralateral landmarks are missing (Figs 16a-d). This mock-up should be removable to allow for an intraoral try-in.

During this mock-up try-in, all aspects of esthetics and function are evaluated as accurately as possible, including tooth positions and angulations, tooth widths and lengths, occlusal interactions, and cervical/interproximal relationships between the teeth and soft tissue.

Existing soft-tissue defects are masked with pink wax on the try-in device. In this way, the clinician can evaluate whether pink ceramics would make for an adequate substitute or whether more invasive surgical modes of hard- or soft-tissue augmentation are required. Especially in patients with a low or moderately high smile line, the issue of how to approach soft-tissue replacement is an important one and can be optimally discussed with the patient at chairside with the help of a diagnostic mock-up (Figs 17a-d).

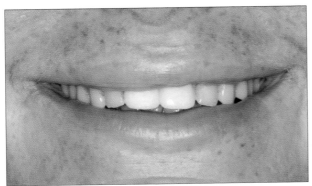

Fig 16c   Diagnostic mock-up try-in.

Fig 16d   Mock-up try-in with low smile line.

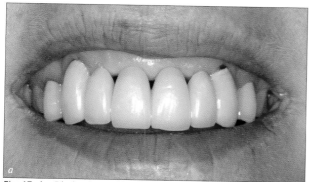
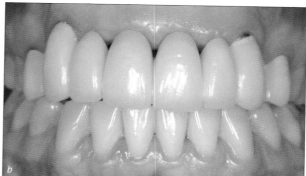

Figs 17a-b   Displeasing and failing fixed prosthesis associated with a high smile line.

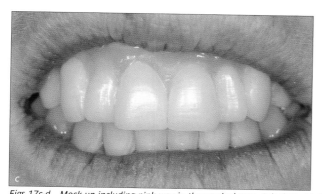
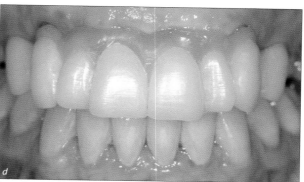

Figs 17c-d   Mock-up including pink wax in the cervical area. It is desirable to have the transition zone between the artificial gingiva and the underlying ridge mucosa covered by the lip to determine if, and to what extent, ridge augmentation is desirable. (Images courtesy of Dr. Kenneth Malament.)

3.5.3   Implant Selection from a Prosthodontic Viewpoint

Spaces of two or more adjacent missing teeth to be treated with implant restorations should ideally encompass the total mesiodistal width of the natural teeth that normally belong there. The diagnostic setup is important for the proper design of the planned dental units and, ultimately, for selecting the appropriate implants and their locations with regard to the proposed prosthodontic design. A mesiodistal tooth width of 7 mm or more, which generally applies to central incisors and canines, will allow insertion of standard-platform (Regular Neck) implants, if the buccolingual bone width is also adequate for this choice. Narrow-platform (Narrow Neck) implants should normally be used for teeth featuring a mesiodistal width less than 7 mm such as the upper lateral incisors.

Indications in the maxillary anterior area exist for implants placed at the soft-tissue level or at the bone level (i.e. tissue-level or bone-level designs). In either case, esthetic success can only be achieved with correct three-dimensional placement. For tissue-level implants, the local mucosa should be 3 mm deep or deeper to avoid having to sink the implant too deep into the alveolar crest, which results in more circumferential crestal bone loss around the implant as part of the "biologic width" formation during remodeling (Hermann and coworkers 2000) (Figs 18a-d). Bone-level implants should be preferred if the mucosa is thinner than that and whenever simultaneous bone augmentation procedures are required (Figs 19a-d).

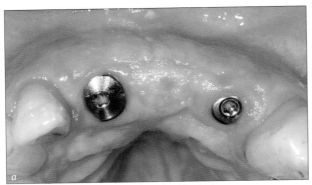

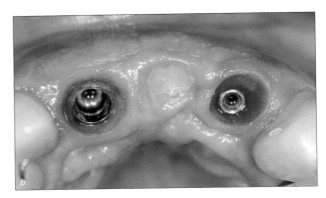

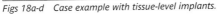

Figs 18a-d   Case example with tissue-level implants.

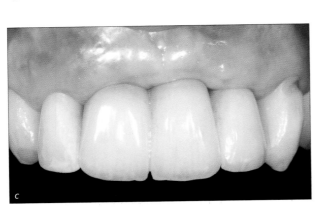

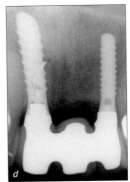

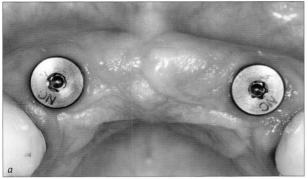
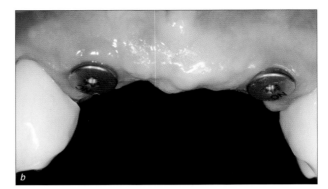

Figs 19a-d   Case example with bone-level implants.

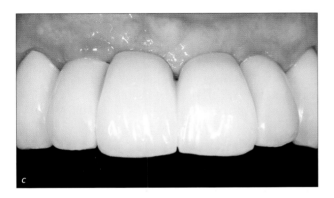
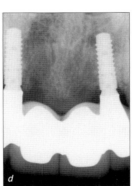

3.6 Surgical Planning

Esthetically and functionally desirable implant restorations in the maxillary anterior segment depend on optimal surgical implant placement in accordance with the detailed diagnostic and prosthodontic plan outlined above. Surgical planning includes additional radiographic diagnostics to be performed on CBCT scans. Some patients may still be hesitant to undergo these CBCT scans because they are afraid of any added radiation exposure and because of the costs involved. They need to be informed, however, of the benefits gained in terms of helping the surgeon arrive at a diagnosis or in facilitating treatment, especially in an esthetically demanding area such as the anterior maxilla. Three-dimensional imaging lets the clinician visualize internal anatomical features that cannot be diagnosed by any other means. The location and orientation of vital structures such as nerves, adjacent tooth roots or implants, the maxillary sinus and the nasal floor can be readily visualized and potential risks of infringing on these structures assessed.

For optimal prosthodontically driven surgical planning, it is most beneficial to fabricate a radiographic template for the patient to wear during the imaging procedure. This template is a duplicate of the mock-up discussed above, which was tried and verified in the patient's mouth and subsequently duplicated with radiopaque teeth. For optimal reproducibility, it is important that the patient's residual dentition offer stable support for this template during radiographic imaging. In this way, the axes and contours of the planned teeth can be viewed in relation to the underlying alveolar bone, allowing the clinician to determine if appropriate implant locations and angulations can be attained at the sites considered and to assessed if bone augmentation procedures are necessary either prior to implant placement in a staged procedure or in a simultaneous procedure. Based on this information, the patient can be provided with an appropriate treatment plan and a listing of the treatment steps involved, as well as an accurate cost estimate.

Another advantage of CBCT scans is that the data files can be imported into implant-planning software. Many of these software systems are now available on the market. The selected implant designs (length, diameter, and platform), their three-dimensional placement, and their angulation can be previsualized and adjusted to achieve the most favorable combination of prosthodontically driven and surgically attainable parameters of implant placement (Figs 20a-c).

The use of planning software to optimize implant positioning and selection will also allow the surgical and prosthodontic colleagues to discuss various options and to decide on the best possible solution by sharing the planning images online without having to meet physically.

Once the implant placement planning is complete, the diagnostic template is modified into a surgical guide. The choice is between a surgical guide that will still allow some freedom in placing the implant(s) within the landmarks defined by the template (Fig 21a), or actual drilling guides with sleeves that allow no deviation from the guided path (Fig 21b). The latter can only be trusted—and is only worth the additional cost—if the intraoral positions of the diagnostic and surgical templates are identical and stable. The essential criterion for the successful execution of guided surgical procedures is whether the drilling guide will end up accurately in the same stable position as the diagnostic template used for CBCT scanning. This is more likely the case in partially edentulous indications with an adequate number of stable teeth to support the template.

More in-depth details on surgical planning and procedures are given in the following chapters of this Treatment Guide.

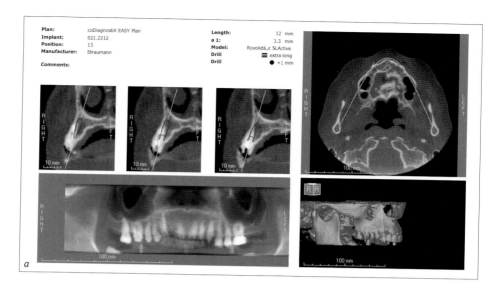

Figs 20a-c Example of a digital plan for guided surgery in the anterior maxilla.

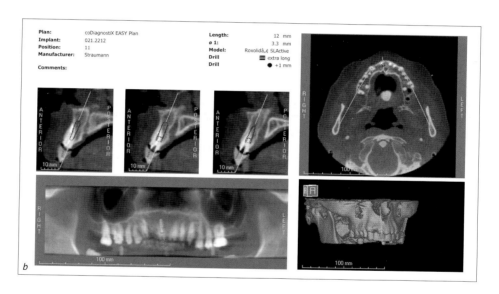

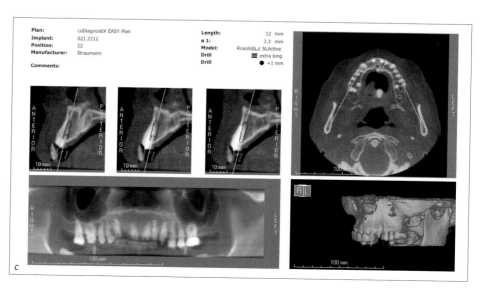

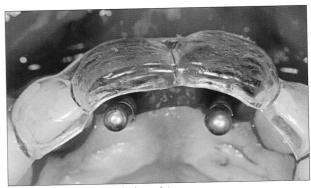

Fig 21a   Conventional surgical template.

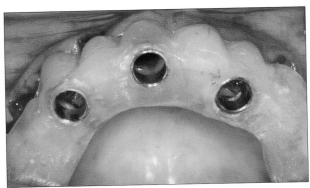

Fig 21b   Guided-surgery guide.

4 Surgical Considerations and Treatment Procedures for Extended Edentulous Spaces in the Esthetic Zone

S. Chen, D. Buser

4.1 Introduction

The primary objective of implant surgery is to attain successful and highly predictable outcomes with a low risk of complications. Secondary objectives include minimizing the number of surgical procedures, reducing patient morbidity, and reducing the healing times after surgery. Numerous improvement efforts have been made over the past 15 years in order to make implant therapy more attractive to patients. However, these improvements should never compromise the primary objectives of implant surgery.

The replacement of multiple missing teeth in the anterior maxilla counts among the greatest challenges in implant dentistry. The implant-supported prosthesis must meet functional and phonetic requirements and satisfy patients' high esthetic demands in this visually exposed area. In the anterior maxilla, tooth loss invariably results in rapid and significant resorption of the alveolar bone, leaving behind an alveolar crest that is reduced in width and height. The surgical requirements therefore extend beyond simply maintaining or reconstructing bone volume to accommodate the planned implants; the surgical management must also—as discussed later in this chapter—include steps toward restoring an appropriate ridge contour. Clinicians therefore need a sound understanding of the tissue biology and underlying biologic events following tooth extraction, the functional and esthetic requirements for replacing teeth in the maxillary anterior region, the surgical steps required to place implants, and any associated augmentation procedures.

4.2 Ridge Alterations Following Tooth Extraction

4.2.1 Histological Changes

Following the extraction of a tooth, a dynamic series of events take place during the tissue healing process, leading to bone regeneration within the socket and to external resorption, which is most evident on the facial aspect of the alveolar ridge (Araújo and Lindhe 2005). A blood clot forms within the socket that is converted to a provisional connective-tissue matrix within a matter of days. The bundle bone lining the extraction socket undergoes resorption and loses its continuity, allowing blood vessels to proliferate from the surrounding marrow space into the provisional matrix. Osteogenesis follows angiogenesis, with newly formed woven bone initially deposited at the socket periphery, eventually extending centrally to fill the socket. As the bone is being remodeled, the socket entrance eventually corticalizes and becomes continuous with the cortical bone of the surrounding alveolus. Centrally, the bone is remodeled to form trabecular bone. Early in the healing process, epithelial cells migrate from the surrounding mucosa to create a soft-tissue barrier over the socket entrance. The supracrestal soft tissue eventually organizes to form mucosa indistinguishable from the surrounding oral mucosa (Cardaropoli and coworkers 2005).

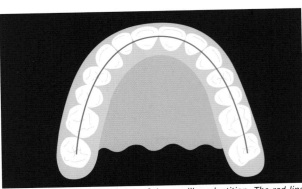

Fig 1a   Schematic occlusal view of the maxillary dentition. The red line represents the curvature of the dental arch.

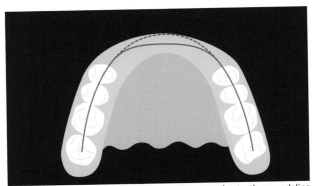

Fig 1b   Following extraction of the maxillary anterior teeth, remodeling changes, and bone resorption lead to the ridge curvature being flattened. The ridge crest migrates toward the palatal aspect (continuous line) compared to its pre-extraction outline (dotted line). The flattened ridge crest is less convex and therefore has a reduced linear dimension compared to the pre-extraction situation. This has implications for the number of implants that can be placed and the proximity to each other.

4.2.2   Dimensional Changes of the Alveolar Ridge

During healing, the external surface of the alveolar ridge also undergoes changes particularly on the facial aspect. Initially, the bundle bone lining the socket undergoes resorption through intense osteoclastic activity. The coronal portion of the facial socket wall is often thin or even absent (Januario and coworkers 2011; Braut and coworkers 2011). In most patients it is composed entirely of bundle bone that is resorbed within 4 to 8 weeks of extraction (Araújo and Lindhe 2005), resulting in vertical and horizontal bone loss on the facial aspect of the coronal third of the ridge. Subsequent remodeling of the facial bone adds to a loss in orofacial crest width, combined with a facial flattening of the ridge contour. The net result is ridge resorption toward the palatal aspect and a loss of vertical crestal bone height on the facial aspect. The normal curvature of the ridge (when teeth are present) changes to yield a flatter profile (Figs 1a-b).

The linear dimension of the arch is reduced because of this flattening of the ridge curvature. Multiple adjacent implants carry a risk of ending up too close to each other, thus encroaching into embrasure areas. Implants separated by at least a single-tooth gap can usually be placed into the correct restorative position (Fig 1c). At the alveolar crest, ridge height is generally reduced, and the bone that originally formed the interproximal bone peaks is flattened (Figs 2a-b).

The oral mucosa overlying the crestal bone in extended maxillary tooth spaces is between 2 and 4 mm thick (Turck 1965; Uchida and coworkers 1989).

In single-tooth extraction sites, this resorption is limited by the presence of adjacent tooth roots. When multiple adjacent teeth are extracted, however, the influence of retained teeth in maintaining the bone decreases as the edentulous span increases. Ridge resorption can be significant in extended edentulous spaces in the anterior maxilla with serial extraction of multiple adjacent teeth (Figs 3a-c).

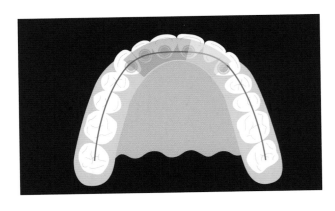

Fig 1c   Multiple adjacent implants (red zone) risk ending up too close to each other, encroaching into the embrasure spaces (as illustrated for the site of the maxillary right lateral incisor). Implants separated by at least a single-tooth gap (green zone) can usually be placed at the correct restorative position.

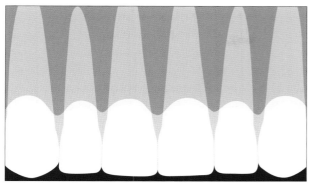

Fig 2a   Schematic anterior view of the maxillary anterior teeth.

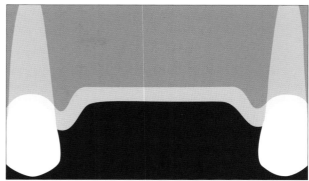

Fig 2b   Following extraction of the four maxillary incisors, vertical resorption of the ridge takes place. The overlying mucosa is 2 to 4 mm thick.

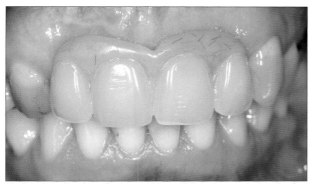

Fig 3a   Anterior view of a removable partial denture replacing the four maxillary incisors. A pink flange replaces missing hard and soft tissue.

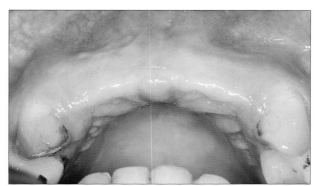

Fig 3b   Occlusal view of an anterior maxillary ridge with evident flattening of the facial bone following resorption of the bony ridge.

In a study of over 200 maxillary diagnostic casts of partially edentulous ridges, more than 90% presented with ridge deformities (Abrams and coworkers 1987). That study was based on Seibert's classification (Seibert 1983) and revealed 55.8% of all ridges to be class III defects (combined loss of ridge width and height). Class I defects (loss of orofacial contour with normal apical coronal ridge height) accounted for 32.3% of the ridge defects observed, while class II defects (loss of coronoapical ridge height in the presence of normal orofacial ridge width) were rare.

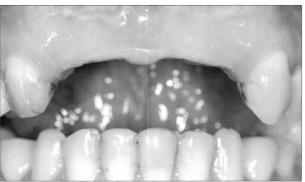

Fig 3c   Anterior view of an anterior maxillary ridge showing vertical resorption. The combined horizontal and vertical resorption falls into the category of Seibert class III ridge defects.

The rate of ridge resorption may be influenced by the following factors:

Integrity of socket walls upon extraction. Damage to the facial bone wall of an extraction socket will accelerate ridge resorption. As a general observation, wide dehiscences of the facial bone are associated with more rapid resorption of the alveolar ridge than with narrow dehiscences.

Cause of tooth loss. Traumatic loss of maxillary anterior teeth often leads to significant ridge resorption both vertically and horizontally. Teeth lost to chronic periodontitis may also be associated with significant vertical and horizontal resorption of the residual alveolar ridge.

Number of teeth. The potential for ridge resorption increases with the number of adjacent teeth extracted. Where more teeth are removed, the bone-preserving effect of natural teeth is increasingly lost.

Surgical trauma. Elevation of surgical flaps to extract teeth will accelerate resorption due to disruption of the blood supply to the superficial bone through periosteal vessels. To minimize this effect, teeth should be extracted without elevating a flap whenever possible.

Post-extraction healing time. The greatest dimensional change to the alveolar ridge usually occurs within the first 3 months after extracting the teeth. The timing of implant placement is therefore critical. Late implant placement (type 4) should ideally be avoided, as this strategy increases the risks of advanced resorption and of staged bone augmentation being required. In addition, patients today do not readily accept treatment strategies that involve extended healing periods.

Bone loss between implants. Frequently, the bone between adjacent implants will assume a flat profile as physiological bone remodeling takes place around the implant necks. Different implant systems are associated with different patterns of crestal bone remodeling. External-hex and tissue-level implants, for example, give rise to bony "saucer" shapes. Even with implants designed to preserve the crestal bone, bone peaks between adjacent implants are not predictably maintained. It is therefore very difficult to create peri-implant papillae between adjacent implants.

4.2.3   Soft-Tissue Thickness in Edentulous Areas of the Anterior Maxilla

The dimensions of the peri-implant mucosa are relatively stable. In single-tooth implants, the supracrestal dimension (apicocoronal height) of the soft tissue covering the midfacial aspect of implants is 3.5 to 4 mm (Berglundh and Lindhe 1996; Cochran and coworkers 1997). The supracrestal dimension of the tooth-to-implant papillae is slightly larger (5 to 6 mm) due to support from the periodontal attachment of the adjacent natural teeth (Kan and coworkers 2003). The mucosa in extended edentulous spaces, by contrast, has no support from adjacent teeth. Mucosal thickness is therefore similar both between implants and on the midfacial aspect of implants, both ranging from 2 to 4 mm (mean 3.4 mm) in coronoapical height, as verified in a study of interimplant soft-tissue height (Tarnow and coworkers 2003).

Consequently, as the height of the interimplant papillae cannot exceed biologically determined levels, these papillae are relatively short in the majority of implant-supported reconstructions spanning extended edentulous spaces in the anterior maxilla (Figs 4a-e). More often than not, pink ceramic needs to be added to the prosthesis to replicate the missing papillae (Fig 5a).

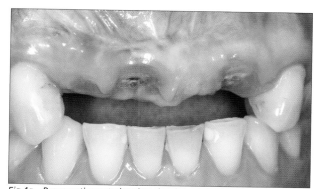

Fig 4a   Preoperative anterior view showing retained roots at sites 11 and 22. Note the height of the ridge in relation to the mandibular incisors.

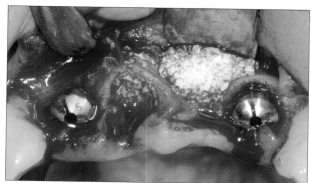

Fig 4b   Intraoperative view showing implants at sites 12 and 22. Socket 11 has been grafted with DBBM, and so has the facial bone surface at site 21.

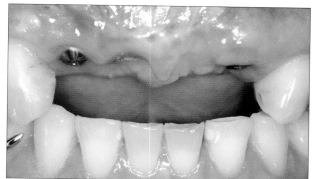

Fig 4c   Situation after 8 weeks of healing. Note the loss of ridge height relative to the mandibular incisors due to bone remodeling.

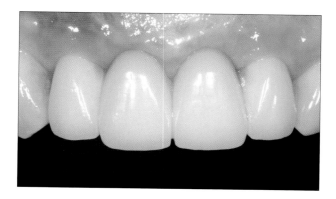

Fig 4d   View of the completed implant-supported fixed partial denture 4 years after implant surgery. The interproximal "papillae" are relatively short. The contact areas between the tooth units are elongated to compensate for the postoperative vertical loss of ridge height. The pontics at sites 11 and 21 overlap the ridge on the buccal aspect.

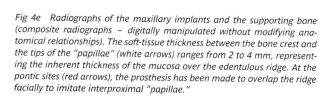

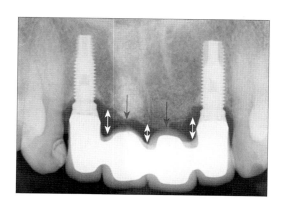

Fig 4e   Radiographs of the maxillary implants and the supporting bone (composite radiographs – digitally manipulated without modifying anatomical relationships). The soft-tissue thickness between the bone crest and the tips of the "papillae" (white arrows) ranges from 2 to 4 mm, representing the inherent thickness of the mucosa over the edentulous ridge. At the pontic sites (red arrows), the prosthesis has been made to overlap the ridge facially to imitate interproximal "papillae."

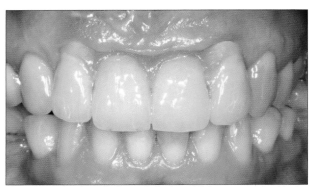

Fig 5a Anterior view of a four-unit fixed partial denture supported by implants at sites 12 and 22. Pink ceramic has been added to the prosthesis to replace the missing soft tissue including the papillae.

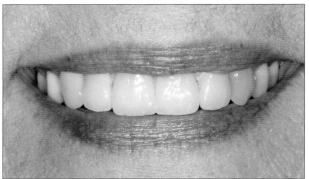

Fig 5b The transition zone between the implant-supported fixed partial denture and the alveolar mucosa is not visible in the patient's smile.

4.2.4 Surgical and Esthetic Implications

Maxillary ridge resorption in extended edentulous spaces may render the bone volume insufficient for implant placement. These volume deficits have a coronoapical and an orofacial dimension.

Orofacial resorption leads to flattening of the anterior ridge and reduces its orofacial dimension. The following complications may ensue:

- Bone volume can be insufficient for appropriately dimensioned implants to be placed into the residual ridge such that correct restorative positioning is achieved. Simultaneous or staged bone augmentation procedures may be required.
- If the ridge is resorbed, but sufficient bone volume remains, implants may be positioned too far palatally, resulting in an anterior cantilever and a ridge-lap design of the fixed dental prosthesis. This may encumber proper maintenance of plaque control by the patient.
- In the presence of vertical crestal resorption, natural papilla form and mucosal height are lost as the ridge is resorbed. In many cases, the papillae cannot be reconstructed with mucosa alone; the clinician must add pink ceramics as a flange to the fixed dental prosthesis to reproduce the missing papillae and soft-tissue volume. In doing so, it is important to note the position of the lip and smile line. The surgery and subsequent restorative steps should be carried out with a view to concealing the transition zone between the alveolar mucosa and the flange of the fixed dental prosthesis behind the lip (Fig 5b). The esthetic consequences of a visible transition zone in the smile can be quite negative. Vertical augmentation procedures should therefore be avoided if they bring the transition zone into view.

4.3 Surgical Procedures in Extended Edentulous Spaces

4.3.1 Simultaneous versus Staged Approach

Based on the above biologic and anatomical considerations, implant placement is more often than not combined with bone augmentation, using either a simultaneous or a staged approach. To minimize the number of surgical interventions, simultaneous guided bone regeneration (GBR) is preferred whenever possible, as this is associated with lower morbidity and expenses. A predictable regenerative outcome of bone augmentation should only be expected if the defect morphology with the exposed implant surface inside the alveolar crest covers at least two walls (Figs 6a-b). The bony walls and adjacent bone marrow will provide the osteogenic elements for new bone formation (Bosshardt and Schenk 2009). In addition, new bone formation can be accelerated with locally harvested autologous bone chips, which will be discussed later.

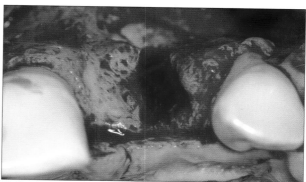

Fig 6a   Intraoperative view of the alveolar ridge at site 21. Note the loss of facial bone.

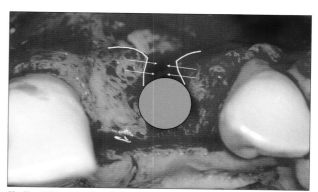

Fig 6b   With an implant in its correct three-dimensional position (gray circle), a defect on the facial aspect of the implant is anticipated. This defect will have two bone walls, one mesial and one distal (white lines). The bone walls and the adjacent bone marrow will provide the osteogenic elements for new bone formation in the defect area (white arrows depict the path of migration of the osteogenic cells).

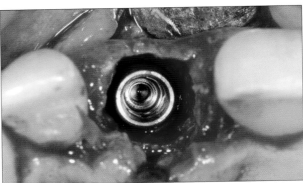

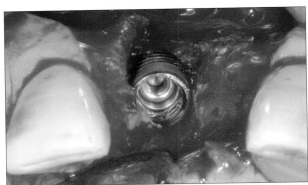

Fig 7a   Intraoperative view of an implant placed immediately into an extraction socket (type 1 placement) with intact walls. As the implant is placed toward the palatal aspect of the socket, the resultant bony defect is on the facial aspect of the implant. This defect has three bone walls (mesial, distal, and facial).

Fig 7b   This implant was placed 8 weeks following removal of the tooth. At the time of extraction, the facial bone was missing due to chronic infection from the fractured tooth root. The bony defect on the facial aspect of the implant has two bone walls (mesial and distal).

Implants placed in extraction sites are routinely associated with a three- or two-wall defect morphology if an immediate or early placement protocol has been followed (Figs 7a-b).

In healed sites with facial flattening of the ridge, defects with a two-wall morphology are seen much less frequently. Bone augmentation at sites with a one-wall defect morphology is much more demanding and less predictable in terms of regenerative outcomes (Figs 8a-b).

Potential implant sites at which the alveolar crest is less than 4 mm thick are extremely challenging. It is very difficult to prepare implant beds in these locations, and correct three-dimensional positioning of an implant such that stability is ensured is often impossible. A staged GBR approach is therefore recommended, using cortico-cancellous block grafts covered by a barrier membrane (Buser and coworkers 1996; von Arx and Buser 2006; Cordaro and coworkers 2002). These grafts are routinely harvested in the mandible either from the chin or retromolar area (von Arx and Buser 2006). This does not change the fact, however, that they increase the morbidity for patients (Chiapasco and coworkers 1999).

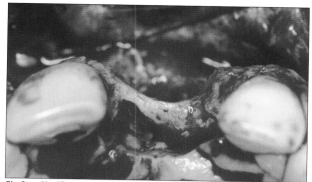

Fig 8a   Significant horizontal resorption has occurred in this bony ridge. An extended period has elapsed since the tooth was extracted. The occlusal view reveals a concavity in the facial bone; the bone width is not adequate for implant placement.

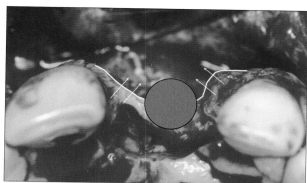

Fig 8b   With an implant in its correct three-dimensional position (gray circle), the defect on its facial aspect is not delimited by bone walls. This represents a one-wall defect (wall outlined in white). Osteogenic cells for new bone formation need to migrate from the facial bone surface (white arrows) into the defect area. One-wall defects are much more demanding and less predictable than two- or three-wall defects in terms of regenerative outcomes.

Recently, a titanium zirconium (Ti-Zr) alloy (Roxolid, Straumann AG, Basel, Switzerland) has been introduced as an implant material (Thoma and coworkers 2011; Barter and coworkers 2011). This α-phase titanium alloy offers enhanced mechanical strength, allowing clinicians to use narrower implants without increasing the risk of fracture (Bernhard and coworkers 2009). Simultaneous

GBR procedures can be performed more frequently with reduced-diameter implants (3.3 mm), as these improve the two-wall morphology of peri-implant defects (Fig 9). While the experience available for Ti-Zr alloy implants of this type is currently confined to short-term data (Barter and coworkers 2011; Chiapasco and coworkers 2011), their introduction has added an interesting perspective.

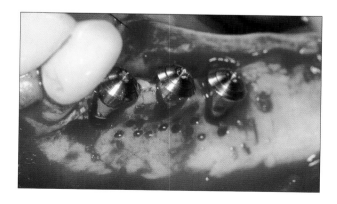

Fig 9   Two reduced-diameter (3.3 mm) Ti-Zr alloy implants (Roxolid; Straumann AG, Basel, Switzerland) placed in a bony ridge of reduced dimensions in the posterior mandible. As these implants could be placed entirely within the bony envelope, the resultant defects on their facial aspect included two bone walls. The use of reduced-diameter designs improved the two-wall morphology of the peri-implant defects.

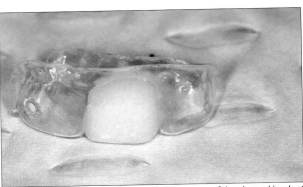

Fig 10a   Radiographic stent derived from a wax-up of the planned implant site. Barium sulfate has been incorporated into the acrylic.

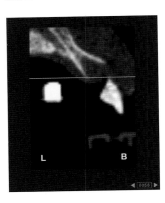

Fig 10b   CT scan of the site with radiographic stent in place at the time of acquisition. The outline of the prosthetic tooth is clearly visible against the cross-sectional representation of the hard and soft tissues constituting the ridge.

4.3.2   Preoperative Radiographic Examination

As outlined above, a detailed knowledge of the underlying bone anatomy in the anterior maxilla is important for surgical treatment planning. A three-dimensional (3D) radiographic examination is therefore needed in the majority of cases. Cone-beam computed tomography (CBCT) is the state of the art and should be preferred to multi-slice dental CT scans as they offer much better resolution and expose patients to less radiation (Hirsch and coworkers 2008). Radiographic guides (also known as "radiographic stents") derived from a wax-up are routinely used to visualize the correct position and axis of the future tooth restorations (Figs 10a-b).

In addition to evaluating the width of the crest and the shape of the ridge at each potential implant site, the location and size of the nasopalatine canal must be examined. This canal can vary considerably in size and location (Bornstein and coworkers 2011) and often causes problems with correct implant positioning. A detailed radiographic analysis will help decide if a given clinical situation can be handled with a simultaneous GBR procedure or if a staged approach is necessary. If a simultaneous approach is possible, the data obtained by CBCT will offer assistance in determining the number, position, diameter, and length of the implants required. The past few years have seen the emergence of planning software as a useful adjunct to implant planning.

4.3.3 Esthetic Risk Assessment (with Special Consideration of the Smile Line)

An assessment of the esthetic risk is mandatory whenever implant-supported reconstructions are planned in the anterior maxilla. The relationship between the mucosal crest of the edentulous area and the lip in repose and with the patient smiling must be evaluated carefully. If the crest is visible during normal speech or in the smile, the transition zone between the implant-supported fixed prosthetic denture and the mucosa will likely be visible also. Such visibility raises the stakes for the prosthodontist and dental technician to create an esthetically pleasing transition zone that will be acceptable to the patient. Sometimes the crest of the ridge may have to be reduced to conceal the transition zone behind the upper lip. Clinicians should also be aware that augmentation procedures elevating the vertical ridge could bring a previously hidden transition zone into view, thus detracting from the final esthetic outcome. It is important that any potential esthetic risks and outcomes be carefully discussed with patients before seeking their consent and initiating treatment.

4.3.4 Timing of Implant Placement

Implants may be placed at certain critical times following tooth extraction. A classification system for postextraction timing of implant insertion based on desired biologic outcomes of wound healing was proposed at two ITI Consensus Conferences in 2003 and in 2008 (Hämmerle and coworkers 2004; Chen and Buser 2009; Chen and coworkers 2009c). Immediate placement (type 1) refers to implant placement into a fresh extraction socket when no healing of bone or soft tissues has occurred. Early placement with soft-tissue healing (type 2) typically takes place 4 to 8 weeks after tooth extraction, the desired healing outcome being soft-tissue healing over the socket in the absence of clinically significant bone fill within the socket. Early implant placement with partial bone healing (type 3) is usually undertaken 12 to 16 weeks after tooth extraction, at a time when both soft-tissue healing and substantial bone fill within the socket has occurred. Late implant placement (type 4) refers to insertion of an implant into a fully healed alveolar ridge.

Type 1 placement. Although immediate placement (type 1) of implants has been strongly advocated in the maxillary anterior region to enhance esthetic outcomes, great care should be taken when recommending this approach. In a recent series of experimental studies, Araújo and coworkers demonstrated that immediate placement into fresh extraction sockets did not prevent resorption of the surrounding alveolar bone (Araújo and coworkers 2005; Araújo and coworkers 2006; Araújo and coworkers 2006). The thin facial bone underwent vertical and horizontal resorption similar to an undisturbed extraction socket. Recent clinical studies have corroborated these findings. Immediate placement carries an increased risk of mucosal margin recession. A recent review of immediate implant studies showed that approximately 30% of sites exhibited recession of 1 mm or more (Chen and Buser, 2009), thus exceeding the visual threshold of detecting a difference (Kokich and coworkers 2006). Several risk factors have been identified:

- There is a lack of keratinized soft tissue following the extraction of a tooth. Additional procedures (e.g. flap advancement, soft-tissue grafting, or socket-seal techniques) are often required to achieve primary wound closure or to partially submerge the implant. At sites characterized by thin gingiva, an elevated risk of mucosal recession will remain even when supplementary procedures of this type are performed.

- Thin facial bone is susceptible to vertical and horizontal resorption. This susceptibility may result in dehiscence defects and exposure of the implant surface at the level of the implant neck, which reduces the volume of bone support to the facial mucosa and increases the risk of mucosal recession. It should be noted that thin bone is much more commonly encountered than thick bone on the facial aspect of maxillary anterior tooth sockets (Braut and coworkers 2011; Januario and coworkers 2011). Also, the thickness of the gingiva (tissue biotype) correlates poorly with the thickness of the facial bone (Fu and coworkers 2010).

- Damage inflicted to the facial bone will adversely affect the bone's regenerative potential. With bone regeneration being compromised, less volume will be present to support the midfacial mucosa. The risk of mucosal recession increases proportionately with the extent of damage inflicted to the facial bone (Kan and coworkers 2007).

- Bone regeneration adjacent to immediately placed implants is unpredictable. Even in the presence of a bone substitute with a low substitution rate, a complete fill of the extraction site is not always achieved (Botticelli and coworkers 2004; Chen and coworkers 2007).

- Technical errors during placement of implants into extraction sockets may complicate outcomes. It has been shown that implants placed too far facially within extraction sockets are associated with mucosal recession (Evans and Chen 2008). The difficulty of preparing a correctly positioned osteotomy is increased by the high density of the palatal bone in extraction sockets, which may also cause the implant to be deflected toward the facial at the time of insertion. Facially placed implants offer less space for the prosthetic components of the restoration in the transmucosal zone, thus exerting pressure and thinning of the mucosa with subsequent recession. Oversized implants, too, have been shown to be associated with mucosal recession for similar reasons (Small and coworkers 2001).

Immediate implant placement (type 1) should therefore be restricted to experienced clinicians and ideal clinical situations. Favorable conditions include a thick facial gingiva, a thick and intact facial wall of the socket, and a patient with low esthetic demands. As far as the anterior maxilla is concerned, this combination of factors is relatively uncommon. Furthermore, even in the presence of ideal tissue conditions, clinicians and patients should be prepared to accept 1 mm of soft-tissue recession on average. A flapless surgical approach may be considered when these conditions are met, but appropriate 3D imaging should be obtained during the planning phase. The gaps between implants and the internal facial bone wall should be filled with a bone substitute offering a low substitution rate, such as deproteinized bovine bone mineral (DBBM). A collagen plug or a small connective-tissue graft should be used to protect the bone graft.

Type 2 placement. Early implant placement with soft-tissue healing (type 2) is recommended in the majority of cases. With the soft tissues having substantially healed, an enhanced volume of keratinized soft tissue will be present by this time. Gingiva that was initially thin will have converted to thicker tissue once the mucosa has healed over the socket. This conversion facilitates flap closure to protect the implant and its related biomaterials and results in preservation of a thick and wide band of keratinized mucosa, which is essential for

achieving good esthetic outcomes (Buser and coworkers 2008). At the time of implant placement, bone defects present usually with two or three walls, which is conducive to GBR procedures. Additionally, softening of the palatal bone during normal bone remodeling after extraction allows the palatal side of the alveolar bone to be prepared and the implants to be placed in their correct three-dimensional position with less risk of deflection toward the facial side. With type 2 placement, some flattening of the facial bone occurs during the early stages of healing. The clinician is able to reconstruct the entire facial bone using bone substitutes with a combination of autologous bone chips and a superficial layer of low-substitution filler. This concept of contour augmentation is essential to the reconstruction and long-term maintenance of a proper ridge contour in esthetic areas. It is described below in Section 4.3.6.

Type 3 placement. Early implant placement with partial bone healing (type 3) may be indicated in extended apical defects that require longer periods of healing and bone regeneration. It should be noted, however, that the bone resorption encountered with this approach may be quite extensive. There is an increased risk of peri-implant defects presenting with only one wall, which may require correspondingly larger grafting procedures for contour augmentation. For this reason, the type 2 approach is clearly favored over the type 3 approach.

Type 4 placement. It is generally agreed that late implant placement (type 4) should be avoided whenever possible due to its potential risk of extensive ridge resorption (Chen and coworkers 2009a). This is particularly relevant in the maxillary anterior region. Ridge resorption may be extensive after removal of multiple adjacent teeth. To avoid late placement, extractions should be planned in conjunction with subsequent implant treatment whenever possible.

4.3.5 Correct Three-Dimensional Implant Placement

It is mandatory to correctly position the implant shoulder or implant platform in the mesiodistal, coronoapical and orofacial planes. This principle is commonly referred to as "three-dimensional" implant positioning. At the 3rd ITI Consensus Conference in 2003, the concept of comfort and danger zones was introduced (Buser and coworkers 2004). This concept is still valid and applies not only to single-tooth restorations but also to the reconstruction of extended edentulous spaces. Whenever surgical flaps are elevated in these procedures, normal anatomical landmarks that may guide implant placement in all three dimensions are usually missing. The use of a surgical stent allowing for proper positioning and alignment of implants is strongly recommended. These stents should offer landmarks for correct implant placement.

Two types of surgical stents are generally used in implant dentistry. The first type is vacuum-formed from a translucent material and does not include guide sleeves.

These stents have a completely open configuration on the palatal aspect of the incisal edge, allowing the surgeon to modify the entry points and axes of the preparations in accordance with bone conditions (Figs 11a-e). By incorporating the shape of the future crowns in the stent, the surgeon is able to determine the correct mesiodistal position of the implants, their apical insertion depth in relation to the anticipated mid-mucosal margins, and their proper orofacial axis, thereby facilitating correct three-dimensional positioning of the implant platform.

The second type of stent incorporates a drilling guide that offers fixed surgical guidance. Both the entry point at the bone crest and the axis of the osteotomy are predetermined. These stents are manufactured with the aid of planning software that utilizes raw DICOM data of CT scans of the patient's jaws. They are usually made from acrylic or a thick inflexible vacuum-form material. Interchangeable sleeves with diameters matching the surgical drills assist with the preparation of the osteotomy (Figs 12a-e).

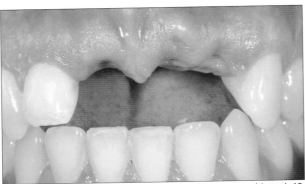

Fig 11a   *Preoperative view of a maxillary anterior segment with teeth 12, 11, and 21 missing.*

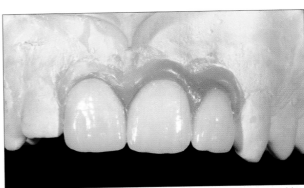

Fig 11b   *Setup of acrylic teeth in their ideal three-dimensional positions on a diagnostic cast.*

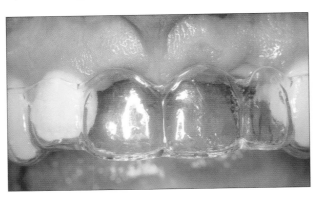

Fig 11c   *A surgical stent derived from the setup on the diagnostic cast has been manufactured from translucent vacuum-form material. The main feature of this stent type is its open configuration on the palatal aspect of the incisal edge. It also indicates the position of the mid-facial mucosal margin of the anticipated prosthesis.*

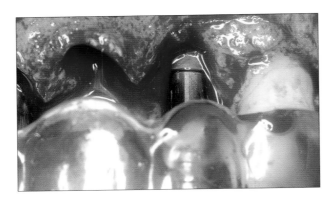

Fig 11d   *Intraoperative facial view of the stent against the implant shoulder at site 22. The shoulder of the implant has been ideally placed 3 mm apically of the mid-facial mucosal margin, as indicated by the stent.*

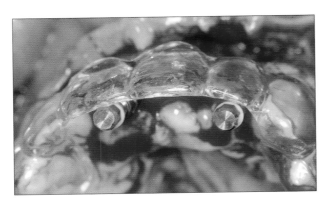

Fig 11e   *Occlusal view of the surgical stent in place, confirming the correct orofacial position of the two implants. The open configuration on the palatal aspect gives the surgeon freedom to alter the position of the entry point and axis of the preparation, depending upon the condition of the bone.*

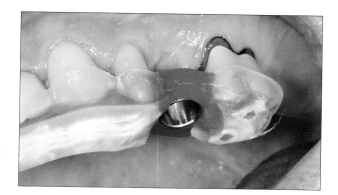

Fig 12a   Intraoral view of a surgical stent incorporating a metal tube that serves as a drilling guide. Both the entry point at the bone crest and the axis of the osteotomy were predetermined by planning software. The stent is manufactured from acrylic or an inflexible vacuum-form material.

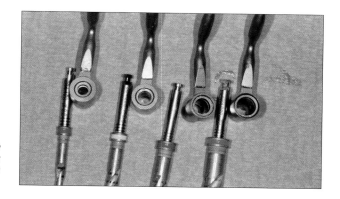

Fig 12b   Interchangeable sleeves of different diameters corresponding to the drills to be used at the time of surgery. The sleeves are inserted into the surgical guide during surgery. This type of surgical stent does not allow the surgeon to modify the position or axis of the osteotomy.

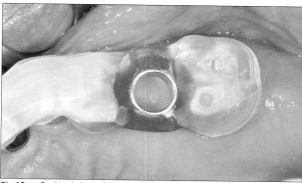

Fig 12c   Occlusal view of the surgical stent in place.

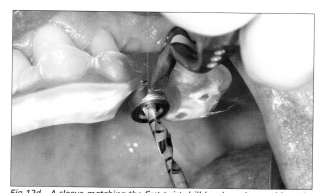

Fig 12d   A sleeve matching the first twist drill has been inserted into the guide.

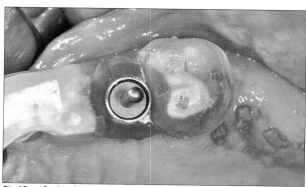

Fig 12e   Occlusal view of a guide pin that has been inserted into the osteotomy following preparation with the first twist drill. Note the accuracy of the osteotomy as shown by the fit of the guide pin in the stent.

4.3.6 Number of Implants

Care should be taken during treatment planning that adjacent implants are avoided whenever possible, since the bone between two adjacent implants will always flatten to a certain extent, resulting in a short interproximal papilla (Tarnow and coworkers 2003). Ideally, any two implants should be separated by at least one pontic unit. This can easily be achieved in areas of three to six missing teeth. In the anterior maxilla, up to four teeth can be supported by two implants.

Areas of two missing adjacent teeth are more problematic. If two central incisors are missing, two adjacent implants are placed, carefully ensuring that a minimum distance of 3 mm is respected between the implant shoulders (Figs 13a-b). In areas including a missing lateral incisor, only one implant is placed in either the central incisor or the canine position, with the restoration taking the form of a crown with a small cantilever unit (Figs 14a-b).

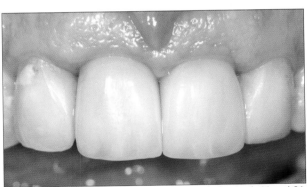

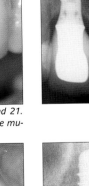

Fig 13b Periapical radiograph showing two tissue-level implants placed with shoulders 3 mm apart. This separation ensures that the interimplant bone level will be preserved.

Fig 13a Anterior view of adjacent implants replacing teeth 11 and 21. The midline papilla, although relatively short, is in harmony with the mucosal contour of the anterior teeth at large.

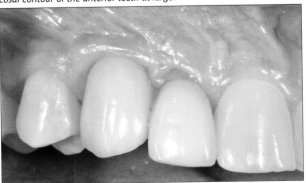

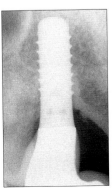

Fig 14b Radiographic view of the implant supporting the cantilever fixed partial denture.

Fig 14a The missing teeth 12 and 13 have been replaced with a cantilever fixed partial denture supported by a single implant at the canine site.

4.3.7 Contour Augmentation Using Guided Bone Regeneration (GBR)

In addition to grafting to create sufficient bone volume for an implant, bone augmentation is required almost invariably to restore a proper orofacial ridge contour in the anterior maxilla. It is important that the augmented ridge offers a maximum degree of dimensional stability over time. The concept of contour augmentation based on the principle of GBR as described by Buser and coworkers (2008) hinges on the following surgical requirements:

Locally harvested autologous bone chips should be used to cover any exposed implant surfaces. Autologous bone chips are rich in bone morphogenetic proteins and other non-collagenous proteins, thereby enhancing new bone formation (Bosshardt and Schenk 2009). In addition, osteocytes are embedded in grafted bone chips that seem to have a beneficial effect on new bone formation and bone remodeling (Bonewald 2011). In this way, autografts will expedite bone regeneration and offer shorter healing periods than bone substitutes alone (Buser and coworkers 1998; Jensen and coworkers 2006), and they offers reduced healing periods.

On top of the applied bone chips, a layer of hydroxyapatite-based (HA-based) bone filler is used to overcontour the external surface of the facial bone. The grafting material is used to reconstruct the facial contour of the bone to its pre-extraction arch form. HA-based bone fill-

ers with a low substitution rate should be selected to ensure longterm graft stability and to avoid dimensional changes over time. Suitable products include DBBM and biphasic calcium phosphate (BCP) (Jensen and coworkers 2006; Jensen and coworkers 2007).

The grafting material is covered by a barrier membrane in accordance with the GBR principle (Nyman and coworkers 1990; Schenk and coworkers 1994). The presence of a barrier membrane will exclude soft-tissue cells of the overlying mucosa from participating in the events of early wound healing inside the secluded space. Resorbable collagen membranes are generally preferred today because they carry a low risk of complications, are easy to handle, and do not require a second surgical procedure for removal (von Arx and Buser 2006; Hürzeler and coworkers 1998; Zitzmann and coworkers 1999; Bornstein and coworkers 2009). The membrane acts as a temporary barrier and prevents the particulate filler material from migrating.

The buccal flap is released and advanced to ensure tension-free primary wound closure, thus ensuring that the biomaterials are protected from the oral environment to avoid bacterial contamination.

The transitional prosthesis needs to be carefully adjusted to prevent pressure over the augmented ridge. In extended edentulous areas, Essix retainers are mainly used because they offer good stability in the surgical area and protect the wound during the initial healing phase. Figures 15a-i show an illustrative procedure.

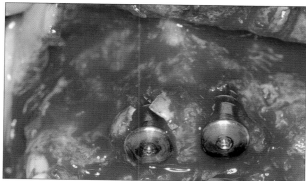

Fig 15a   Intraoperative view of two implants at sites 11 and 21. Due to resorption of the ridge, the facial surfaces of the implants are exposed at the coronal level.

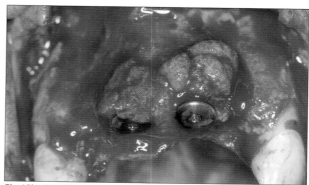

Fig 15b   Locally harvested autologous bone chips have been applied to cover the exposed implant surfaces.

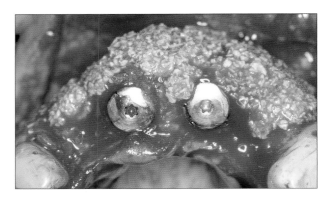

Fig 15c Occlusal view following application of a thick DBBM layer to over-contour the external surface of the facial bone. The grafting material has been used to reconstruct the facial contour of the bone to its original pre-extraction arch form.

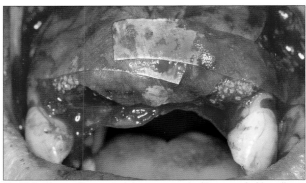

Fig 15d The grafting materials are covered with a resorbable collagen membrane, which acts as a temporary barrier and prevents the particulate filler material from migrating.

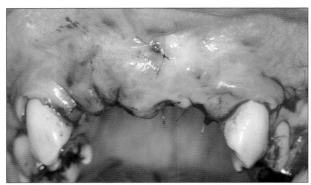

Fig 15e The buccal flap is released and advanced to ensure tension-free primary closure of the wound.

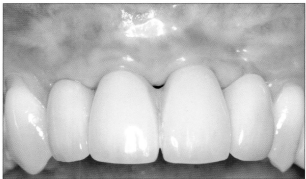

Fig 15f Anterior view of the definitive four-unit fixed partial denture supported by implants at sites 11 and 21. The image was taken 8 years after placing the implants.

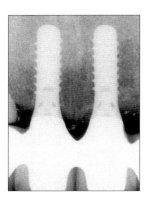

Fig 15g Periapical radiograph obtained after 8 years. Bone conditions are stable around both implants.

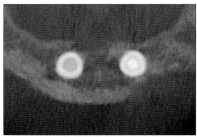

Fig 15h Axial CBCT slice obtained after 8 years, illustrating the bone graft on the facial aspect of both implants. A mild loss of contour is noted on the implant at site 21.

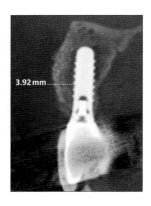

3.92 mm

Fig 15i Orofacial CBCT view obtained after 8 years. The implant at site 11 reveals 4 mm of facial bone thickness in its coronal segment.

4.3.8 Soft-Tissue Grafting

Soft-tissue grafting may be considered if there is a lack of keratinized mucosa, which is important for long-term tissue health and esthetic outcomes. In cases involving contour augmentation, this is preferably achieved by correcting the local bone anatomy using a bone substitutes as previously described. If performed correctly, the ridge of an extended maxillary space can be augmented with no need for adjunctive soft-tissue grafting in the majority of cases. Enhancing the ridge contour exclusively by soft-tissue grafting would usually require harvesting a substantial soft-tissue graft from the palate and there-

fore should be avoided. While substitutes to autologous soft tissue like cellular dermal matrix may be considered (Harris 2003), clinical evidence for their long-term efficacy is limited.

At fresh extraction sites, soft-tissue grafts may be used to seal the socket opening after implant placement (Landsberg 1997; Gelb 1993; Edel 1995) to augment the soft tissue in thickness (Kan and coworkers 2005; Grunder and coworkers 1996) and to protect any applied biomaterials by flapless implant placement (Chen and coworkers 2009a).

4.4 Conclusions

Replacing multiple missing teeth in the anterior maxilla is one of the most challenging tasks in implant dentistry. A detailed clinical and radiographic examination is required to establish a proper diagnosis. Close collaboration between the surgical and restorative clinicians involved is mandatory to set out a treatment plan that satisfies the patient's functional, phonetic and esthetic requirements. Surgical management needs to consider the most appropriate time to place implants after tooth extraction, the esthetic objectives, the degree of ridge resorption, the conditions for either staged or simultaneous bone augmentation, and the number and location of implants appropriate for the case.

5 <u>Prosthodontic Considerations and Treatment Procedures</u>

J.-G. Wittneben, H. P. Weber

5.1 Loading Protocols for Extended Edentulous Spaces in the Esthetic Zone

The esthetic zone represents an especially sensitive restorative region where multiple risk factors have to be considered. Predictable esthetic outcomes rely on the selection of the appropriate treatment approach, and in particular the selection of the loading protocol. Multiple factors are capable of influencing the quality and/or predictability of loading protocols in extended edentulous areas. These may be related to the patient, the biomaterials, and the clinician. Patient-related factors including health, intraoral condition (e.g. periodontal conditions, parafunction, bruxism, occlusion), and the implant site itself. Factors related to biomaterials include the size, shape, material, and surface characteristics of selected implants. Procedures for bone grafting are frequently required, which adds another biomaterials component. Clinician-related factors include education, clinical skills, experience, and selection of treatment (e.g. timing and methodology of implant placement, primary implant stability, choice of biomaterials) (Weber and coworkers 2009) (Fig 1).

While an early loading protocol is defined as 1 week to 2 months after implant placement, established clinical protocols suggest that loading be delayed until at least the third week. Studies on the latest generation of implant surface modifications have demonstrated adequate bone-to-implant contact after 3 weeks (Bornstein and coworkers 2010). The use of simultaneous bone grafting would be an exception (Weber and coworkers 2009; Grütter and Belser 2009). If the need for bone grafting is not overly extensive, an early loading protocol may be considered for the majority of extended edentulous sites in the anterior maxilla.

Immediate loading may be considered under these well-defined clinical conditions:

- Implant placement not combined with simultaneous bone grafting
- No simultaneous sinus floor elevation
- Adequate implant length (8 mm or more) and diameter (4 mm or more)
- Good primary stability of the implant
- Only implant-supported provisionalization
- Provisional restoration without static or dynamic occlusal contact(s)
- Screw retention preferred

Primary implant stability is a requirement for immediate loading of the implant with a screw-retained provisional restoration. It depends on bone density and quality, implant design and surface characteristics, as well as on the preparation technique and resultant accuracy of the osteotomy (Cordaro and coworkers 2009). Eligible cases are therefore limited, as a bone quantity close to ideal is required at the implant site. In addition, the clinician should be well educated and experienced with immediate loading protocols (Weber and coworkers 2009). Screw retention is recommended because it eliminates the need for cementation and hence a potential source of interference with the healing process.

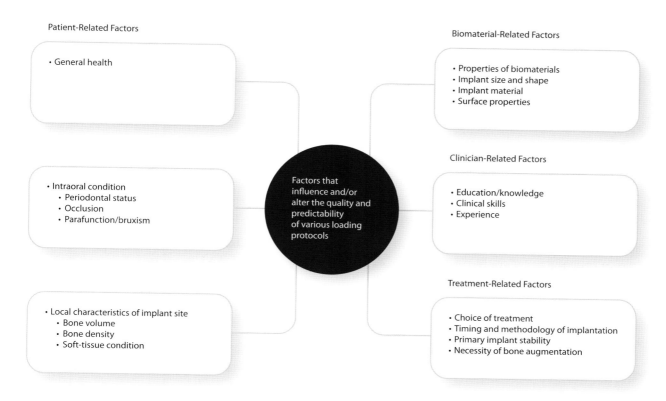

Patient-Related Factors

- General health

- Intraoral condition
  - Periodontal status
  - Occlusion
  - Parafunction/bruxism

- Local characteristics of implant site
  - Bone volume
  - Bone density
  - Soft-tissue condition

Factors that influence and/or alter the quality and predictability of various loading protocols

Biomaterial-Related Factors

- Properties of biomaterials
- Implant size and shape
- Implant material
- Surface properties

Clinician-Related Factors

- Education/knowledge
- Clinical skills
- Experience

Treatment-Related Factors

- Choice of treatment
- Timing and methodology of implantation
- Primary implant stability
- Necessity of bone augmentation

Fig 1   Modifiers of the success and predictability of loading protocols.

Clinicians should exercise caution when considering immediate loading in extended edentulous areas in the anterior maxilla, as the body of available outcome data is limited and primarily based on implant survival. There is a considerable lack of scientific evidence for actual treatment success, including esthetic outcomes and patient satisfaction (Grütter and Belser 2009).

Conventional loading protocols are indicated whenever the stability of an implant is considered inadequate for early or immediate loading an whenever specific clinical conditions enter the equation, including a compromised host status or implant site, the presence of parafunctions, and a need for extensive bone grafting and sinus floor elevation procedures (Weber and coworkers 2009).

5.2 Provisionalization

5.2.1 Pre-Implant Provisional Restorations

The provisional phase of treatment can be the most challenging aspect of implant dentistry (Cho and co-workers 2007). The benefits of a provisional restoration/prosthesis in the esthetic zone include their role in determining the best restorative design and in offering a template around which soft-tissue contours can be evaluated and manipulated (Lewis and coworkers 1995). Implant treatment of extended edentulism in the anterior maxilla includes three provisional phases (Fig 2). The first phase is provisionalization immediately after tooth extraction, the second phase follows implant placement but precedes loading, and the third phase involves an implant-supported fixed provisional prosthesis that loads the implants and develops the emergence and mucosal profile. Patients do not like anyone to notice their tooth loss and therefore rely on being provided with a restoration immediately. The most important requirement for a favorable long-term treatment outcome is that the surrounding tissue is modified and improved by a provisional restoration. The primary indication for provisional restorations is their role as a placeholder to avoid migration of neighboring and extrusion of opposing teeth. Their

secondary role in the esthetic zone is to offer esthetics, function, and stability, in addition to the requirement that they should be easy to fabricate (Cho and coworkers 2007).

Provisionalization remains a challenge in situations of anterior extended edentulism. Patients will attach great importance to provisional restorations especially in this area. Implant surgery in conjunction with guided bone regeneration (GBR) procedures may result in phonetic and functional problems. Several options are available for provisional rehabilitation during the healing period following procedures of tooth extraction or implant placement; these include removable and fixed prosthetic designs. Table 1 summarizes these options, listing descriptions, indications, advantages, disadvantages, and situations in which caution should be exercised.

After implant placement, especially with the use of GBR techniques, the provisional prosthesis may inadvertently apply pressure to the healing site. This pressure, also known as "transmucosal loading," may eventually be detrimental to implant survival (Cho and coworkers 2007) and alter the surrounding tissue. Interim removable partial dentures must be designed with great care and checked for stability in function to avoid any contact and pressure to the underlying tissues. Where this is impossible, an interim removable partial denture might be an inappropriate choice and the use of an Essix retainer (Figs 3a-f) might be indicated, which can be easily modified.

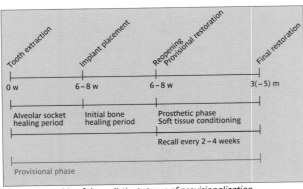

Fig 2   Timetable of three distinct stages of provisionalization

Table 1   Selection of provisional restorations for extended edentulous spaces in the esthetic zone.

Options for removable provisionals	Description	Indication	Advantages	Disadvantages	Caution
Essix retainer	Clear thermo-plastic appliance with incorporated denture teeth or filled acrylic as replacements; should cover all residual teeth	Provisionaliza-tion after tooth extraction and/ or implant placement; for short-term use	– No transmucosal loading of healing sites – Inexpensive – Good esthetics with low lip line – Psychological benefit of not wearing a denture – Can be readily modified before and after surgery – Can be used for soft-tissue conditioning	– Poor esthetics with high smile line – Occlusal wear – Not durable – Accumulates plaque – Chewing difficulties	– High lip line – Requires good compliance with oral hygiene needs
Provisional partial denture	PMMA-based interim removable denture with or without wrought-wire clasps and denture teeth to replace missing teeth	Provisionaliza-tion after tooth extraction and/or implant placement; for long-term use	– Can be readily fabricated, relined and modified – Stable – Inexpensive	– Poor esthetics (especially with high lip line) if clasps are used – Due to transmucosal loading, a partial denture is not recommended for cases involving GBR unless it can be completely relieved of mucosa during healing – Potential gag-reflex issues – May interfere with speech – Psychologically difficult for patients who have never worn dentures (notably young patients)	– In deep over-bite situations, a provisional partial denture is not recommended after implant placement (because of transmu-cosal loading) unless it can be completely relieved of mucosa during healing – Potential for transmucosal loading
Valplast/Flex	PMMA-based interim removable prosthesis with-out metal clasps, softer material	Provisionaliza-tion after tooth extraction; for short-term use	– Softer material for better patient comfort – No metal claps – Good esthetics	– Not very stable – Cannot be readily modified after surgical procedures	– Not indicated after implant placement

Options for fixed provisionals	Description	Indication	Advantages	Disadvantages	Caution
Tooth-supported fixed partial denture	– Long-term temporary resin bridge – Can be reinforced with gold mesh, cast metal or glass fiber for greater stability	– Provision-alization after tooth extrac-tion and/ or implant placement; for long-term use	– No transmucosal loading of healing sites – Good esthetics – Good Stability – Can be readily modified/relined – Good diagnostic tool for esthetic analysis	– Case selective and only indicated if neighboring teeth are restored already – Contraindicated on adjacent natural teeth if these are virgin	– Trauma related to preparing the abutment teeth especially with long-term use

A bonded tooth, a bonded resin bridge, or an orthodontic retainer would not offer adequate stability and are therefore not an option for interim use in these situations. The first choice for fixed provisional use—unless the adjacent natural teeth are virgin—is a tooth-supported partial denture (Figs 4a-b).

5.2.2 Implant-Supported Provisional Restorations and Soft-Tissue Conditioning

Any esthetic implant-supported rehabilitation will depend on both biologically and prosthodontically driven implant placement (Belser and coworkers 1996; Buser and coworkers 2004; Brugnami and Caleffi 2005; Mankoo 2007; Buser 2008), on a pleasing appearance of the pros-

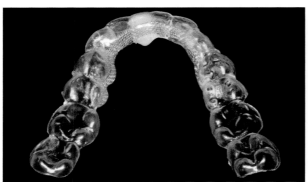

Fig 3a   Essix retainer with reinforcement (gold mesh).

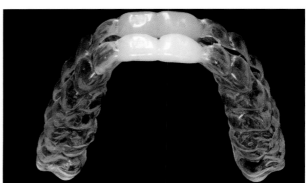

Fig 3b   Essix retainer without reinforcement.

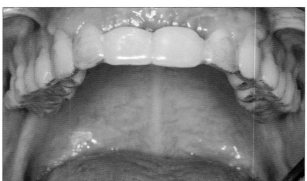

Fig 3c   Essix retainer inserted after surgery.

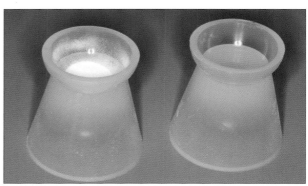

Fig 3d   Light-cured acrylic material.

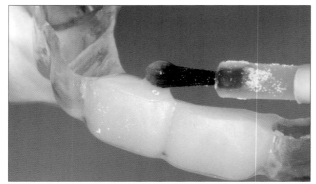

Fig 3e   Material is added to the Essix retainer after intraoral swelling has resolved.

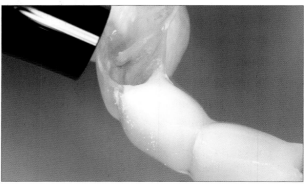

Fig 3f   Light-curing of acrylic material.

thesis itself (Buser 2011; Cooper 2008) and surrounding peri-implant mucosa (Buser 2011; Belser and coworkers 2009; Fürhauser 2005; Weber 1998). Peri-implant tissue architecture is the essence of implant esthetics (Kan 2009). Patient perceptions on the presence of interdental papillae are subjective and depend upon individual interpretation (Kan and coworkers 2003), although a lack of papilla, resulting in an open embrasure, can affect the patient's smile. Kokich and coworkers (1999) demonstrated a threshold for open gingival embrasures (from the tip of the interdental papilla to the interproximal contact point) of 3 mm, at which point both general dentists and lay people started to rate the esthetic relationship as unattractive.

Depending on the amount of (soft and hard) tissue loss and tissue defects and depending on the patient's lip line, it may be important to evaluate in the phase of treatment planning whether pink ceramics imitating the peri-implant mucosa should be incorporated into the final restoration. If so, soft-tissue conditioning via the provisional restoration or prosthesis may not be needed. Details for treatment guidance with pink ceramics are described in Section 5.3.4.

As discussed in Chapter 3, bone-level implants are indicated in the esthetic zone to allow for greater freedom in defining the location of the restorative margin, the final position of the mucosal zenith, the emergence profile, and the soft-tissue architecture.

Endosteal implants differ from natural teeth by their morphology and shape at the mucosal level. Natural anterior teeth, due to their form and emergence profile, have a triangular cross-sectional shape at the gingival level. By contrast, the cross-sectional shape of the peri-implant mucosa at the mucosal level is defined by the (usually round) cross-sectional form of the healing abutment. The peri-implant soft-tissue architecture needs to be thoroughly sculpted via the implant-supported provisional restoration or prosthesis to replicate the form of the natural tooth being replaced.

Heat-polymerized polymethyl methacrylate (PMMA) should be used to make the provisional restoration. The fact that this material stimulates the smallest number of pro-inflammatory cytokines makes it more compatible than other acrylic materials (Labban and coworkers 2008). The implant-supported provisional restoration is needed to create a number of features:

- A papilla of adequate height and width
- A mucosal level in balance with the gingiva of the adjacent teeth

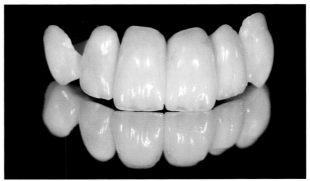

Fig 4a   Fixed provisional prosthesis.

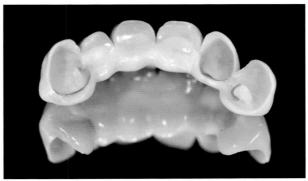

Fig 4b   Reinforcement with wire of fixed provisional prosthesis.

- An established gingival zenith position (Cooper 2008)
- An accurate emergence profile
- A triangular shape of the tissue profile at the mucosal level
- A proximal contact point with the adjacent tooth or restoration (Tarnow 1992)

Scientifically documented techniques for soft-tissue conditioning with implant-supported provisional restorations are lacking in the literature, and only few case reports have been published on this topic. Provisional restorations are used with the intention of creating a defined volume of peri-implant mucosa to establish optimal papillary and sulcular profiles (Priest 2005; Chee 2003).

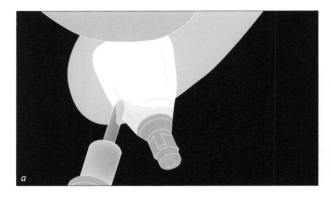

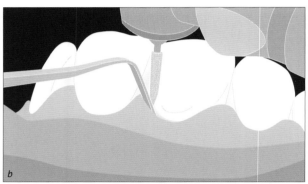

Figs 5a-b   Soft tissue conditioning with the dynamic compression technique: (a) addition of acrylic or resin material extraorally to the provisional restoration to compress the mucosa, and (b) removal of acrylic or resin material intraorally from the provisional restoration to create space for the papillae to fill in.

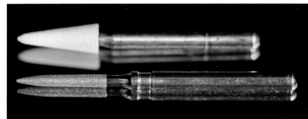

Fig 6a   A fine diamond bur (lower half of image) is used for intraoral shaping of the provisional restoration, which is then polished with white Arkansas stone (upper half of image).

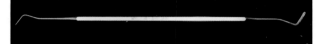

Fig 6b   The mucosa is retracted with a spatula.

Screw-retained provisional restorations should be used, so that they can be modified. Addition of resin to the provisional restorations has been recommended to bring about soft-tissue modifications (Santosa 2007; Priest 2006; Chee 2001). An important step in the initial phase is to add pressure and compress the mucosa in the correct direction. Caution should be exercised in the papillary space as the provisional restoration will be slightly overcontoured and the tissue will not have the space to grow and fill up. The dynamic compression technique is therefore recommended in the esthetic zone, which relies on addition of material to the provisional restorations for initial pressure (Fig 5a) and subsequent modifications by periodically reducing the restoration in the papillary region (Fig 5b), thereby creating space for the soft tissue to fill in (Wittneben and coworkers 2012). These reductions in the papillary areas can be performed intraorally on the provisional restorations, using a fine diamond bur to remove acrylic material (Fig 6a) followed by polishing the restorations with a white Arkansas stone (Fig 6a) while retracting the mucosa with a spatula (Fig 6b). This process can be carried on over several appointments.

In addition, the provisional restoration serves both as a communication tool to discuss patients' desires and esthetic expectations and, especially in situations of multiple missing teeth, as a diagnostic tool for esthetic analysis. Here the temporary prosthesis facilitates evaluation of the following parameters:

* Positions of the dental and facial midline
* Final position of the incisal edge
* Anterior tooth widths, lengths, and axes
* Tooth-to-tooth proportions (Figs 7a-b)

After completion of soft-tissue conditioning, it is important to transfer the newly developed emergence profile and soft-tissue architecture to the final master cast by fabricating a customized impression coping that features the same tissue profile as the provisional restoration in its final form. This is accomplished either by using the provisional restoration as impression coping or by injecting an impression material around a provisional restoration seated on a master cast (Elian and coworkers 2007). To fabricate a customized impression coping, the provisional crown is first attached to an implant analog, taking a silicone impression to capture the developed emergence profile (Figs 8a-b). Subsequently the provisional restoration is removed and the impression coping screwed onto the analog (Fig 9). The space between the copied emergence profile and the impression coping is filled in with a resin material (Figs 10a-b) and is then finished and polished with disks (Figs 10c-d). The result can then be used as an impression coping for a regular implant level impression using either an open-tray or closed-tray technique (Figs 11a-c).

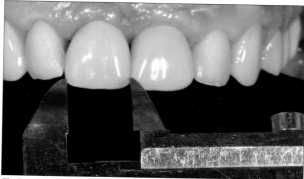

Fig 7a   Evaluation of tooth-to-tooth proportions: Measuring the width of the provisional restoration.

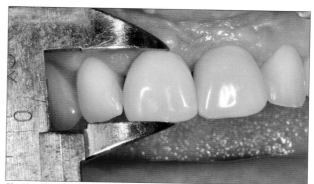

Fig 7b   Evaluation of tooth-to-tooth proportions: Measuring the length of the provisional restoration.

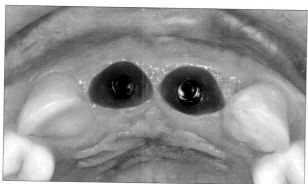

Fig 8a   The triangular shape of the mucosal profile needs to be captured in the final impression.

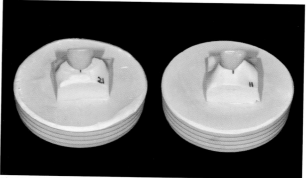

Fig 8b   With the provisional restorations connected to the implant analogs, silicone impressions of the emergence profiles are taken.

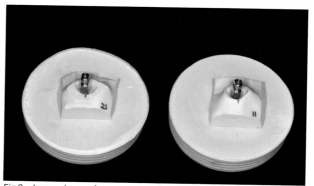

Fig 9   Impression copings are screwed to the implant analogs.

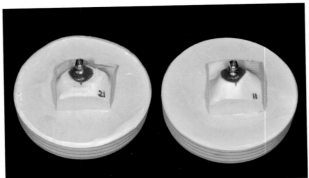

Fig 10a Pattern resin is used to fabricate the customized impression copings.

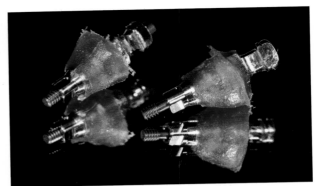

Fig 10b Customized impression coping before polishing.

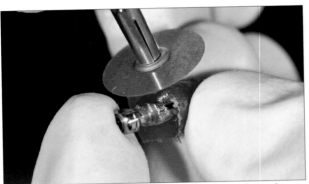

Fig 10c Finishing and polishing of the customized impression coping.

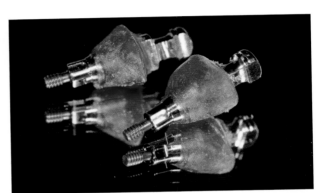

Fig 10d Final impression copings.

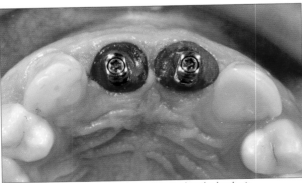

Fig 11a Final impression copings connected to the implants.

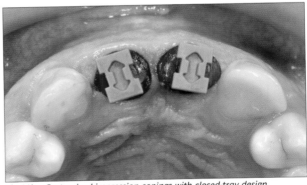

Fig 11b Customized impression copings with closed-tray design.

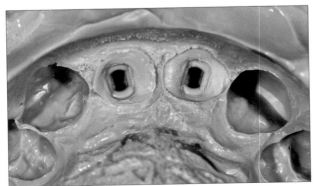

Fig 11c Final closed-tray implant impression.

5.3 Permanent Prostheses

5.3.1 Cementation versus Screw Retention

The connection of the final restoration to the implant may be accomplished via a screw connection or by cementation. Both methods have their benefits and shortcomings and should be selected on a case-by-case basis. Limited scientific evidence is available on cementation versus screw retention (Michalakis and coworkers 2003).

In the anterior zone, screw retention is easier if the position of the screw access hole is planned below the incisal edge position on the lingual aspect (Figs 12a-b). In addition, the implant should be placed in a correct prosthodontic position.

Extended edentulous areas are usually an indication for fixed partial dentures. What matters in this case is the prosthodontic position of the implant. Standard abutments can be used for cemented restorations, which simplifies the procedure from a technical point of view and reduces costs. The advantages of cementation are simplicity, passivity of fit, improved esthetics, easier control of occlusion, and economy (Wilson 2009). Cement can also act as a shock absorber and enhance the transfer of load throughout the prosthesis-implant-bone system (Guichet 1994). A major disadvantage of cementation is the difficulty of removing excess material, residual cement having been implicated in the development of peri-implant mucositis and peri-implantitis (Wilson 2009). It is recommended to position the cement margins at the level of the mucosa or up to 2 mm below this level to make any excess cement accessible for removal.

Lack of retrievability is another disadvantage of cementation with permanent cement. An adequately tapered (ideally 6 degrees) abutment will usually suffice for effective retention of the restoration by temporary cement. The use of temporary cement may also be indicated for cementing permanent restorations. Hebel and Gajjar (1997) suggested the use of temporary cement mixed with petroleum jelly for multiple units and of non-modified temporary cement for single-unit implant-supported restorations. This consideration is particularly relevant for posterior restorations, where screw access holes may interfere with occlusion.

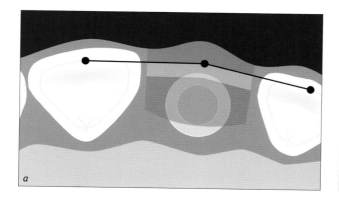
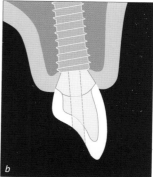

Figs 12a-b Prosthetic correct position of implant, with the future screw access hole below the planned incisal edge position.

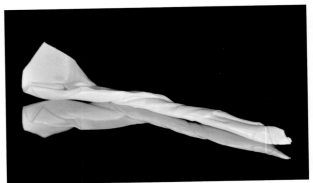

Fig 13   Polytetrafluoroethylene (PTFE) tape.

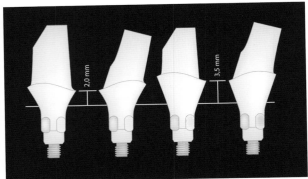

Fig 14   The collars of prefabricated zirconia abutments should follow the contour of the mucosal margin.

Screw-retained restorations are recommended as the method of choice in the esthetic zone where screw access holes do not interfere with occlusion as commonly as in posterior sites. Furthermore, screw retention eliminates the risk of mucositis or peri-implantitis due to the absence of cement residues.

Screw-retained prostheses will invariably require the use of customized abutments, thus involving technique-sensitive and demanding fabrication steps (Michalakis 2003). It is important that all screws be torqued according to their manufacturers' instructions. Subsequently the screw holes are obturated with a suitable material — as with a polytetrafluoroethylene (PTFE) tape (Moráguez and coworkers 2010) (Fig 13) and composite resin.

If the interocclusal space is limited, screw-retained restorations are the technique of choice, as these restorations can be screwed directly to the implants and thus require the smallest amount of interocclusal space.

In a recent long-term evaluation of implant-supported restorations retained by either screw connections or cementation in the anterior maxilla, the patients reported perceiving no differences between the two retention types. Five-year implant survival in the anterior maxilla was 96% overall, with no differences between screw and cement retention (Sherif and coworkers 2010). The authors concluded, however, that soft-tissue health might be better around screw-retained restorations, judging from lower mean sulcular bleeding index (SBI) and modified plaque index (MPI) values compared to cemented restorations.

5.3.2   Abutment Selection

Abutment selection is a quintessential aspect of implant treatment in the esthetic zone. The advantage of bone level-type implants in this area is that they offer prosthodontic freedom of creating custom emergence profiles, of defining the final position of the restorative margin, and of leveling out divergences of up to 60 degrees in cemented bridge reconstructions.

Eligible materials for final abutments include titanium, gold, zirconia, and alumina-based ceramics. Clinical studies have shown that both titanium and zirconia abutments are well tolerated by the peri-implant soft tissue and that both offer similar soft-tissue integration. Gold-alloy abutments may, however, be disadvantageous. In a study comparing titanium, gold-alloy and zirconia abutments inserted in six Labrador dogs, the hard and soft tissues were histologically analyzed 2 and 5 months after insertion. While soft-tissue dimensions were found to be stable around titanium and zirconia abutments, apical shifts of the barrier epithelium and marginal bone were noted around gold-alloy abutments after 2 to 5 months (Welander and coworkers 2008).

Dental implant abutments may be prefabricated or customized. Prefabricated abutments are indicated for use with implants that are placed in a prosthodontically ideal position. They are advantageous for being time-efficient within the overall context of treatment because the abutment only needs to be modified by the dental technician and the crown or FDP can be immediately finalized. In the esthetic zone, it is important that the collar height of a prefabricated abutment is not a uniform 360 degrees, as the interproximal position of the crown margin would be placed too far submucosally.

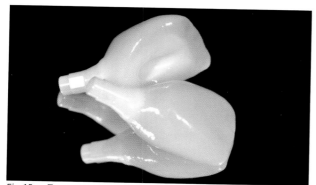

Fig 15a Two screw-retained implant-supported all-ceramic crowns with CAD/CAM manufactured zirconia abutments.

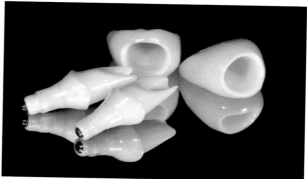

Fig 15b Two cemented implant-supported all-ceramic crowns with CAD/CAM manufactured zirconia abutments.

Therefore, an ideal shape of a standard or prefabricated abutment should be similar to a tooth preparation—following the contour of the gingival margin (Giglio 1999) (Fig 14).

For cemented reconstructions, clinicians should always use prefabricated or customized abutments that place the restorative margin between the level of the mucosa (Michalakis and coworkers 2003) and not more than 2 mm below the mucosal margin. Prefabricated abutments should be available in various gingival heights and should be readily reshaped if necessary.

In contrast to using prefabricated abutments, customizing an abutment gives the clinician freedom to tailor the position, angulation, and future margin of the restoration to individual requirements. The same philosophy also allows abutments to be specifically designed for optimal support of veneering ceramics (Figs 15a-b). Methods of customization include CAD/CAM technology or traditional lost-wax casting.

According to clinical studies, ceramic abutments exhibit high survival and low complication rates similar to those of metal abutments. Systematic reviews have been conducted to evaluate the available body of evidence. The observation periods of the studies included did not exceed 5 years (Kapos and coworkers 2009; Sailer and coworkers 2009). Zirconia abutments have better outcomes than alumina abutments. No fractures of zirconia abutments were reported in studies with up to 4 years of follow-up (Sailer and coworkers 2009). More long-term clinical studies and randomized clinical trials are needed.

There are several patient and intraoral site-dependent factors influencing the choice of abutment. The mucosal thickness presents a determining factor. In an animal study comparing different dental materials under different mucosal thickness (1.5, 2, and 3 mm), it was concluded that titanium yielded the most pronounced color changes. Zirconia did not induce visible color changes under mucosal tissue 2 or 3 mm thick. Covered by 3 mm of mucosal tissue, the color of the material did not matter because changes of color were no longer detectable by the human eye (Jung and coworkers 2007). It should be emphasized that a patient's biotype may thin with age, which means that any use of titanium or gold abutments may potentially have late consequences in terms of visible color changes.

Another important parameter is the depth of implant placement. Bone-level implants should ideally be placed 2–3 mm below the cementoenamel junction of the prospective crown, while the shoulder of tissue-level implants should be placed approximately 1 mm apical to the cemento enamel junction of the contralateral tooth in esthetic sites (Buser and coworkers 2007b).

Implants placed too deep will frequently preclude the use of prefabricated abutments, whose length may end up being inadequate (too short), especially for screw-retained restorations in this situation. Also, the abutment collar should be positioned at an excessively apical level, thus resulting in an overly deep restorative margin. Even the abutment lengths attainable by CAD/CAM are limited and might cause problems when these abutments are used on deeply inserted implants. Some computer-assisted design (CAD) systems may not be able to handle the manufacturing process if an implant has been inserted beyond a critical depth level.

If implants are placed too shallow, ceramic abutments are usually the only alternative offering an esthetically acceptable outcome. Titanium or gold would be visible at the crown margin.

Caution should be exercised in the event of screw loosening with zirconia abutments. Clinical observations have shown that whenever patients or clinicians have waited too long before the abutment is retightened to torque, the implant-abutment connection may have worn out in the meantime.

Implant abutments may be engaging or non-engaging. A connection engaging the interior of the implant (internal connection) will preclude all rotational movement and is therefore indicated for single restorations or cemented short-span fixed partial dentures. Non-engaging abutments are indicated for screw-retained fixed partial dentures to ensure stable seating without tension inside the connection. Multi-base standard titanium abutments are indicated for screw-retained porcelain-fused-to-metal (PFM) implant-supported bridges (Fig 16).

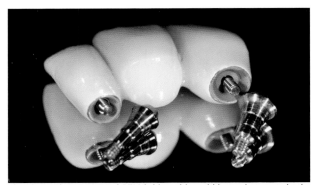

Fig 16   Implant-supported PFM bridge with multi-base abutments in the extended edentulous esthetic site.

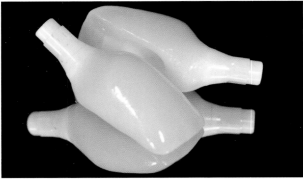

Fig 17   Two implant-supported screw-retained all-ceramic restorations replacing two missing teeth.

5.3.3   Treatment Procedures

In the esthetic zone, patient expectations of the definitive prosthodontic esthetic outcome are the highest compared to other regions of the dentition. Important concerns include the overall duration of treatment, morbidity, cost considerations, and the psychological stress of having lost anterior teeth. Compensation for these concerns should be offered in the form of a final prosthodontic design that will ensure a satisfactory esthetic outcome.

The final phase of prosthodontic treatment is challenging. Difficult decisions are required with regard to retention type, abutment selection, prosthodontic design, and restorative materials. The prosthodontic design depends on the selected material and mode of retention.

In the esthetic zone, the selected material should be optimal from the esthetic as well as functional viewpoints. Both all-ceramic and PFM reconstructions should be considered. Which of these is selected will depend on each patient's individual situation. Some of the factors to be considered would include bruxing habits, space requirements for the abutments and the superstructure, and posterior support. If the patient is a bruxer, the occlusal or incisal contact areas should be fabricated in gold, thus indicating that a metal-ceramic design should be selected. If space is limited, a metal-ceramic design is also recommended because an all-ceramic solution requires more space for the veneering ceramic and the abutment. And, regardless of materials and designs, posterior support must be present to equalize the load distribution evenly throughout the dental arch.

All-ceramic restorations offer excellent esthetic outcomes. In a randomized clinical trial, color differences between midfacial peri-implant mucosa and the gingival margins of the corresponding neighboring teeth were evaluated in a group of patients with all-ceramic crowns on alumina-based abutments and compared to a group of patients with PFM crowns on titanium or gold abutments (Jung and coworkers 2008). The color changes in the mucosa were considerably less obvious prominent in the all-ceramic than in the PFM group (Jung and coworkers 2008).

With posterior support ensured and no history of bruxism, implant-supported all-ceramic restorations are therefore recommended in the esthetic zone. Screw retention is the first choice, depending on the restorative positions of the implants. If screw retention is precluded by these positions, cementation is an option and can be used with prefabricated abutments. If two missing teeth are replaced by two implants, screw-retained single restorations with the implant abutments covered by no more than 2 mm of veneering ceramic are recommended (Fig 17).

Once the phase of soft-tissue conditioning has been completed and the surrounding peri-implant mucosa conditioned to its final shape via the implant-supported fixed provisional restoration (Fig 18), the time has come to take the final impression with customized impression posts as explained previously in this chapter.

As discussed, the provisional restoration offers esthetic guidance by helping to evaluate the final prosthetic design. An additional mock-up is recommended if the patient is dissatisfied with the provisional restoration or if more esthetic analysis is necessary, or if the framework will be implemented by CAD/CAM. The case illustrated here was planned with a CAD/CAM framework and a pressable veneering ceramic, therefore requiring a wax-up to be performed in the dental laboratory. With a mock-up of the final design, the patient gets a chance to preview the shape of the final prosthesis (Figs 19a-e). The opportunity can be seized to evaluate the facial and dental midline, the tooth axes, the tooth-to-tooth proportions, the width/length ratio of teeth, the position and length of the incisal edges with phonetics (S and V/F sounds), and vertical height with profile analysis and nasolabial angle assessment (Figs 19c-e).

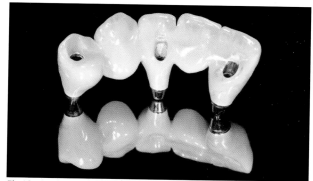

Fig 18   Implant-supported fixed provisional restoration.

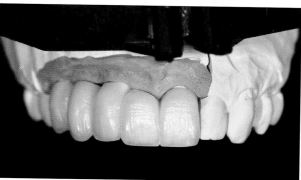

Fig 19a   Mock-up on a master cast.

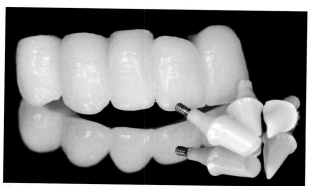

Fig 19b   Mock-up with final CAD/CAM zirconia abutments.

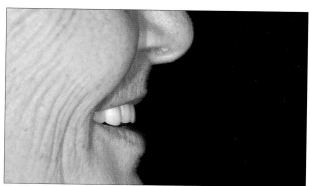

Fig 19c   Profile analysis with mock-up in situ.

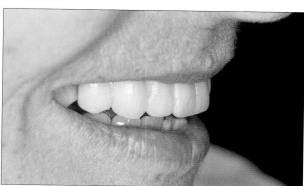

Fig 19d   Esthetic assessment with mock-up in situ.

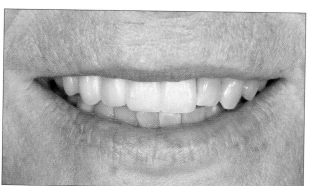

Fig 19e   Esthetic assessment with mock-up in full smile.

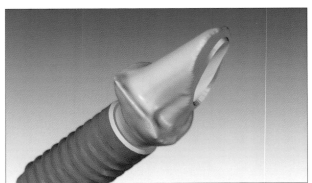

Fig 20a   Digital scanning prior to designing the implant abutments via CAD. (CAD design by CDT T. Furter, Bern.)

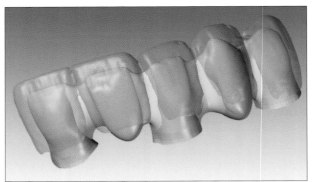

Fig 20b   Second scanning of the waxed framework and designing zirconia framework via CAD.

One way of fabricating the final reconstruction is by CAD/CAM technology. Both the abutments and the framework design can be scanned and planned using CAD/CAM software. For all-ceramic frameworks, the use of transformation-toughened zirconia is recommended. At a fracture toughness at least twice that of alumina ceramics, this material yield high-strength frameworks (Hannink and coworkers 2000; Kelly and Benetti 2011). Zirconium dioxide can be transformed from one crystalline state to another during firing. In the late 1980s, ceramic engineers learned how to stabilize the tetragonal form at room temperature by adding small amounts of calcium initially and by further adding yttrium or cerium later. The main advantage of the tetragonal form is that, in the presence of a highly localized stress inside the zirconia material (e.g. a starting crack), it can be transformed back to the monoclinic state with a 4.4% volume increase. This volume increase offers the benefit of changing the material around the crack tip, shielding it from the outside material (Kelly and Benetti 2011).

Problems with zirconium dioxide ceramics may include long-term instability in the presence of water, issues of porcelain compatibility, and some esthetic limitations related to their opacity (Kelly and Benetti 2011).

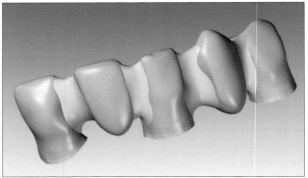

Fig 20c   Customization of connector areas.

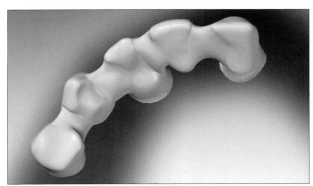

Fig 20d   Occlusal view of the future framework and connector areas.

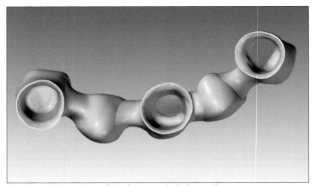

Fig 20e   Bottom view of the framework design and connector areas.

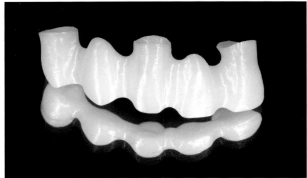

Fig 20f   Final zirconia framework.

Complications of "porcelain chipping" have been reported repeatedly in recent years. They may result from a number of factors, including (1) a non-anatomical substructure design; (2) unsupported porcelain; (3) weaker porcelain; (4) mismatches between thermal expansion and contraction; and (5) poor porcelain-zirconia bonding (Kelly and Benetti 2011). It is further hypothesized that residual stress within the porcelain may have developed as a result of too rapid cooling (Kelly and Benetti 2011). Long-term clinical studies are needed to verify the validity of these proposed etiologies.

In-vitro studies have shown that the fracture toughness of veneering ceramics used on zirconia restorations is lower than the fracture toughness of veneering ceramics used on PFM restorations (0.73 ± 0.02 MPa versus 1.10 ± 0.2 MPa) (Quinn and coworkers 2010).

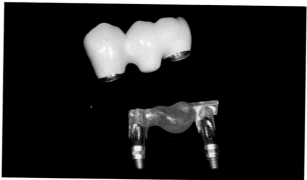

Fig 21   Insertion guide with standard abutments. The implant-supported PFM fixed partial denture is also shown.

For the framework design, it is important to provide enough supporting anatomic structure to the final reconstruction to avoid chipping problems in the future. The framework should not be covered by more than 2 mm of veneering ceramic. The overall bridge design and its geometric features are important as they define the maximum stress and the corresponding failure risk (Quinn and coworkers 2010).

In multiple-unit restorations, another highly relevant factor with regard to fracture strength is the size of the connectors. An in-vitro study compared the levels of fracture strength attained by four-unit zirconia frameworks that featured connectors of different diameters (Larsson and coworkers 2007). Five groups of restorative cores were investigated (connector dimensions: 2.0, 2.5, 3.0, 3.5, 4.0 mm). The levels of fracture strength were found to increase significantly with each diameter increment, except for the increment from 2.0 mm to 2.5 mm, as all fractures in these groups occurred in the preload phase. Furthermore, all core fractures occurred in connector areas. The authors therefore recommended that all-ceramic zirconia-based restorations covering extended spans and/or replacing molars should have a minimum diameter of 4.0 mm (Larsson and coworkers 2007).

Zirconia frameworks are invariably designed in digital CAD environments (Figs 20a-f). The dental technician will still be able to define and customize the connector area (Figs 20 c-f).

After evaluating the framework extraorally for its design and integrity, an intraoral try-in is performed. If the reconstruction has a cemented design, the try-in is started by inserting the abutments into the implants, using the same insertion path as previously on the master cast. An insertion guide is always helpful in finding the correct position (Fig 21).

The framework should fit passively without any rocking. The best way to verify the accuracy of fit is to use a fine dental probe. Also, a silicone material such as Fit Checker should be used to detect inaccuracies.

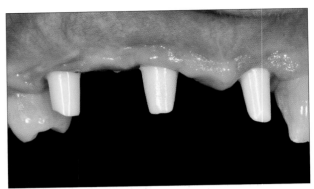

Fig 22a   Zirconia abutments in situ.

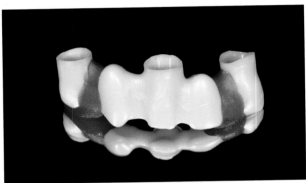

Fig 22b   Zirconia framework with verification record.

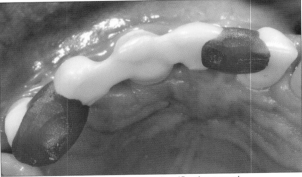

Fig 22c   Zirconia framework try-in and verification record.

A bite-verification record should be obtained (e.g. with pattern resin) in combination with the framework try-in (Figs 22a-c).

If the reconstruction is screw-retained, the framework try-in should not involve any friction. An effort should be made to find the insertion path without damaging the implant-abutment interface. Once the screw-retained framework has been found to fit passively, the screws can be tightened to full torque.

Inaccuracies of fit in the framework may induce inadequate load distribution and possibly increase load transfer to the bone. Also, there may be an increased risk of microleakage from the gap between the implant and the abutment. Screw loosening or fracture of an abutment screw is more frequently observed in the presence of a non-passive fit.

The bisque try-in offers an ideal communication tool to evaluate the final result with the patient. The same (esthetic-phonetic profile analysis) parameters are evaluated as in the mock-up phase. Additional parameters in this stage include color and occlusion, as well as the ways in which the restoration interacts with the underlying or adjacent soft tissue and teeth.

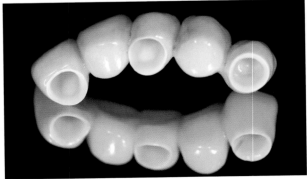

Fig 23a   Final all-ceramic restoration.

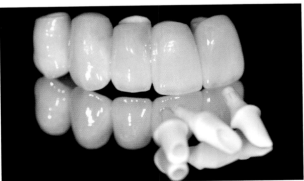

Fig 23b   Frontal view of the final restoration and the CAD/CAM zirconia abutments.

Once the final prosthesis has been completed and accepted by the patient, it is either screwed or cemented to the implants (Figs 23a-b; Figs 24a-d; Fig 25). Definitive cements are used to optimize retention and the quality of the marginal seal (Michalakis and coworkers 2003). As discussed previously in this chapter, even temporary cements can be used to retain final implant-supported restorations, since implants carry no risk of dental decay. Cements of this type, being considerably weaker than definitive cements, can be used to maintain retrievability of the prosthesis (Michalakis and coworkers 2003). During the cementation process it is important to avoid excess cement for the reasons explained in Chapter 5.3.1. As little cement as possible should therefore be used. It is recommended that the cement margins be located at or up to 2 mm below the level of the mucosa. Ligatures placed on the mucosal margin are beneficial but should be used with caution in patients with a thin tissue biotype. Upon completion of treatment, a periapical radiograph is needed to evaluate the final reconstruction for its accuracy of fit and, unless retained by screws, for any residual cement. There are, however, limitations to detecting excess cement in radiographs, as any remnants on the facial and lingual implant surfaces will not be visible.

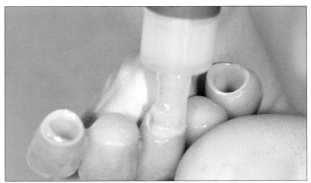

Fig 24a   Application of a try-in paste to the final restoration.

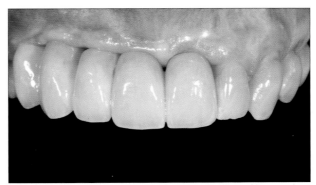

Fig 24b   Insertion of the final implant-supported all-ceramic reconstruction.

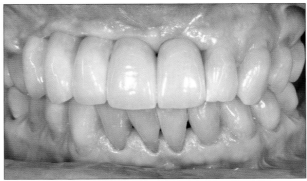

Fig 24c   Frontal view of the final restoration in centric occlusion.

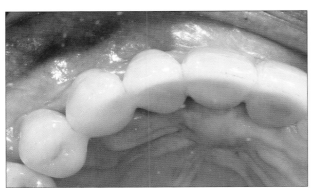

Fig 24d   Occlusal view of the final restoration.

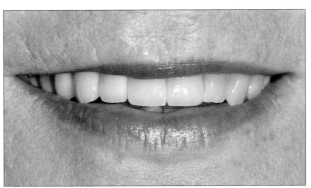

Fig 25   Perioral view of the patient's full smile with the implant-supported restoration in situ.

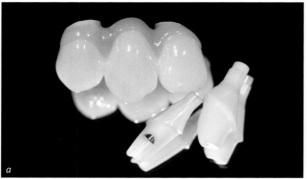
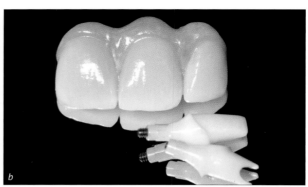

Figs 26a-b   Implant-supported all-ceramic reconstructions with pink ceramics.

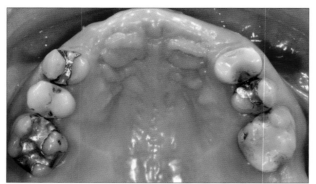

Fig 27   Initial situation with inadequate restorations and extended edentulism in the anterior maxilla.

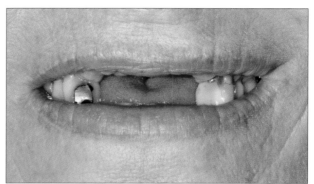

Fig 28   The patient presents with a medium smile line.

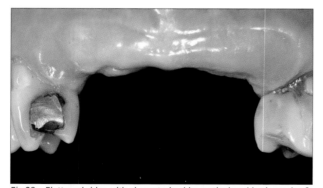

Fig 29   Flattened ridge with characterized by vertical and horizontal soft-tissue and bone deficiencies.

5.3.4   Use of Pink Ceramics in the Extended Edentulous Space

The prosthetic design of the final restoration depends on the preexisting situation, the outcome of the surgical procedures, and the risk factors involved. If a vertical and horizontal deficiency of the partially edentulous ridge is present, gingiva-colored pink ceramics are an option to optimize the esthetic result (Coachman and coworkers 2009) (Figs 26a-b).

They may be indicated whenever patients with a low or medium-high smile line present with vertical and horizontal hard- or soft-tissue defect. In patients with a very high lip line, the use of pink ceramics is not always an option (Salama and coworkers 2009). Bone augmentation may need to be performed horizontally in these situations, with vertical bone reduction and gingival reshaping to flatten the ridge (Salama and coworkers 2009) so that the junction between the pink ceramics and the mucosa can be concealed under the lip line (Figs 27 to 29).

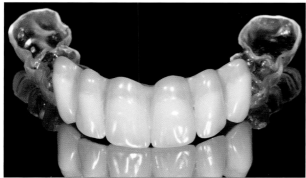

Fig 30a   Mock-up appliance.

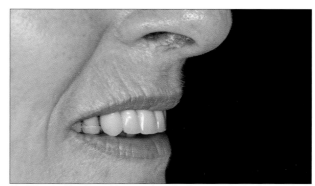

Fig 30b   Profile view with a mock-up in situ to evaluate the prosthetic tooth position, the nasolabial angle, and lip support.

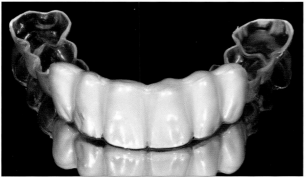

Fig 31a   Radiographic template.

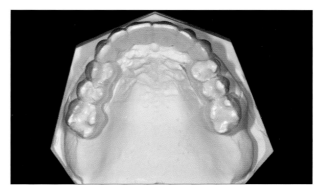

Fig 31b   Radiographic template on the cast.

Since the decision to use artificial gingiva is highly case-sensitive, proper treatment planning is essential. As discussed in Chapter 3, a careful preoperative assessment is needed to analyze each patient's risk profile for treatment planning. The prosthetic aspects of using pink ceramics will be discussed in this section.

Once the initial examinations are completed, a decision must be made as to the prosthetic positions and the number of implants to place depending on the existing bone architecture.

A radiographic template is needed to evaluate bone height and width and to correlate these parameters with the desired prosthetic position. A diagnostic mock-up helps determine this prospective position of the restoration and may consist, for example, of denture teeth embedded in a thermoformed appliance made of clear plastic material (Fig 30a). A major focus of this mock-up should be on correct incisal and labial positions of the future restorations through phonetic and profile analysis (Fig 30b).

This information is then transferred to a radiographic template (Figs 31a-b) and a cone-beam computed tomography (CBCT) scan obtained (see Chapter 3.3.7, Figs 11a-h).

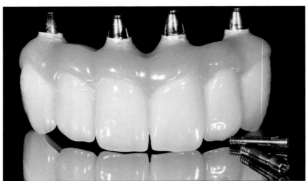

Fig 32a Implant-supported screw-retained provisional with non-engaging titanium abutments.

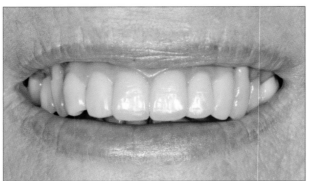

Fig 32b Full smile with implant-supported provisional.

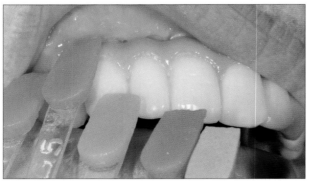

Fig 33 Evaluation of shade for pink ceramics.

The provisional restoration serves to replace the missing teeth on an interim basis (Figs 32a-b). The position of the mucosa and the soft-tissue morphology observed by the end of the provisional phase are important guide for designing the final prosthesis. The provisional restoration does not offer any information about the position of the transition line, which needs to be collected during the mock-up and bisque try-ins. The provisional restoration must be designed to offer easy access for hygiene, and the patient should be given instructions on how to perform home maintenance.

Before the prosthesis can be finalized, gingival and dental shade-taking is required (Fig 33). The gingival shade most precisely matching the surrounding mucosa is selected.

An intraoral diagnostic wax-up/set-up is strongly recommended to determine three important aspects relative to the prosthetic design (Figs 35a-c):

- Morphology of the future pink portion of the implant supported prostheses by evaluating the exact position of the transition zone between the planned pink ceramic and the existing mucosa.
- Cervical height of the planned gingival level.
- Maintenance of and access to the future restoration by oral hygiene devices such as proximal brushes or Superfloss.

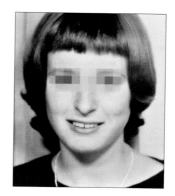

Fig 34   Picture of the patient at a younger age. Diastema in the esthetic zone.

In addition, the intraoral diagnostic wax-up/set-up it is a diagnostic tool to evaluate the overall dental esthetic appearance, including tooth length, width, and form, as well as other intraoral and extraoral parameters such as the facial and dental midline, vertical dimension of occlusion, and smile.

Finally, the intraoral diagnostic wax-up/set-up helps elicit the patient's esthetic expectations and acceptance of the suggested design. Patients should be encouraged to furnish any pictures showing their former teeth (Fig 34). It is important to discuss the patient's interpretation of dental esthetics, e.g. a geometric/symmetric versus a more natural tooth arrangement.

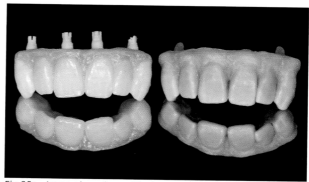

Fig 35a   Intraoral mock-up with denture teeth and simulated pink ceramic in wax.

The teeth in the wax-up of the present case were arranged in a personalized fashion (Figs 35a-c). The patient, dental technician, and prosthodontist decided to develop a personalized esthetic design with a straighter tooth alignment than in the wax-up.

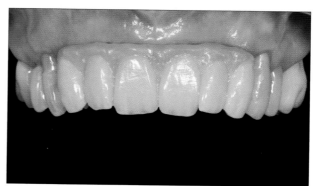

Fig 35b   Intraoral mock-up with individualized tooth positions.

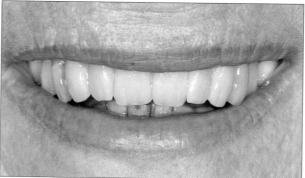

Fig 35c   Smile line with mock-up in situ.

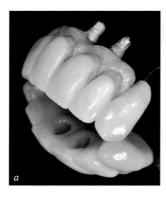
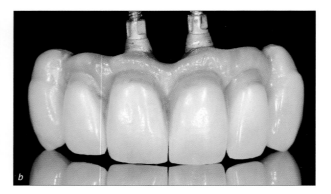

Figs 36a-b Bisque balle stage of porcelain try-in.

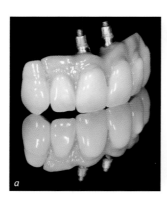
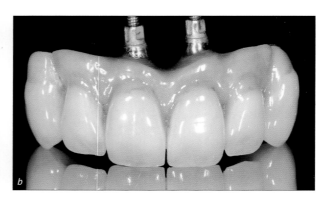

Figs 37a-b Final implant-supported restoration.

The bisque try-in with the use of pink ceramics can be divided into two steps (Figs 36a-b):

1. ***Elaboration of exact tooth forms.*** Only if the correct tooth forms are evident can decisions on the dimension of the future pink portion of the restoration be made. Pink ceramics is therefore not finalized at the first bisque try-in, so that the position and thickness of "pink" and the planned transition line can be assessed directly with the patient. It is also important to evaluate accessibility of the restoration for cleaning and maintenance by the patient.

2. ***Elaboration of pink ceramics after first try-in.*** This step is accomplished in accordance with the tooth forms and the neighboring teeth. The decision exactly where the transition line should be placed is key to a successful esthetic outcome. One can readily visualize the correct level during smile and phonetic movements, the present case being a good example. An excessively large proportion of pink ceramics would have been visible in the patient's full smile through exposure of the transition between the artificial and natural mucosa. The transition line was placed mesially instead of distally on the canine, and the canines replicated the shape and recessions of the neighboring natural teeth (Figs 36a-b, 37a-b, and 38a-b). With the transition line moved to the mesial aspect, it was no longer visible in the patient's full smile (Figs 38c-e).

The shape of the prosthesis should offer good access for hygiene, in the absence of any concavities underneath, and should allow Superfloss to pass through the entire interface between the artificial and natural mucosa and along the abutments (Coachman and coworkers 2010). It must be ensured that the patient can use the floss without assistance and that the pressure level between the natural and artificial mucosa is similar to the one inside an interproximal tooth contact, i.e. the Superfloss should be able to pass through the area by overcoming mild resistance (Coachman and coworkers 2010). Oral hygiene instructions should be given and explained in front of a mirror.

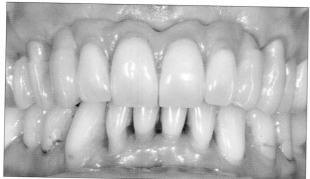

Fig 38a   Delivery of final restoration.

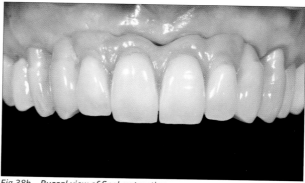

Fig 38b   Buccal view of final restoration.

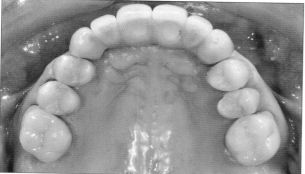

Fig 38c   Occlusal view of final restoration.

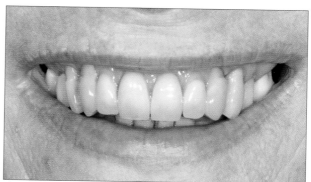

Fig 38d   Lip line during full smile with the final restoration in situ.

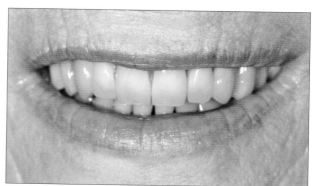

Fig 38e   Lip line during normal smile with the final restoration in situ.

5.4 Occlusion

Occlusion continues to be a controversial issue in prosthodontics generally and in implant dentistry specifically (Carlsson 2009). Insufficient evidence from studies focusing on the occlusion of implant-supported restorations is currently available, and different occlusal concepts have never been compared in randomized controlled clinical trials (Carlsson 2009; Taylor and coworkers 2000).

The most important biophysiological difference between a natural tooth and a dental implant is that the natural tooth is connected to the surrounding alveolar bone via the periodontal ligament. Dental implants, by contrast, are in contact with the bone directly by osseointegration. As a consequence, natural teeth are subject to a mean axial displacement of approximately 25–100 µm while dental implants get displaced by only 3–5 µm (Kim and coworkers 2005; Schulte 1995). Periodontal ligament can function like a shock absorber that transfers occlusal stresses along the axes of natural teeth, thus ensuring that they get distributed. Occlusal loads acting on implants are concentrated at the crest of the surrounding bone without being absorbed. Another advantage of periodontal ligament is its neurophysiologic receptor function, whereby information of proprioceptive nerve endings is transmitted to the central nervous system (Taylor and coworkers 2005; Kim and coworkers 2005). The presence or absence of periodontal ligament accounts for a significant difference in tactile sensitivity between implants and natural teeth (Taylor and coworkers 2005; Schulte 1995). Hämmerle and coworkers (1995) found that the mean threshold values of tactile sensitivity perception were 8.75 times higher for implants than for teeth.

To adjust and re-evaluate the occlusion with implant supported reconstructions is therefore of fundamental importance, as the absence of a periodontal ligament significantly detracts from their load-sharing ability, occlusal-force adaptation, and mechanoperception (Kim and coworkers 2005).

A mutually protected occlusion, with slightly more contacts on the adjacent natural dentition, is the recommended occlusal concept in treatments dealing with extended edentulism in the esthetic zone.

Since fixed reconstructions supported by implants are generally preferred in these situations, the presence of posterior support is essential. A mutually protected occlusion is selected to protect the anterior reconstruction during centric (habitual) static occlusion and to provide anterior guidance in lateral and protrusive excursion movements. To distribute the occlusal force in static occlusion evenly to the posterior teeth, the implant-supported fixed reconstruction in the anterior maxilla should be in light contact with the opposing mandibular dentition when tested with an 8-µm Shimstock foil (Hanel, Langenau, Germany) during forceful jaw closure, while no contact should be present during light bite (Fig 39a).

Bilateral stability in centric (habitual) occlusion is important. Therefore, the following guidelines should be respected: evenly distributed occlusal contacts and forces (centered contacts) and absence of interference in dynamic occlusion (lateral and protrusive excursive movements). If a slide in centric is present between centric and habitual occlusion, no interferences in static occlusion should be present (Kim and coworkers 2005) (Fig 39b).

Cantilever extensions are commonly used on implant-supported restorations but should be regarded with caution. A higher overall incidence of technical complications has been reported in implant-supported reconstructions with than in those without cantilever extensions (Kreissl and coworkers 2007; Salvi and Brägger 2009). It is therefore recommended that cantilever extensions should be limited in length and placed slightly below the occlusal level (0.1 – 0.2 mm). An important requirement for cantilever units is disclusion during lateral and protrusive excursive movements with an absence of premature contacts (Carlsson 2009).

Another risk factor is bruxism, which has been discussed in Chapter 3 to be associated with mechanical and technical complications (Salvi and Brägger 2009).

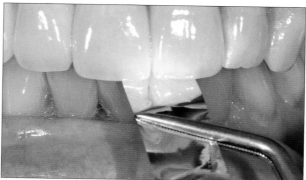

Fig 39a   Occlusal evaluation under light and heavy bite force with Shimstock foil.

Recommended occlusal design for implant-supported fixed multi-unit prostheses in the maxillary anterior zone

a   Static occlusion:
- Evenly distributed and centered occlusal contacts in posterior areas.
- No detectable contacts under light bite force and light contact under heavy bite force, on the anterior units.
- No interferences or premature contacts.

b   Dynamic occlusion:
- Mutually protected occlusion with canine guidance or anterior group function during lateral movements.
- Incisal guidance during protrusive movements.
- No interferences on the working and non-working sides.

→   **Minimize occlusal contacts on cantilevers.**
→   **Periodically reevaluate occlusion during recall visits.**

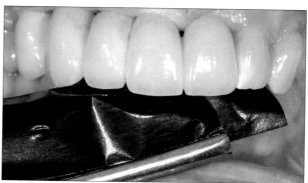

Fig 39b   Occlusal evaluation with thin articulating paper to determine static and dynamic occlusion.

Acknowledgments

Surgical procedures
Prof. Daniel Buser – Professor and Chair, Department of Oral Surgery and Stomatology, University of Bern, Switzerland

Laboratory procedures
MDT Tom Furter (Art Dent, Dental Laboratory, Bern, Switzerland) performed all laboratory procedures related to the case presented in Section 5.3.3 and in Figures 26a-b and 30a, 31a, 32a (Section 5.3.4).

MDT Alwin Schönenberger (Dental Ceramics, Zürich, Switzerland) performed all laboratory procedures for the implant-supported restoration with pink ceramics presented in Section 5.3.4 (Figs 35a to 39b).

6 Clinical Case Presentations

6.1 Replacement of Two Central Incisors with Non-Splinted Crowns on Bone-Level Implants

U.C. Belser, D. Buser

A 27-year-old female patient was referred to the Clinic of Oral Surgery and Stomatology of the University of Bern due to acute pain in the region of her two maxillary central incisors. The patient was in good general health. She reported a bicycle accident approximately 5 years earlier in which teeth 11 and 21 had been traumatized but neither fractured nor displaced. Several weeks after the accident, endodontic treatment was performed on both central incisors, although the patient did not recall the precise reasons for this decision. About 2 years ago, non-vital bleaching had been conducted, in accordance with the "walking-bleach" principle, due to progressive discoloration of teeth 11 and 21.

Minor discoloration of tooth 11 was observable at the time of clinical examination (Figs 1a-b). The intraoral radiographs, by contrast, revealed major external root resorption in the cervical area of both teeth that originally had been traumatized (Figs 1c-d). Root 11 was clearly affected by more advanced disease. In the literature, this type of pathology has been described in the context of both dental trauma and internal bleaching. The treat-

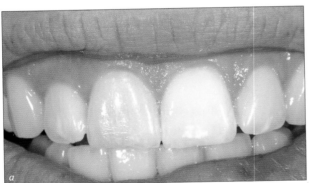
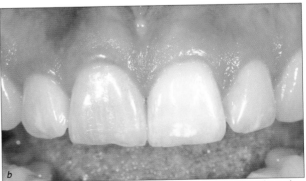

Figs 1a-b   Initial clinical close-up views of a 27-year old woman who sought treatment because of acute pain in the area of teeth 11 and 21. The patient had a high smile line completely exposing both the papillary and the cervical gingiva (left). No problems other than moderate discoloration of the clinical crown of tooth 11 were noted; in particular, there were no open embrasures or disturbances in the scalloped course of the gingival line (right).

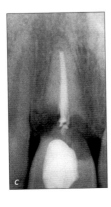
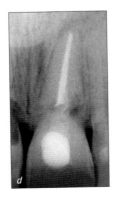

Figs 1c-d   Initial radiographs showing advanced external root resorption in the cervical areas of teeth 11 and 21. The bone height at the mesial aspect of the two lateral incisors, and between the two central incisors, had been maintained at a physiological distance apical to the cementoenamel junction (CEJ).

ment of choice with advanced external resorptive lesions of this type is to extract the tooth, which, in the present case, was going to result in a clinical situation characterized by two adjacent missing maxillary incisors. This is widely considered to be therapeutically problematic, especially in terms of esthetic outcome. The clinical examination therefore had to include a comprehensive esthetic risk assessment, following the guidelines defined by Martin and coworkers (2006). The relevant 12-item checklist for the patient revealed three items that clearly belonged in the high-risk category:

- High smile line
- High esthetic expectations
- Two adjacent missing maxillary incisors

All other potential risk parameters were considered favorable, including the presence of a thick gingival biotype, a rectangular form of the anatomical tooth crowns, intact neighboring teeth, and no current or anticipated tissue deficiencies. Based on the SAC classification (Dawson and Chen 2009), the clinical situation fell into the "advanced" category (level A). Only two treatment options were looked at more closely: either tooth extraction followed by insertion of two adjacent bone-level implants with a standard diameter (Straumann Bone Level, diameter 4.1 mm, length 12 mm) or a tooth-supported four-unit metal-ceramic fixed prosthesis covering sites 12 to 22. In the brief discussion that ensued, the patient opted for the implant-supported restoration without hesitation. After carefully extracting the two central incisors without elevation of a flap, a removable partial denture was inserted as temporary restoration. In accordance with the concept of early implant placement (Buser and coworkers 2008), implant surgery was to be performed after 8 weeks of uneventful soft-tissue healing (Fig 2a). A simple surgical guide was fabricated that defined the future incisal edge position and the mucosal emergence line of the two planned implant crowns (Fig 2b).

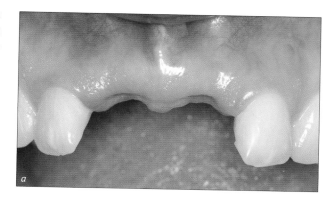

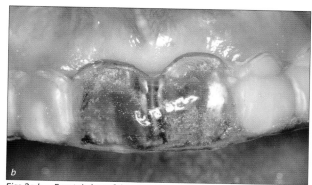

Figs 2a-b   Frontal view of the anterior maxilla 8 weeks after extraction of teeth 11 and 21 (left). A simple surgical stent was fabricated to visualize the mucosal emergence line of the future implant crowns.

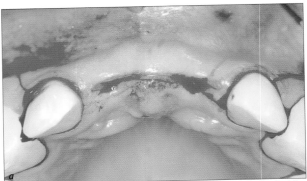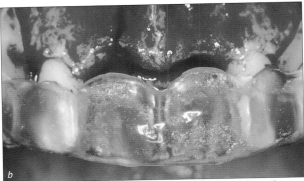

Figs 3a-b   A midcrestal incision with two distovestibular relieving incisions was used (left) prior to elevating a mucoperiosteal flap (right). Note the presence of a dehiscence-type bone defect at site 11.

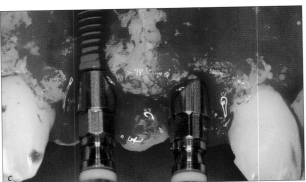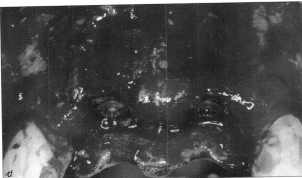

Figs 3c-d   After insertion of two implants (Straumann Bone Level, Regular CrossFit, length 12 mm), the implant at site 11 was exposed on its labial aspect (left), requiring coverage with autologous bone chips (right) harvested from the same surgical site (i.e. from the nasal spine and apical portion of the vestibulum).

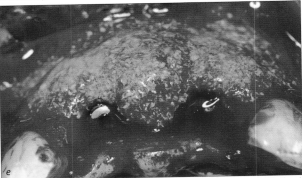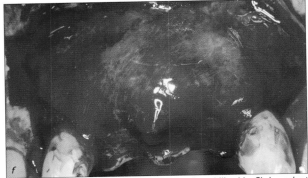

Figs 3e-f   Contour augmentation was performed with a low-substitution bone filler (BioOss; Geistlich, Wolhusen, Switzerland), stabilized by fibrin sealant (Tissue Col; Baxter, USA) and then covered by two layers of a bio-absorbable collagen membrane (BioGide; Geistlich).

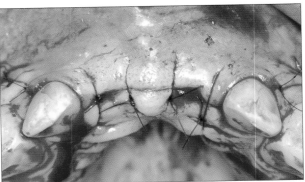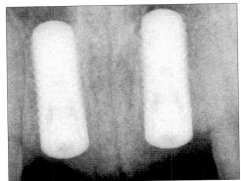

Fig 3g   Tension-free primary wound closure was achieved with interrupted sutures after sectioning the periosteum at the base of the flap (left).

Fig 3h   Intraoral radiograph taken immediately after implant placement.

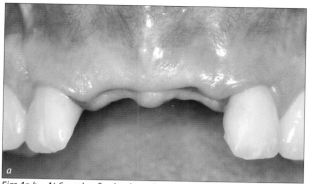 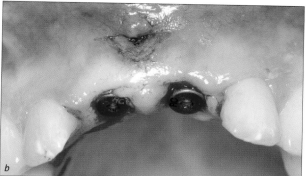

Figs 4a-b   At 6 weeks after implant placement, the surgical site presented with healed soft tissue (left). The low-inserting central frenulum was excised with a CO_2 laser at this stage, and the short healing caps were replaced with two longer ones to make the implant shoulders accessible (right).

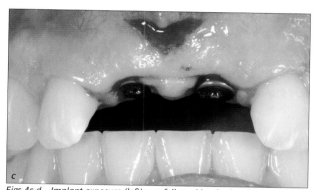 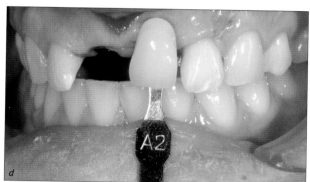

Figs 4c-d   Implant exposure (left) was followed by shade selection (right) for a laboratory-made, screw-retained, temporary prosthesis.

At this stage, a midcrestal incision was performed and complemented by two relieving incisions at the distal line angles of teeth 12 and 22 (Fig 3a). Following elevation of a mucoperiosteal flap, the surgical guide was repositioned both to verify the distance between the alveolar bone crest and the future line of emergence from the alveolar mucosa (Fig 3b) and to decide whether "bone scalloping" was indicated. Two bone-level implants (Straumann Bone Level, diameter 4.1 mm, length 12 mm) were inserted in a correct three-dimensional position, carefully respecting the parameters of existing danger and comfort zones as previously reported in detail by the present authors (Buser and coworkers 2006). As anticipated, this resulted in site 11 presenting with a marked dehiscence-type defect (Fig 3c) that required a contour augmentation procedure, which was accomplished by first placing autologous bone chips harvested from appropriate locations of the same surgical site in direct contact with the exposed implant surface (Fig 3d) and completing the procedure by applying a low-substitution bone filler (BioOss; Geistlich, Wolhusen,

Switzerland) (Fig 3e) and covering it with two layers of a bioabsorbable membrane (BioGide; Geistlich) (Fig 3f). Finally, tension-free primary wound closure was obtained with interrupted sutures after splitting the periosteum at the base of the flap (Fig 3g). A postoperative radiograph (Fig 3h) confirmed that the interimplant distance exceeded 3mm and that an adequate volume of contour augmentation had been attained.

After 8 weeks of uneventful healing following implant placement, after confirming that complete soft-tissue coverage was present (Fig 4a), access to the implant shoulder was established through a minimally invasive punch procedure to preserve a maximum of keratinized mucosa on the vestibular aspect of the implants (Fig 4b). Simultaneously, the low-inserting central frenulum was excised with a CO_2 laser. The same appointment also included an open-tray impression and shade selection for the implant-supported screw-retained temporary crowns (Figs 4c-d).

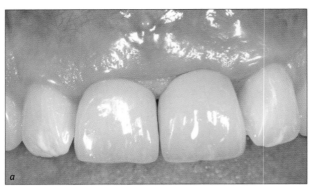

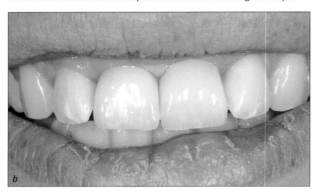

Figs 5a-b   Clinical views obtained shortly after insertion of the two implant-supported screw-retained temporary crowns at sites 11 and 21. The altered length-to-width ratios gave the restorations an unnatural appearance. For visual harmony, the mesial and distal transition line angles needed to be accentuated and the cervical aspects modified into a triangular shape.

These were inserted 2 weeks later (Figs 5a-b). It became apparent that the normal length-to-width ratio of the two clinical crowns was significantly altered by the facts that interproximal volume had been added to close the embrasures and that the line of emergence was located at a slightly too coronal level due to an excess of soft tissue at the implant sites.

Several modifications in form, outline, and contour were required to improve the esthetic appearance of the two implant-supported restorations. The esthetically pertinent elements of an intact anterior maxillary dentition are schematically represented in Fig 6a. They refer to a harmoniously scalloped mucosal line and interproximal closure with soft tissue. Following loss of the two central maxillary incisors and their replacement by implant-supported single crowns that precisely replicate the original forms and volumes, esthetic harmony is disturbed by open embrasures between the implant sites (Fig 6b). To make the "black triangles" narrower, the interproximal contact zone needs to be elongated in a cervical direction, and the cervical crown volume has to be increased mesially and distally (Fig 6c). Figure 6d illustrates a summary of restorative design parameters that can be utilized to enhance esthetics, including the position of the mesial and distal transition line angles, the relative extension (weight) of the midlabial crown compartment, and the cervical "wings." These modifications had been implemented during the temporary phase, which took approximately 3 months, with an esthetically acceptable outcome (Figs 7a-b). In fact, stable and esthetic peri-implant soft-tissue contours had been established by the end of the temporary phase of restorative treatment, with harmonious scalloping of the mucosal line also extending through the highly critical area between both implants.

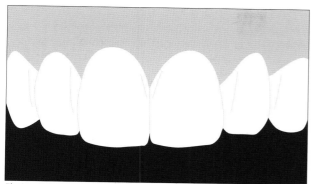

Fig 6a   Schematic representation of an intact anterior maxillary dentition, with harmonious scalloping of the mucosal line and complete closure of the interproximal spaces by soft tissue.

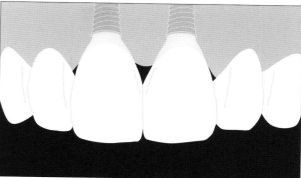

Fig 6b   Schematic representation of the same anterior maxilla following virtual loss of both central incisors and replacement by two implant-supported crowns. Note the evident visual tension caused by marked flattening of the mucosal line, notably between the two implant sites, resulting in unsightly open embrasures ("black triangles").

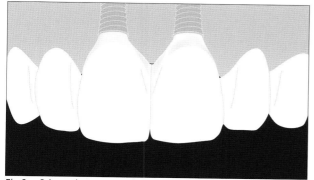

Fig 6c   Schematic representation of the same implant-supported crowns after contour modification, which included elongation of the interproximal contact in an apical direction and addition of crown volume in the cervical area. These simple measures were taken to reestablish visual harmony.

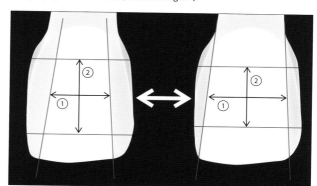

Fig 6d   Labial outline of a maxillary central incisor. The red lines illustrate the key parameters influencing visual perception of (1) the length-to-width ratio (i.e. positions and inclinations of the mesial and distal transition line angles) and (2) the length of the midcentral labial compartment. These parameters can be adjusted to visually compensate for an overly short and large appearance (right), making it seem more elongated and narrower (left) without modifying the outline of the clinical crown. This effect, combined with the options of vertically increasing the interproximal contact (located distinctly further palatally) and of adding cervical volume, can be utilized to compensate for minor discrepancies between existing and ideal space conditions.

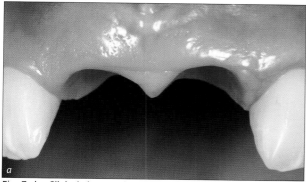

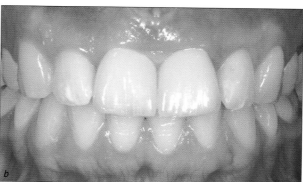

Figs 7a-b   Clinical close-up views 3 months after delivery of the temporary restorations, without and with the finalized implant-supported temporary crowns in place (left and right). Crown contouring was the key both to obtaining a triangular cervical appearance and to eliminating open embrasures.

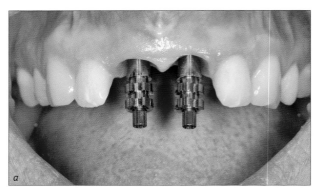

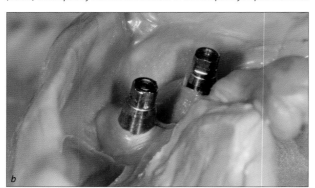

Figs 8a-b   At this stage, a final open-tray type impression was taken with the aid of screw-retained impression posts (above). It is recommended to proceed without delay to pick up as much as possible of the sulcular profile (below) developed by the cervical contour of the temporary implant crowns.

This tissue profile is largely the result of adequate submucosal and supramucosal axial contours and an adequate volume of the implant-supported temporary restorations themselves. There are several ways to transfer this valuable information from the patient's mouth to the master cast for the definitive implant-supported crowns, the most predictable option being to customize the impression post before taking the impression (as discussed in Chapter 5).

As an acceptable alternative, the authors proposed to first take an alginate impression with the temporary restorations still in place. The cast derived from this impression would also be mounted in the articulator to serve as a well-defined three-dimensional reference. Following removal of the screw-retained temporary restorations, the impression posts were immediately attached and the impression taken without delay to minimize the ensuing collapse of soft tissue (Fig 8a). The resultant impression in polyvinyl siloxane (Fig 8b) included an adequate representation of both the intrasulcular area and the interproximal sides (without air inclusions), which in turn is critical to the future establishment of accurate interproximal contacts.

Using silicone indices, the dental technician fabricated the final crowns such that the positions, forms, and volumes previously defined by the temporary restorations were respected and reproduced (Fig 9a).

CAD/CAM-generated zirconia substructures (CARES; Straumann, Basel, Switzerland) were veneered using a pressable ceramic system (Figs 9b-h).

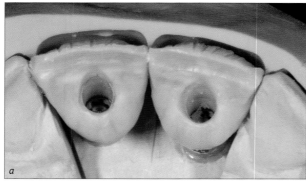

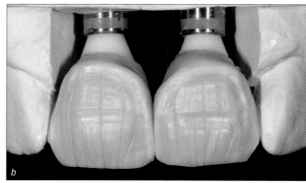

Figs 9a-b   After creating two directly screw-retained anatomic zirconia abutments by CAD/CAM (CARES; Straumann, Basel, Switzerland), the laboratory technician completed the crown volumes in wax to be replaced by pressed veneering ceramics later. A minimum amount of space was reserved on the labial aspect (left) for completion during the final stage of esthetic characterization.

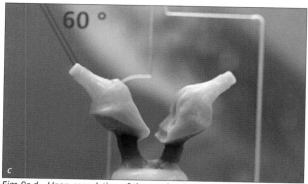
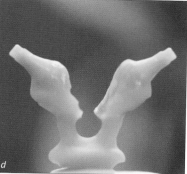

Figs 9c-d   Upon completion of the previously described wax-up, the two elements were sprued (left) and then invested. The lost-wax technique was used for direct pressing of the veneering ceramic to the zirconia substructure (right).

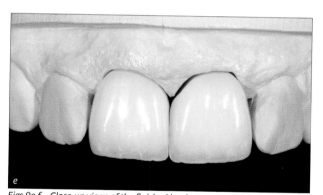
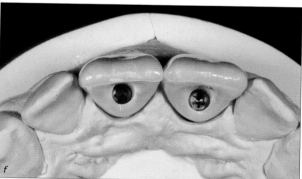

Figs 9e-f   Close-up views of the finished implant-supported all-ceramic crowns. Characterization of the incisal third was performed by manual stratification (left). Due to correct three-dimensional implant positioning in general, and implant axes located palatal to the incisal edge line in particular, direct screw connections could be implemented to retain the crowns (right).

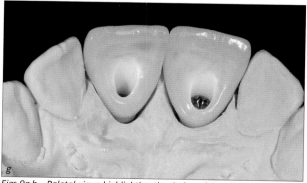
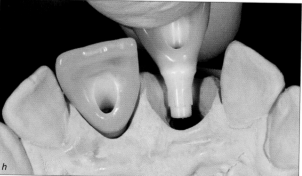

Figs 9g-h   Palatal views highlighting the design of the clinical crowns (left) and the flat emergence profile of the smooth transition between the zirconia substructure and the pressed veneering ceramic (right).

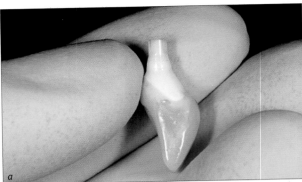

Figures 10a-b illustrate the basic design details of the restoration type selected, and Figures 11a-i present the final clinical and radiographic documentation of the case. Figures 12a-d and 13a-b were taken at the follow-up examinations at 1 and 5 years.

Figs 10a-b Detail views of the implant-supported directly screw-retained all-ceramic crowns.

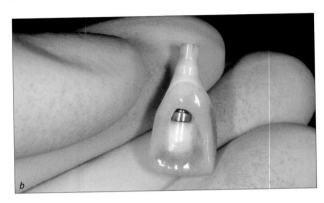

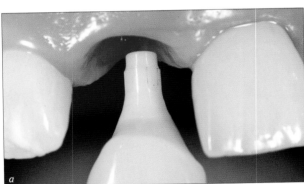
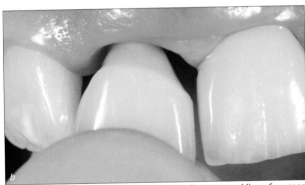

Figs 11a-b During crown insertion, the distinctly distal eccentricity of the triangular neck configuration was apparent, ensuring a natural line of mucosal emergence with the zenith located distally to the longitudinal tooth axis.

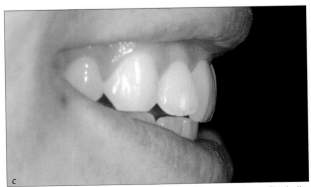
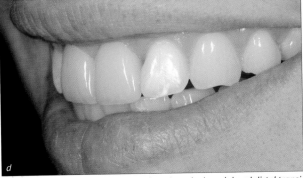

Figs 11c-d Two lateral views showing both a flat emergence profile similar to the one observed at the adjacent teeth and marked mesial and distal transition line angles, which significantly contributed to the natural appearance of the two implant-supported restorations.

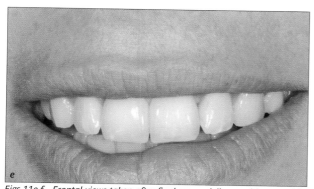

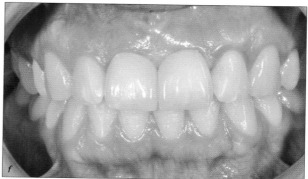

Figs 11e-f   Frontal views taken after final crown delivery, with normal lip coverage (left) and with the lips retracted (right). Note the acceptable esthetic integration.

Fig 11g   Follow-up radiograph after delivery of the final implant-supported directly screw-retained zirconia-based restorations.

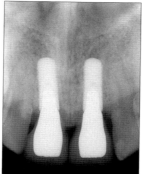
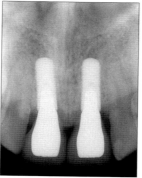

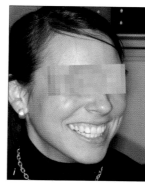

Figs 11h-i   Views of the patient's natural (left) and forced smile (right) at the end of active treatment documenting that her high esthetic expectations could be satisfied despite a high smile line.

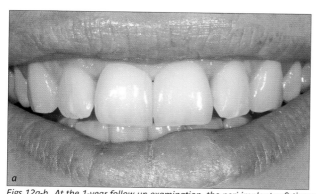

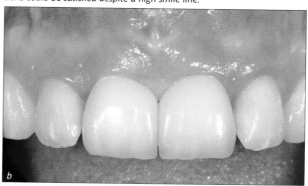

Figs 12a-b   At the 1-year follow-up examination, the peri-implant soft-tissue contours were stable and esthetically pleasing.

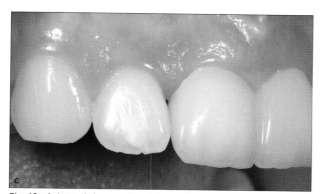

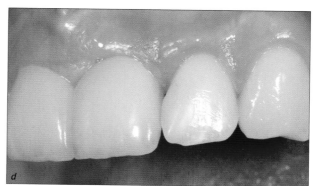

Figs 12c-d   Lateral close-up views taken at the 1-year follow-up, confirming the successful integration of the two implant-supported crowns.

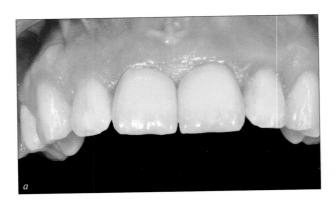

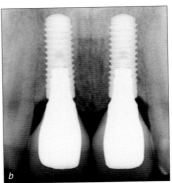

Figs 13a-b Clinical close-up view taken at the 5-year follow-up confirming that the soft tissue continues to be stable (left). A radiograph obtained at the same time reveals favorable bone conditions, especially between the implants (right).

Conclusion

This case study has illustrated the substantial challenge, particularly from an esthetic viewpoint, of implementing adjacent implant-supported restorations in the anterior maxilla. It has reemphasized the importance of a structured preoperative esthetic risk assessment and the validity of early implant placement in combination with vestibular contour augmentation. Design criteria, prosthetic guidelines, and tips and tricks to master the esthetic implications of anterior implant restorations have been described in detail. Finally, this case report confirmed the favorable potential, especially from an esthetic viewpoint, of implant concepts relying on "platform switching."

Acknowledgments

The authors wish to thank Dental Technician and Master Ceramist Dominique Vinci (Geneva, Switzerland) for his expertise and outstanding performance once again reflected in the laboratory work that has been presented in this case study. They also acknowledge the contributions made by Dr. Francesca Vailati (Senior Lecturer at the School of Dental Medicine, University of Geneva, Switzerland) to some of the clinical photography shown.

6.2 Replacement of Two Central Incisors with Non-Splinted Crowns on Tissue-Level Implants

W. Martin, J. Ruskin

A 28-year-old female patient presented to our clinic in 2000 with failing teeth 11 and 21. She reported no general medical conditions that would prevent routine restorative and surgical procedures. She was experiencing no pain, but reported that the teeth were mobile and would like to replace them with something more permanent.

Upon an extraoral and intraoral clinical examination and radiographic review, teeth 11 and 21 exhibited external and internal resorption, class II mobility, and periapical pathology (Figs 1 to 4). Given their poor prognosis for long-term survival, it was determined that they should be extracted. Several treatment options were considered, ranging from a conventional fixed dental prosthesis to single (cantilevered restoration) or multiple dental implants. Considering the patient's desire to have individual teeth and the available architecture of the hard and soft tissue, it was determined that adjacent implant-supported restorations should be explored.

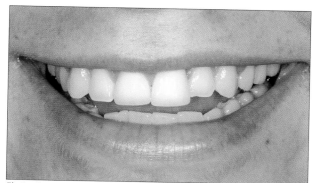

Fig 1   Pretreatment smile.

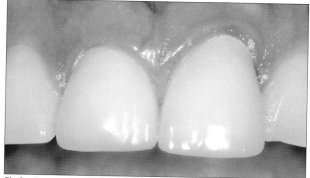

Fig 2   Frontal view of teeth 11 and 21.

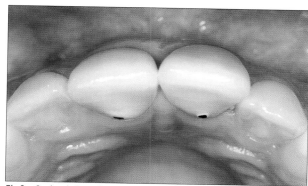

Fig 3   Occlusal view of teeth 11 and 21.

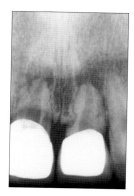

Fig 4   Pretreatment periapical radiograph.

Table 1   Esthetic Risk Assessment (ERA).

Esthetic Risk Factor	Level of Risk		
	Low	Moderate	High
Medical status	Healthy, co-operative patient with an intact immune system.		Reduced immune system
Smoking habit	Non-smoker	Light smoker (< 10 cigs/day)	Heavy smoker ≥ 10 cigs/day)
Patient's esthetic expectations	Low	Medium	High
Lip line	Low	Medium	High
Gingival biotype	Low-scalloped, thick	Medium-scalloped, medium thick	High-scalloped, thin
Shape of tooth crowns	Rectangular		Triangular
Infection at implant site	None	Chronic	Acute
Bone level at adjacent teeth	≤ 5 mm to contact point	5.5 to 6.5 mm to contact point	≥ 7 mm to contact point
Restorative status of neighboring teeth	Virgin		Restored
Width of edentulous span	1 tooth (≥ 7 mm)	1 tooth (≤ 7 mm)	2 teeth or more
Soft-tissue anatomy	Intact soft tissue		Soft-tissue defects
Bone anatomy of alveolar crest	Alveolar crest without bone deficiency	Horizontal bone deficiency	Vertical bone deficiency

An Esthetic Risk Assessment (ERA) was generated and reviewed with the patient (see ITI Treatment Guide, Volume 1). Table 1 highlights the key factors for an esthetic outcome. Based on these factors, the esthetic risk profile was determined to be "moderate" to "high."

The planned treatment for this patient required placement of adjacent implants in the esthetic zone. Several challenges arise when placing implants adjacent to each other, and while evidence-based information in this area is scarce, several articles have addressed limitations to this treatment based upon clinical experience. The main limitation lies in the ability to maintain or create an interimplant papilla. This factor is closely related to the maintenance of the interimplant bone crest, which pro-

vides the support for the papilla. It has been reported that 3.4 mm of interimplant papilla can be expected on average when implants are placed in an ideal relationship to each other, i.e. if the distance between the implant bodies is 3 mm (Tarnow and coworkers 2000). Detailed planning and placement of the dental implants would be critical to achieving esthetic success.

The textbook "SAC Classification in Implant Dentistry" was compiled by the ITI to assist treatment teams in determining the complexity of implant rehabilitations based on several normative and modifying factors expressed by the clinical situation. Table 2 highlights some of the key factors in the treatment of this patient and the complexity associated with them.

Table 2   Modifying factors for treatment of anterior extended edentulism.

Anterior Extended Edentulous Spaces	Notes	Straightforward	Advanced	Complex
Esthetic risk	Refer for ERA (Treatment Guide 1)	Low	Moderate	High
Intermaxillary relationship	Refers to horizontal and vertical overlap and the effect on restorability and esthetic outcome	Class I and III	Class II Div 1 and 2	Non-restorable without adjunctive preparatory therapy due to severe malocclusion
Mesiodistal space		Adequate for required tooth replacement	Insufficient space available for replacement of all missing teeth	Adjunctive therapy necessary to replace all missing teeth
Occlusion/ articulation		Harmonious	Irregular, with no need for correction	Changes of existing occlusion necessary
Interim restorations during healing		RDP	Fixed	
Provisional implant-supported restorations	Provisional restorations are recommended		Restorative margin < 3 mm apical to mucosal crest	Restorative margin ≥ 3 mm apical to mucosal crest
Occlusal parafunction	Risk of complication is to the restoration, not to implant survival	Absent		Present
Loading protocol	To date, immediate restoration and loading procedures are lacking scientific documentation	Conventional or early		Immediate

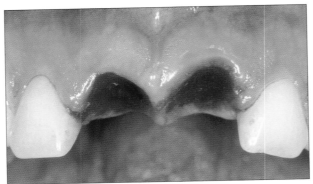

Fig 5   Frontal view after extraction.

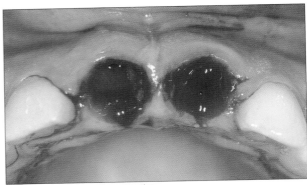

Fig 6   Occlusal view after extraction.

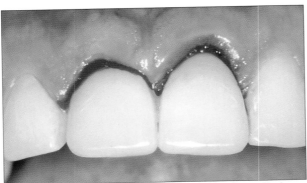

Fig 7   Frontal view after placement of the bonded interim prosthesis.

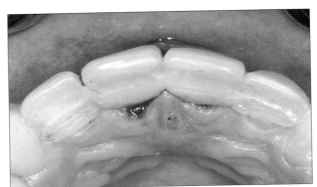

Fig 8   Occlusal view after placement of the bonded interim prosthesis.

Treatment

The first phase of treatment required that the teeth be extracted and the infection be allowed to resolve. A periotome approach was used to remove the teeth and minimize trauma to the sites (Figs 5 and 6). A fixed interim prosthesis with ovate pontics was fabricated utilizing denture teeth (Ivoclar Vivadent, Buffalo, NY, USA) and fiber reinforcement (Kerr Sybron Dental, Orange, CA, USA). The ovate pontics were designed to extend 2 mm beyond the mucosal margin into the extraction sockets. The interim prosthesis was bonded into place with a spot-etch and flowable composite resin on the fiber and adjacent teeth (Figs 7 and 8).

The patient was unable to return to the clinic for continued care for 12 months. Upon clinical examination, it was determined that the area had fully healed and that minimal alteration in ridge height and width had occurred over this period (Figs 9 to 11).

Diagnostic impressions of the interim restoration in place and removed were made for fabrication of a radiographic and surgical template (Figs 12 to 14). The template(s) were utilized to place the implants in an ideal three-dimensional position based upon the planned restorations and in relation to each other.

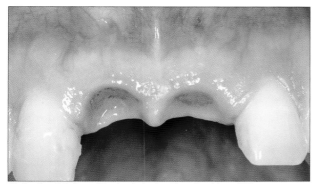

Fig 9   Frontal view of the healed extraction sites 11 and 21.

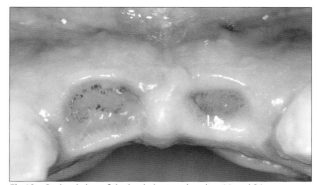

Fig 10   Occlusal view of the healed extraction sites 11 and 21.

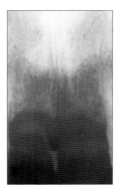

Fig 11   Periapical radiograph 12 months after extraction.

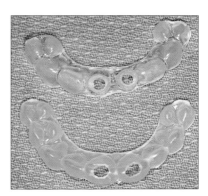

Fig 12   Surgical templates for placement of implants 11 and 21.

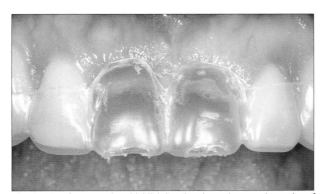

Fig 13   Vacuform template highlighting the planned mucosal margins of the definitive restorations.

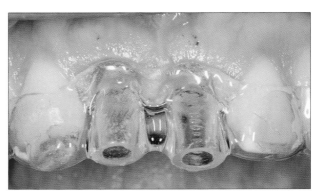

Fig 14   This 2-mm sleeve template was used to dictate mesiodistal and orofacial positioning.

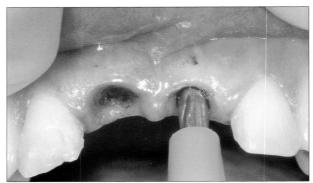

Fig 15   A 4.0-mm tissue punch was used to expose the alveolar crest.

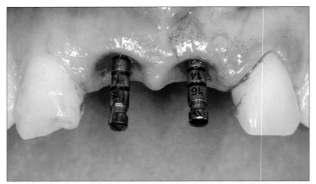

Fig 16   Situation with 2.2-mm guide pins in place, confirming proper depths and angulations of the osteotomies.

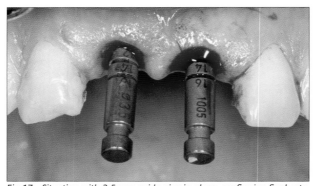

Fig 17   Situation with 3.5-mm guide pins in place, confirming final osteotomy positions.

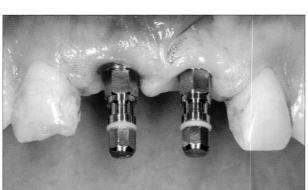

Fig 18   Final implant positioning prior to removing the implant mounts.

The second phase of treatment was dedicated to placement and loading of the dental implants. During the examination process, it was determined that a flapless approach to implant placement would offer the best potential for an esthetic outcome. In today's practice, sectional imaging with guided surgery would provide the best opportunity to position implants such that available bone is maximized in relation to the planned restorations. At the time of this specific surgical procedure, however, the cost of sectional imaging was still prohibitive. It was decided to place the implants based on the surgeon's experience and the surgical templates. The risk experienced during this procedure was the difficulty in ensuring and confirming clinically that the implants were placed entirely within the alveolar bone. Flapless procedures are complex by involving a high risk of complications and should only be undertaken by experienced surgeons. In the present case, the surgeon utilized buccal palpation during the osteotomy procedure to ensure that the cortical bone plate was not perforated. Two dental implants were then placed (Straumann SLA Regular Neck PLUS, diameter 4.1 mm, length 10 mm) (Figs 15 to 17) utilizing the flapless approach.

One critical factor during placement of the dental implants was to assure their proper vertical positioning. The vacuform template highlighting the planned mucosal margins of the restorations was utilized to place the shoulders of the implants exactly 2 mm apically from a midfacial position. This relationship would allow for the establishment of a proper emergence profile of the restorations while maximizing preservation of the interimplant bone crest (Figs 18 and 19).

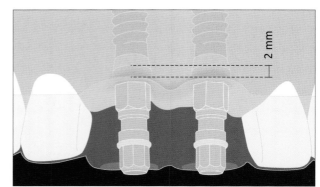

Fig 19   Graphic representation of the implant shoulder position in relation to the planned mucosal margins of the restorations.

After placing the dental implants, it was determined that they offered excellent primary stability. It was decided to fabricate and deliver immediate restorations. Solid abutments (tooth 11: 4.0 mm; tooth 21: 5.5 mm) tightened to 15 Ncm were used to anchor the restorations to the implants and allow for initial healing and shaping of the transition zone (Straumann, Andover, MA, USA) (Fig 20). The temporary restorations were fabricated intraorally utilizing the vacuform template and a bis-GMA temporary material (Integrity; Dentsply, York, PA, USA). All modifications and adjustments to the temporary restorations were performed extraorally. They were delivered with an interim cement, using a venting procedure to minimize cement entrapment (Figs 21 and 22).

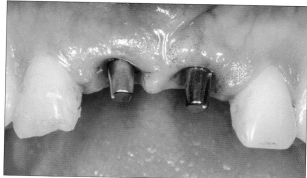

Fig 20   Solid abutments tightened to 15 Ncm.

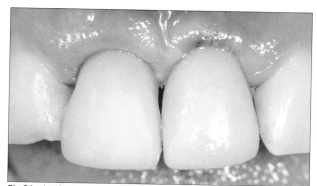

Fig 21   Implant-supported immediate temporary restorations at sites 11 and 21.

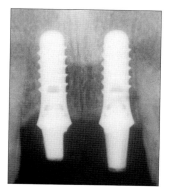

Fig 22   Periapical radiograph after implant placement.

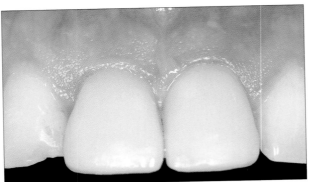

Fig 23   Temporary restorations 6 weeks after implant placement and immediate restoration.

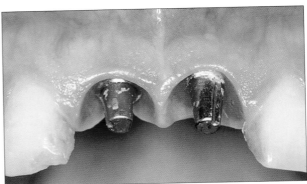

Fig 24   Transition zone prior to removing the solid abutments.

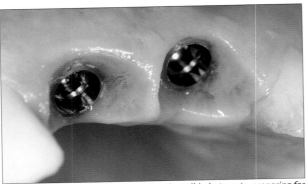

Fig 25   Transition zone after removing the solid abutments, preparing for the synOcta (Straumann, Andover, MA,USA) impression.

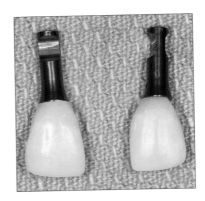

Fig 26   Temporary restorations placed onto implant analogs.

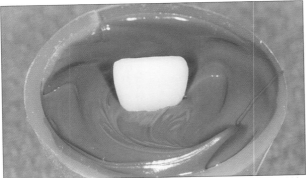

Fig 27   Temporary restoration embedded in a polyvinyl siloxane (PVS) bite registration material.

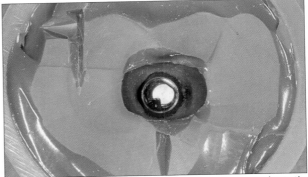

Fig 28   Transition zone transferred from the temporary restoration to the PVS material.

The third phase of treatment was devoted to the final restorations. The patient returned to the clinic for the final impression procedures 6 weeks after implant placement (Fig 23). Following removal of the temporary restorations, it was determined that the implant shoulders in the interproximal areas were more than 2 mm below the mucosal margins (Figs 24 and 25). Custom abutments would be used to bring the cement lines to a more ac-

cessible level. A customized impression of the synOcta connector (Straumann, Andover, MA, USA) was taken to transfer the transition zone of the temporary restorations to the impression copings (Figs 24 to 30). This technique will transfer the clinical contours of the soft tissue to the master cast, providing critical information to the technician so that restorations can be fabricated to support the tissue in an ideal way.

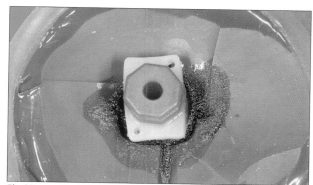

Fig 29   Modified synOcta (Straumann, Andover, MA, USA) impression coping.

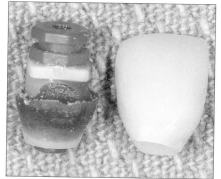

Fig 30   Example of how the contours of the temporary restoration were transferred to the impression coping.

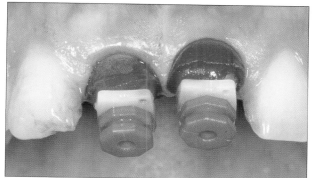

Fig 31   Customized impression copings placed on the dental implants.

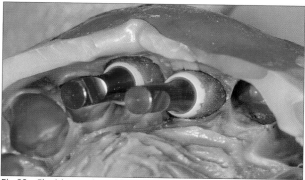

Fig 32   Final impression with synOcta (Straumann, Andover, MA, USA) analogs in place.

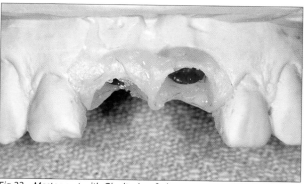

Fig 33   Master cast with Gingitech soft-tissue analog material (Ivoclar Vivadent, Buffalo, NY, USA).

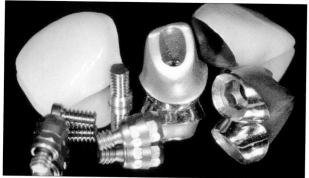

Fig 34   Definitive abutments, copings, and crowns.

A polyvinyl siloxane (PVS) impression was made of the customized impression copings on the implants (Kerr Sybron Dental, Orange, CA, USA) (Figs 31 and 32). Shade selection was performed with Vita tabs and digital photography for communication with the dental technician (Vident, Brea, CA, USA). The impression was poured in a low-expansion die stone for fabrication of the definitive abutments and restorations (Whip Mix, Louisville, KY, USA) (Fig 33).

The restorative plan for this treatment was to use 1.5-mm synOcta abutments, high-noble-alloy custom abutments, and metal-ceramic cemented restorations (Straumann, Andover, MA, USA). The customized impression procedure allowed for the technician to develop circumferential 1-mm submucosal contours in the custom abutments. This allowed for easy access to the cement line upon delivery (Figs 34 to 36).

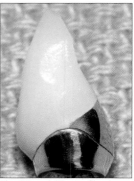 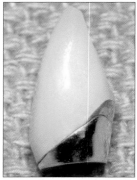 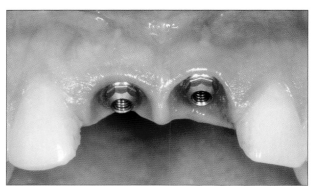

Figs 35 and 36   Profile views of the crowns on the custom abutments, highlighting the cement line.

Fig 37   Frontal view of the 1.5-mm synOcta (Straumann, Andover, MA, USA) abutments tightened to 35 Ncm.

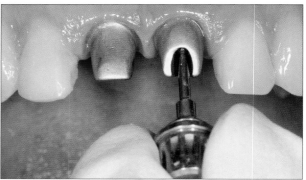 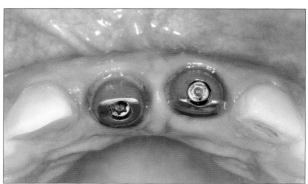

Fig 38   Frontal view of the custom abutments tightened to 20 Ncm.

Fig 39   Occlusal view of the custom abutments.

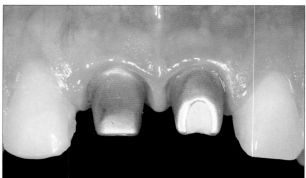 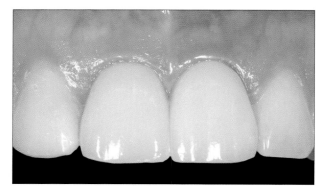

Fig 40   Frontal view of the custom abutments after sealing with cotton and Cavit (3M ESPE, St. Paul, MN, USA).

Fig 41   Frontal view of the definitive restorations.

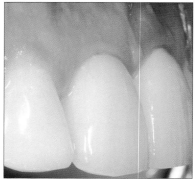 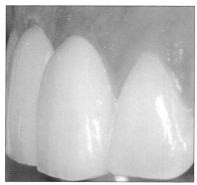

Fig 42   Right profile view.

Fig 43   Left profile view.

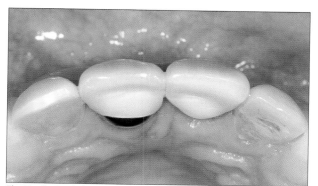

Fig 44   Occlusal view.

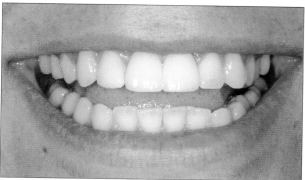

Fig 45   Smile.

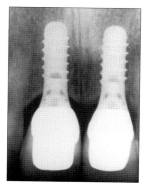

Fig 46   Periapical radiograph obtained after delivery.

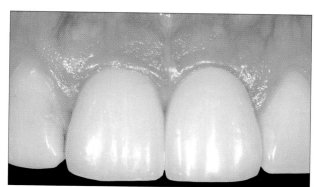

Fig 47   Frontal view at the 5-year follow-up.

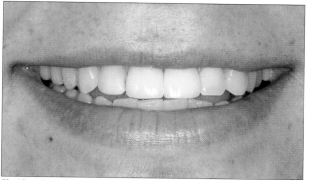

Fig 48   View of the patient's smile at the 5-year follow-up.

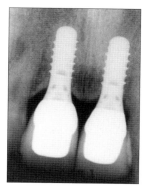

Fig 49   Periapical radiograph at the 5-year follow-up.

At the delivery appointment, all components were tried in to confirm fit, contours, and shade. Upon verification, the 1.5-mm abutments were tightened to 35 Ncm, and the custom abutments were secured with SCS occlusal screws to 20 Ncm and sealed with cotton and Cavit (3M ESPE, St. Paul, MN, USA) (Figs 37 to 40). The metal-ceramic crowns were delivered with a resin-modified cement and the occlusion verified (3M ESPE, St. Paul, MN, USA) (Figs 41 to 46). After obtaining radiographs, the patient was scheduled for a 3-week follow-up visit to reassess occlusal relations and soft-tissue conditions. Then the patient was placed on a yearly recall schedule. She continued to report complete satisfaction with the esthetic and functional outcomes of her implant-supported restorations (Figs 47 to 49).

Acknowledgments

Laboratory procedures
Dental Technician Todd Fridrich, Coralville, IA, USA

6.3   Replacement of an Upper Right Central and Lateral Incisor with an Implant-Supported Crown and a Distal Cantilever

B. Schmid, D. Buser

This 20-year-old woman was referred to our department in July 2006. Four months earlier, she had experienced dental trauma to the anterior maxilla when traveling in South America. The emergency treatment included emergency root canal treatment of teeth 12 and 11. Tooth 21 was also subjected to endodontic treatment later.

At the initial examination, the patient was not in pain but reported increased mobility of tooth 12. The clinical examination revealed a high smile line, medium thickness of the soft tissue, and rectangular tooth forms (Fig 1). Discoloration of tooth 12 was evident (Fig 2). The periapical radiograph provided by the referring dentist indicated a fracture line at both teeth 12 and 11 (Fig 3). A cone-beam computed tomography (CBCT) scan confirmed these fractures (Fig 4). No pathology was found to be associated with tooth 21.

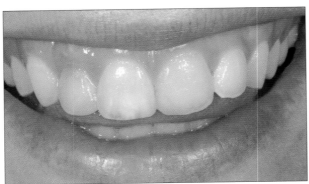

Fig 1   Labial view at the beginning of treatment.

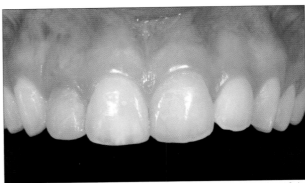

Fig 2   Labial view at the beginning of treatment, with darkening of the anterior teeth due to root canal treatment at sites 12, 11, 21.

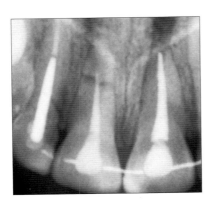

Fig 3   Apical radiograph after emergency treatment in South America. Root fractures in teeth 12 and 11.

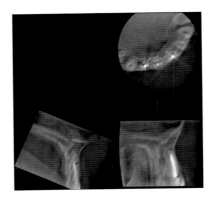

Fig 4   CBCT scan of anterior segment, demonstrating root fractures in teeth 12 and 11.

Table 1   Esthetic Risk Assessment (ERA).

Esthetic Risk Factor	Level of Risk		
	Low	**Moderate**	**High**
Medical status	Healthy, co-operative patient with an intact immune system		Reduced immune system
Smoking habit	Non-smoker	Light smoker (< 10 cigs/day)	Heavy smoker (≥ 10 cigs/day)
Patient's esthetic expectations	Low	Medium	High
Lip line	Low	Medium	High
Gingival biotype	Low-scalloped, thick	Medium-scalloped, medium thick	High-scalloped, thin
Shape of tooth crowns	Rectangular		Triangular
Infection at implant site	None	Chronic	Acute
Bone level at adjacent teeth	≤ 5 mm to contact point	5.5 to 6.5 mm to contact point	≥ 7 mm to contact point
Restorative status of neighboring teeth	Virgin		Restored
Width of edentulous span	1 tooth (≥ 7 mm)	1 tooth (< 7 mm)	2 teeth or more
Soft-tissue anatomy	Intact soft tissue		Soft-tissue defects
Bone anatomy of alveolar crest	Alveolar crest without bone deficiency	Horizontal bone deficiency	Vertical bone deficiency

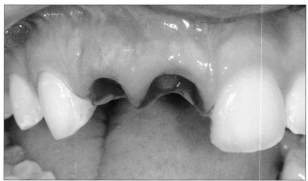

Fig 5 Clinical view immediately after extraction of teeth 12 and 11. This procedure was performed without elevating a mucoperiostal flap.

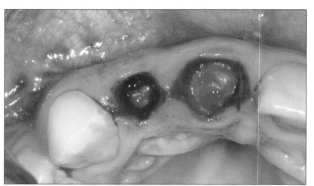

Fig 6 Occlusal view of sites 12 and 11 immediately after tooth extraction. Collagen plugs are used to stabilize the blood clot.

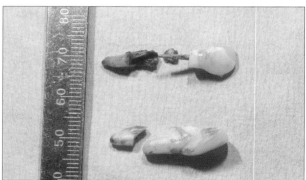

Fig 7 Detailed view of the fractured teeth 12 and 11.

Based on the clinical and radiographic findings, it was decided to extract both fractured teeth (12 and 11) while preserving tooth 21. The resultant situation of an edentulous space at the sites of the central and lateral incisor is a challenge to treat. An Esthetic Risk Assessment (ERA) revealed that 4 of the 12 examined parameters fell into the high-risk category, indicating that the clinical situation had to be regarded as complex (Table 1).

The following treatment plan was selected:

- Extraction of teeth 12 and 11.
- Application of an Essix retainer as removable partial denture.
- Eight week after extraction, placement of a single implant at site 11.
- Implant placement with simultaneous contour augmentation using guided bone regeneration (GBR).
- Augmentation both at the implant site 11 and at the edentulous site 12.
- After healing, delivery of an implant-supported temporary crown at site 11 with a cantilever unit at site 12.
- Full-coverage restoration also of tooth 21 to optimize the esthetic outcome.
- Final metal-ceramic restorations of implant 11 with a distal cantilever and of tooth 21.

Surgical treatment was performed following standard protocols that have been used at the University of Bern for more than 10 years. Teeth 11 and 12 were extracted using a flapless approach (Figs 5 to 7) to avoid unnecessary bone resorption. Following socket debridement, the patient was provided with a removable Essix retainer. Temporary restorations of this type (Fig 8) are today preferred in extended edentulous areas because they offer vertical stability and effectively protect the surgical field notably after implant surgery. Soft-tissue healing progressed without complications after the extraction procedures (Fig 9).

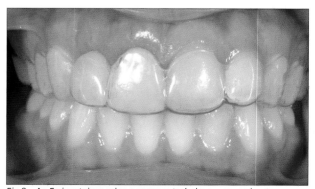

Fig 8 An Essix retainer using a vacuum technique was used as temporary restoration.

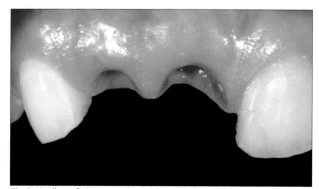

Fig 9 Healing of the extraction sockets 10 days after removing teeth 12 and 11.

Implant surgery was performed 8 weeks after extraction, in accordance with the concept of immediate implant placement (Buser and coworkers 2008). Being conducted as a live demonstration during a master course at the University of Bern, no photographs of the procedure are available. Following flap elevation, a surgical template was used for correct mesiodistal, coronoapical and oro-facial positioning of the implant at site 11 (Buser and coworkers 2004).

A tissue-level implant (Straumann Tissue Level, diameter 4.1 mm, length 12 mm) with a short machined neck was inserted. The facial bone defect present at site 11 after placement was augmented by guided bone regeneration (GBR). Contour augmentation was accomplished following a routine protocol with two bone fillers, locally harvested autologous bone chips to fill the peri-implant bone defect, and a surface layer of deproteinized bovine bone mineral (DBBM) particles (Bio-Oss; Geistlich, Wolhusen, Switzerland). The edentulous site was also augmented with DBBM particles embedded in a collagen matrix (Bio-Oss Collagen; Geistlich). The grafting material was covered with a non-crosslinked collagen membrane (Bio-Gide; Geistlich) to provide a temporary barrier during initial wound healing. Surgery was completed following a tension-free primary wound closure.

Soft-tissue healing progressed uneventfully. After 12 weeks, the surgical site presented with good soft-tissue healing and characteristic flattening of the previous papilla between the sites 11 and 12 (Fig 10). A reopening procedure had been performed at this time to replace the short (2 mm) healing cap on the implant with a longer transmucosal healing cap (Fig 11).

The restorative phase of treatment was initiated 10 days after the reopening procedure (Fig 12) by replacing the healing cap with a screw-retained synOcta impression coping, which was connected to the implant shoulder via its incorporated guide screw (Fig 13). An open-tray technique was used to take a polyether impression (Impregum Penta, 3M ESPE) for the fixed temporary restoration, which consisted in a crown for site 11 with a distal cantilever unit for site 12 and was fabricated in the laboratory using a synOcta regular neck (RN) titanium coping for temporary crowns.

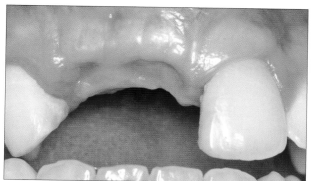

Fig 10   Labial view following implant placement and healing under the removable temporary restoration.

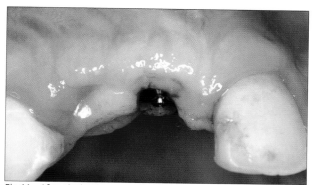

Fig 11   After gingivectomy, a cylindrical healing cap was used to ensure continued access to the implant.

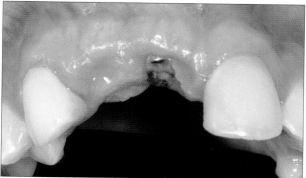

Fig 12   Labial view of the healing cap 10 days after gingivectomy.

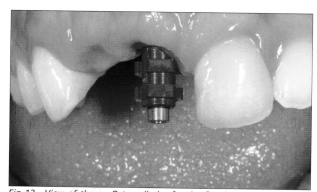

Fig 13   View of the synOcta cylinder for the first impression, using an open-tray technique.

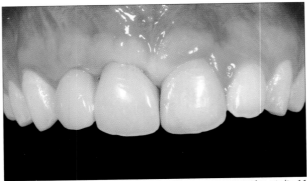

Fig 14   Implant-supported screw-retained temporary restoration at site 11 with a cantilever unit at site 12. Note the tissue blanching immediately after delivery.

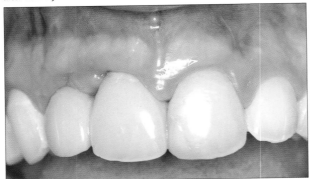

Fig 15   Temporary restoration 1 month after placement.

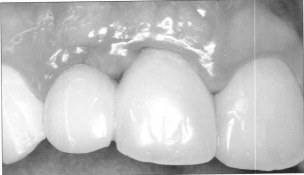

Fig 16   Close-up view of the temporary restoration. Note the scar tissue in the papillary zone between sites 12 and 11.

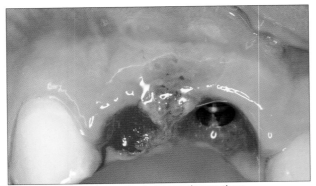

Fig 17   A CO_2 laser was used to freshen up the scar tissue.

Delivery of the temporary restoration was initially associated with soft-tissue blanching (Fig 14) due to its increased volume after adding resin material to the cervical portion. This modification was necessary to establish harmony with the emergence profile of the adjacent natural tooth 21. The temporary restoration was left in place for over 9 months.

One of the main reasons for fabricating an implant-supported temporary restoration is to create stable peri-implant soft-tissue contours. At the same time, the patient's compliance with oral hygiene requirements—which can be demanding for an implant-supported restoration with a cantilever in the esthetic zone—could be monitored and reinforced if necessary (Figs 15 and 16). In an attempt to modify the scar tissue in the papilla-like area distal to the implant-supported crown, the temporary restoration was removed and the soft-tissue surface treated with a CO_2 laser (Fig 17).

Four months after laser treatment, healthy conditions ready to accommodate the final restoration were diagnosed (Fig 18). The endodontically treated tooth 21 was prepared for a crown (Fig 19) and the temporary restoration at sites 11 and 12 removed for final impression. An open-tray technique with a screw-retained impression coping was once again selected, mainly because of the submucosal location of the implant shoulder (Figs 20 and 21).

Care was taken to proceed with the impression immediately after removing the temporary restoration to reproduce the relevant peri-implant soft-tissue contours created by the emergence contours of the temporary restoration as accurately as possible. This immediacy is clinically relevant as the peri-implant soft tissue tends to collapse rapidly toward the impression coping and, once this has occurred, no longer accurately reflects the soft-tissue contours developed by the temporary restoration. A high-accuracy polyether material was used to take the impression (Impregum Penta; 3M ESPE) (Fig 22).

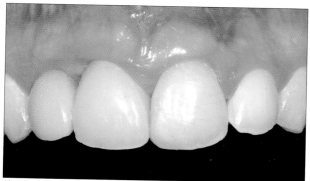

Fig 18 Temporary restoration 4 months after laser treatment of the scar tissue.

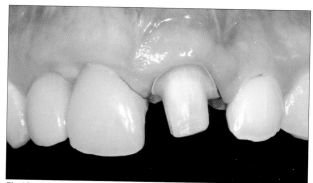

Fig 19 Preparation of tooth 21 for full-coverage restoration.

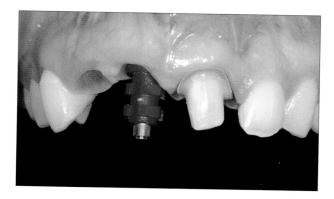

Fig 20 Given the submucosal implant shoulder, an open-tray impression was performed using a screw-retained impression coping. Care was taken to proceed with an impression taken immediately after removing the temporary restoration so as to pick up a maximum amount of the relevant peri-implant soft-tissue contour created by the axial profile of the temporary restoration.

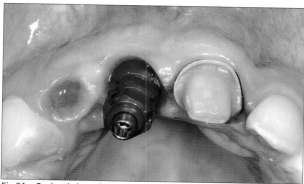

Fig 21 Occlusal view of the cantilever site 12, the screw-retained synOcta impression cylinder at the implant site 11, and the prepared tooth 21.

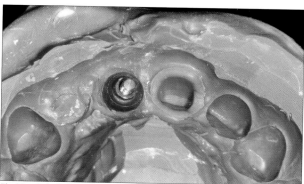

Fig 22 Apical view of the screw-retained impression coping prior to connecting the implant analog.

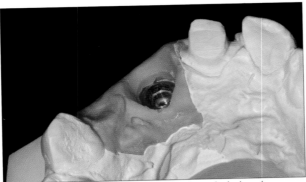

Fig 23   *Palatal view of the stone cast, including a gingival mask.*

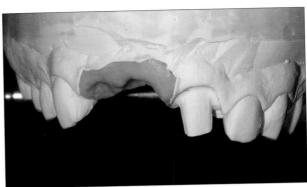

Fig 24   *Labial view of the same stone cast.*

In the laboratory, the master cast was poured with die stone (Figs 23 and 24), including the use of a synOcta implant analog, and mounted in a semi-adjustable articulator, and the definitive metal-ceramic restorations were fabricated.

Due to the scalloped profile of the mucosal margin relative to the uniform height of the implant shoulder, a restoration cemented at the level of the implant shoulder is not recommended. The often deep submucosal location of the implant shoulder, especially on its mesial and distal sides, makes it difficult to remove any residual cement.

In the present case, a screw-retained restoration could be implemented thanks to the favorable axial inclination and positioning of the implant. An RN synOcta gold abutment was used to fabricate a transocclusally screw-retained crown (Fig 25). The metal frameworks of the restorations were modeled in wax (Fig 26) and cast in a precious gold alloy (Esteticor Lumina; Cendres+Métaux) (Fig 27).

A layering technique was used by first applying opaque to the metal and then adding a veneering ceramic. Figures 28 to 30 illustrate the crown restorations ready for insertion.

The tooth-supported crown for site 21 was delivered with a glass-ionomer cement (Ketak Cem, 3M ESPE) and the implant-supported restoration for sites 11 and 12 tightened to 35 Ncm. The screw access hole was obturated by first using a small cotton pellet to protect the retention screw, followed by application of a composite material (Tetric Ceram; Ivoclar Vivadent). The final restorations integrated nicely with the surrounding natural dentition in terms of tooth shape, size, color, and surface texture. The incisal line was harmonious and contributed to the esthetically pleasing outcome (Fig 31). A periapical radiograph obtained after delivery revealed a precise fit of both the implant-supported and the tooth-supported restorations (Fig 32).

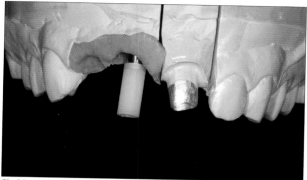

Fig 25   A synOcta gold coping was attached to the implant analog.

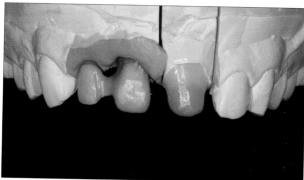

Fig 26   Labial view of the wax-up.

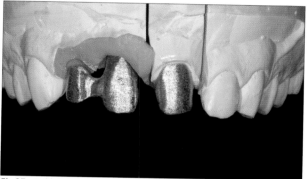

Fig 27   Labial view of the cast metal framework.

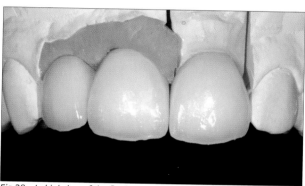

Fig 28   Labial view of the final restoration.

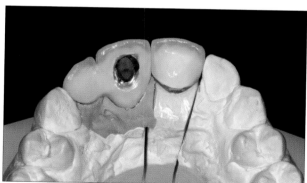

Fig 29   Palatal view of the final restoration. Note the screw access hole of the implant-supported restoration.

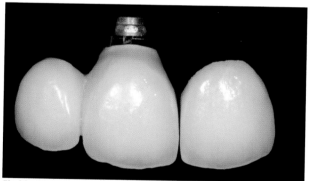

Fig 30   These are the definitive metal-ceramic restorations, including an implant-supported crown for site 11 with a cantilever unit for site 12 and a tooth-supported crown for site 21.

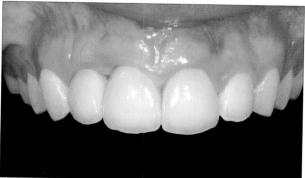

Fig 31   Final restoration in place, including an implant-supported screw-retained (35 Ncm) restoration at site 11 with a distal cantilever at site 12 and a tooth-supported cemented restoration at site 21.

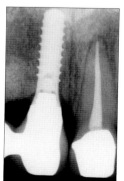

Fig 32   Periapical radiograph obtained after delivery of the final restoration.

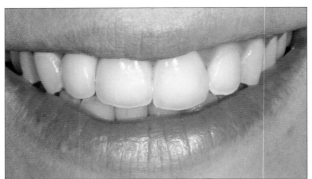

Fig 33   Perioral view of the restorations after 5 years of service.

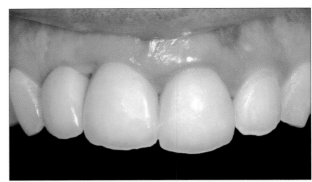

Fig 34   At the 5-year follow-up in April 2012, the soft-tissue contours were found to be stable. Ongoing growth had resulted in a slight difference between the incisal edges of the implant-supported crown at site 11 and the tooth-supported crown at site 21.

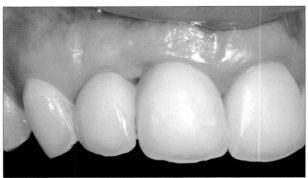

Fig 35   Labial close-up view of the restorations after 5 years of service.

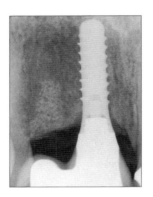

Fig 36   Periapical radiograph after 5 years of service. Note the presence of mild bone resorption around the implant. The probing depths were not increased.

At the 5-year follow-up examination, the clinical situation continued to be esthetically acceptable and included stable soft-tissue conditions (Figs 33 and 34). The peri-implant mucosa was clinically sound and showed no indications of peri-implant disease. However, a step between the incisal edges of the two central incisors was noted, most likely due to some residual growth of the anterior maxilla. The papillary soft tissue between the implant crown and its cantilever unit was roughly 1.5 mm shorter (Fig 35) than the contralateral papilla between teeth 21 and 22. The radiographic examination confirmed stable crestal bone levels around the implant with some evidence of resorption (Fig 36).

Discussion
Situations of two adjacent missing teeth in the esthetic zone still belong to the most challenging clinical situations in implant dentistry. Most of these situations are complex to treat, falling into category C of the SAC Classification (Dawson and Chen 2009).

The main problem is that two adjacent implants will bring about a reduced interproximal height of the bone crest (Tarnow and coworkers 2000; Buser and coworkers 2004). This vertical bone loss is mainly caused by resorption of bundle bone following extraction of teeth, but interimplant distance may also play a role. A minimum distance of 3 mm has been recommended between any two adjacent implants (Tarnow and coworkers 2000).

In addition, the mucosa at edentulous sites is going to flatten out following extraction of teeth. Its thickness will decrease to approximately 3 or 4 mm, which is clearly less than the thickness of a papilla located between an implant and an adjacent tooth (Kan and coworkers 2003). As a result, interimplant papillae will always end up being somewhat shorter, with the consequence of esthetic outcomes being often compromised by disharmonious soft-tissue levels (Belser and coworkers 1998).

These considerations apply to clinical situations involving two missing central incisors, one missing central and one missing lateral incisor, or one missing canine and one lateral incisor. Clinicians are generally left with three options for treatment: (a) placement of two implants to be restored with single crowns, (b) placement of one implant at the site of a central incisor to be restored with a crown and a distal cantilever, or (c) restoration with a tooth-supported prosthesis. Which treatment is preferred should depend on various anatomical parameters to be explored by a thorough preoperative work-up including an esthetic risk assessment (Martin and coworkers 2006). These parameters include the smile line, the mesiodistal size and the location of the edentulous space, the local bone volume measured in width and height, and the presence or absence of bruxism.

The preferred solution for two missing central incisors is to place two implants. Although the resultant interimplant papilla will be slightly reduced in length, the harmony of the soft-tissue margins will not be severely disturbed in most cases, as this papilla is centrally located and does not have a contralateral counterpart. It is important to achieve correct three-dimensional positioning of both implants, ensuring an adequate bone volume between them, and to respect an interimplant distance of at least 3 mm.

Clearly more demanding are edentulous spaces that, like the present case, include one lateral incisor. Here the mesiodistal dimension of the edentulous space is clearly reduced in comparison with two missing central incisors. As a result, the distance between two adjacent implants would fall short of 3 mm in numerous cases. This is why the clinical experience with two adjacent implants was often disappointing back in the 1990s, even though considerable efforts were made to optimize esthetic outcomes surgically by guided bone regeneration (GBR) (Buser and coworkers 2004).

As a consequence, our group started using only one implant in these indications about 12 years ago, and this approach has since remained the preferred approach taken in most cases. After inserting the implant in a correct three-dimensional position at the site of the central incisor (Buser and coworkers 2004), a GBR procedure is used to augment the crestal bone wall at the implant and the cantilever site (Buser and coworkers 2008). At the implant site, this is mainly accomplished by horizontal contour augmentation. At the cantilever site, additional vertical augmentation is beneficial to optimize soft-tissue support in the papilla area.

An essential requirement for contour augmentation is the use of a low-substitution bone filler like deproteinized bovine bone mineral (DBBM) (Jensen and coworkers 2006). This material is combined with locally harvested autologous bone chips to enhance the osteogenic response at the surgical site after implant placement with simultaneous GBR (Buser and coworkers 1998; Buser and coworkers 2008). The resultant soft tissue between the implant-supported crown and the cantilever, while mimicking a papilla, is usually reduced by roughly 2 mm in height. This observation holds true of the case here presented. Two implants are only placed in exceptional cases like those involving a low smile line or in distinct bruxers.

From a restorative viewpoint, the selected treatment modality offers a high degree of flexibility for treatment. To improve the esthetics of the case, the pontic area can be enhanced by connective-tissue grafting even in the phase of temporary fixed restoration. Also, dental technician has more freedom in designing tooth width and form than with single fixed restorations on two implants. The most sensitive aspect is the height of the papilla between the implant-supported crown and its cantilever, as bony support for this papilla is lacking due to the healing pattern of the crestal bone adjacent to the implant.

It remains to be seen whether this shortcoming can be addressed with novel implant designs, e.g. those that feature a horizontally offset implant-abutment interface. Based on numerous years of experience, we still regard tissue-level implants with a regular neck as the implant design of choice in these clinical situations. In patients with a low or moderately high smile line (i.e. in whom the transition between the prosthesis and the alveolar mucosa does not show), the two-unit cantilever design described in the present case would also allow for the use of pink ceramics to lengthen the papilla by prosthetic means. The same would be technically very difficult, if not impossible, with single-unit restorations in the esthetic zone.

In the case here reported, some vertical growth of the maxilla was ongoing although the patient was past 20 by the time the final restoration was delivered. At the 5-year follow-up appointment, a difference in incisal length was observed between the implant-supported restoration at site 11 and the tooth-supported restoration at site 21. This phenomenon has been described in the literature (Bernard and coworkers 2004). Occlusal patterns could not have accounted for the hypereruption of tooth 21, as the restorations at sites 12 and 11 were never in contact with the opposing dentition during maximum intercuspation or protrusion. Also, the tooth was perfectly healthy from a periodontal viewpoint.

Acknowledgments

Laboratory procedures
Master Dental Technician René Schätzle – Unterseen, Switzerland

6.4 Replacement of Two Central Incisors and One Lateral Incisor with a Fixed Dental Prosthesis on Two Bone-Level Implants

R. Jung

A 38-year-old woman presented with an esthetically unacceptable fixed partial denture replacing teeth 11, 21, 22 (Figs 1a-b). She had lost these teeth due to trauma when she was a child.

The patient was not in pain but very concerned based on her previous experience that dental treatments had never satisfied her esthetic expectations. She was in good general health and reported no regular medications.

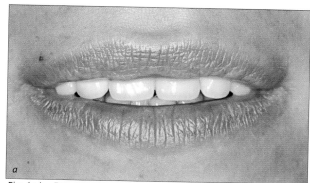

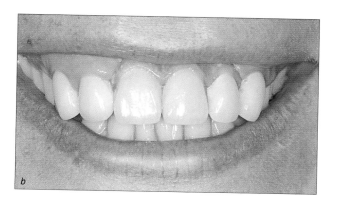

Figs 1a-b   Exposure of teeth in different lip positions.

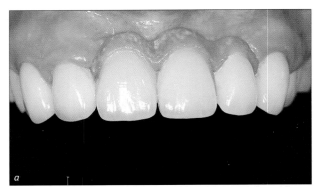

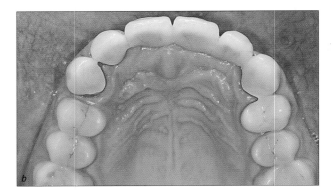

Figs 2a-b   Existing fixed partial denture with a pink ceramic buccal flange.

No periodontal disease was noted despite the fact that the buccal flange of the prosthesis impeded cleaning of the tooth abutments. The patient did not smoke and complied with home maintenance requirements, as evidenced by her good oral hygiene status.

The prosthesis was a seven-unit fixed partial denture supported by four natural abutments (teeth 13, 12, 23, 24). The patient's full smile was associated with a high lip line displaying the mucosal margins in addition to the entire crowns. The transition between the natural gingiva and the esthetically unacceptable pink ceramic material was evident (Figs 2a-b). The crowns had a rectangular shape, and the gingival biotype could be classified as moderately thick with medium scalloping of the papillae.

The preoperative periapical radiographs and orthopantomograph exhibited poorly fitting restorative margins (Figs 3a-d and 4).

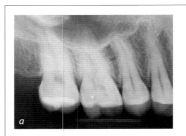 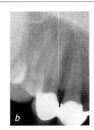 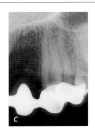 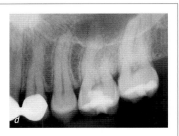

Figs 3a-d   Preoperative periapical radiographs.

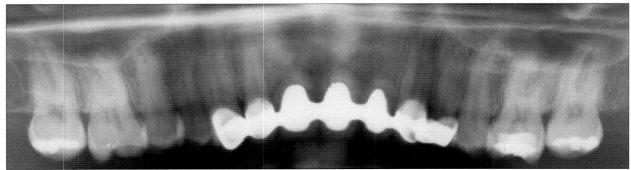

Fig 4   Sectional view of the preoperative orthopantomograph.

Case analysis, preoperative planning, and implant selection

To evaluate the condition of the abutment teeth, the fixed partial denture was removed.

While the abutments adjacent to the edentulous space only showed localized gingivitis on their mesial aspects, the distal abutments presented with extensive tooth decay (Figs 5a-b) and required root canal treatment and restoration (Figs 6a-b).

Teeth 13, 12, 23 were used as abutments for a tooth-supported fixed temporary restoration, while the residual structure of tooth 24 was restored with a temporary single crown (Figs 7a-b).

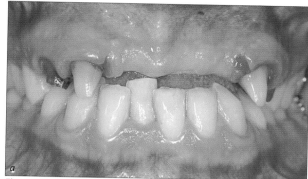

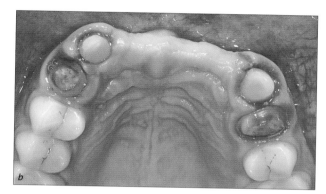

Figs 5a-b   Condition of tooth abutments following removal of the fixed partial denture.

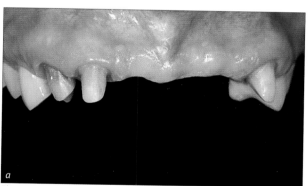

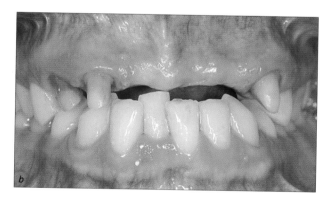

Figs 6a-b   Composite buildups of the decayed abutments.

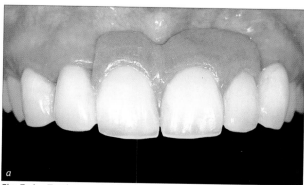

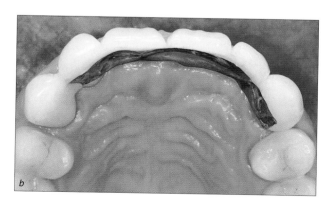

Figs 7a-b   Tooth-supported fixed temporary restoration.

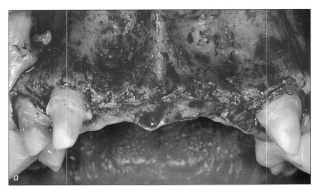

Figs 8a-b   Residual anatomy of the alveolar bone, exposed by flap elevation.

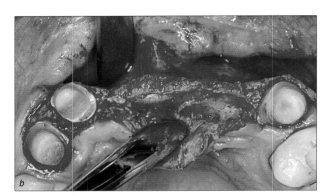

The patient exhibited class III interarch relations with dental compensation of the mandibular anterior teeth, resulting in a deep overbite that limited the restorative space available.

The edentulous area presented with a severe horizontal bone deficiency, which indicated that any placement of implants would have to be preceded by a bone augmentation procedure. The soft-tissue volume was also deficient and featured a reduced band of keratinized tissue.

A pleasing appearance of the temporary restoration demonstrated that enough mesiodistal space was available for the future restoration. Due to the existing ridge deficiency, however, the temporary restoration needed to feature a buccal flange. There were no indications of parafunction.

Based on the information collected during the clinical and radiographic examination, a surgical and restorative analysis was performed (Table 1).

The deficient bone volume and the high esthetic requirements of the patient made this a complex case. The tooth positions in the temporary restoration yielded information on the amount of tissues in need of regeneration.

Horizontal bone grafting using autologous bone blocks from the mental area was planned in a separate surgical stage prior to the implant procedure.

Surgical procedures
A triangular flap was raised to expose the surgical field, also using a single release incision distal to tooth 23 to ensure optimal access without compromising blood supply to the flap (Figs 8a-b).

The residual alveolar ridge had undergone significant (mostly horizontal) resorption.

Table 1   *SAC Complexity Classification.*

Standard SAC criteria			
Esthetic Risk Factor	**Low**	**Moderate**	**High**
Medical status	Healthy, cooperative patient with an intact immune system		Reduced immune system
Smoking habit	Non-smoker	Light smoker (< 10 cigs/day)	Heavy smoker (≥ 10 cigs/day)
Patient's esthetic expectations	Low	Medium	High
Lip line	Low	Medium	High
Gingival biotype	Low-scalloped, thick	Medium-scalloped, medium thick	High-scalloped, thin
Shape of tooth crowns	Rectangular		Triangular
Infection at implant site	None	Chronic	Acute
Bone level at adjacent teeth	≤ 5 mm to contact point	5.5 to 6.5 mm to contact point	≥ 7 mm to contact point
Restorative status of neighboring teeth	Virgin		Restored
Width of edentulous span	1 tooth (≥ 7 mm)	1 tooth (< 7 mm)	2 teeth or more
Soft-tissue anatomy	Intact soft tissue		Soft-tissue defects
Bone anatomy of alveolar crest	Alveolar crest without bone deficiency	Horizontal bone deficiency	Vertical bone deficiency

White: not assessed

Supplementary criteria			
Oral hygiene and compliance	Good	Sufficient	Insufficient
Craniofacial/skeletal growth	Completed		In Progress
Visibility of treatment area upon smiling	No		Yes
Zone selection	Posterior		Anterior
Loading protocol	Conventional	Early	Immediate
Soft-tissue contour and volume	Ideal	Slightly compromised	Significantly deficient
Intermaxillary relationship	Angle Class I and III	Angle Class II Div. 1 and 2	Severe malocclusion
Occlusion	Harmonious	Irregular	Occlusal modifications necessary
Interim restoration	Non required	Removable	Fixed
Bruxism	Absent		Present
Retention	Cemented		Screw-retained

Assessment	
Esthetic risk	High
Normative SAC classification	Complex

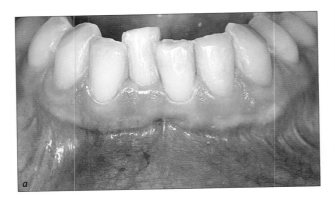
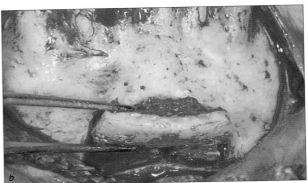
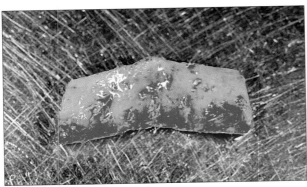
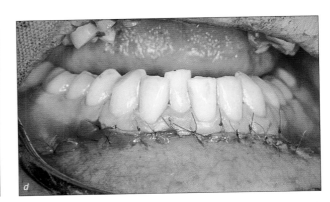

Figs 9a-d   Harvesting of bone block.

A trapezoidal flap was elevated in the mental area, including two vertical relief incisions distal to the canines, with the horizontal incision performed across the keratinized mucosa to avoid any gingival recession (Figs 9a-b).

Next, a rectangular corticocancellous bone block was harvested from the central portion of the symphysis (Fig 9c).

After obtaining hemostasis of the surgical field, primary wound closure was achieved (Fig 9d).

The primary block was divided into two smaller blocks, to be placed on the buccal concavities of the residual ridge using bone-fixation screws (Figs 10a-b).

The blocks were covered with deproteinized bovine bone mineral (DBBM) to render the grafted area homogeneous and to prevent bone resorption. The entire graft was covered with a resorbable collagen barrier membrane (Figs 11a-b).

To ensure primary wound closure without tension, periosteal release incisions were performed at the base of the flap. Two horizontal mattress sutures were created to close the wound borders and reduce tension at the incision line. Single interrupted sutures were created using a non-resorbable material to ensure a hermetic seal (Figs 12a-b).

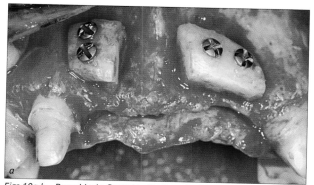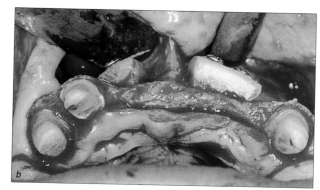

Figs 10a-b   Bone blocks fixated to the bony bed.

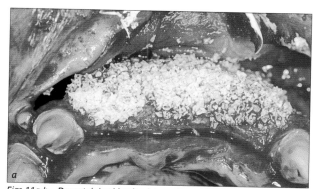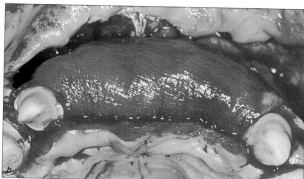

Figs 11a-b   Deproteinized bovine bone mineral (DBBM) and a collagen membrane placed over the bone blocks.

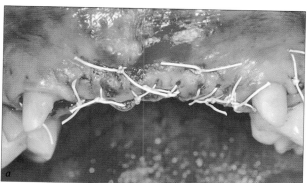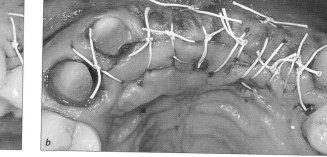

Figs 12a-b   Primary wound closure.

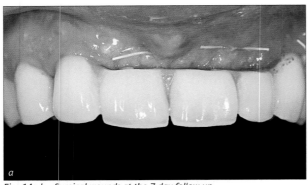

Fig 13 Postoperative view of the provisional restoration.

The provisional prosthesis was cut back to avoid any interference with the augmented tissues (Fig 13).

No wound dehiscences were seen during the postoperative appointments (Figs 14a-b).

The grafted area was allowed to heal for 5 months. By that time, the bone had sufficiently matured to receive the implants (Figs 15a-b).

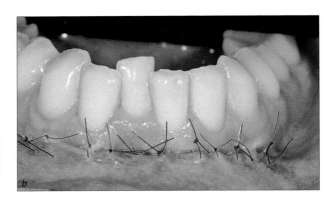

Figs 14a-b Surgical wounds at the 7-day follow-up.

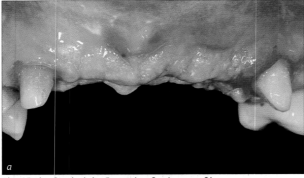

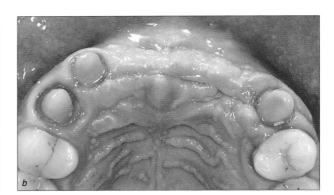

Figs 15a-b Surgical site 5 months after bone grafting.

An identical flap design was selected for the re-entry procedure. Bone regeneration had proceeded successfully and resulted in a considerable volume gain. Direct contact between the screw head and the cortical wall of the grafted block demonstrated that minor resorption of the autologous blocks had occurred (Figs 16a-b).

The four fixation screws were removed to allow placement of the implants (Fig 17).

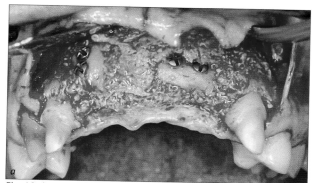

Figs 16a-b   Bone anatomy upon surgical re-entry after 5 months.

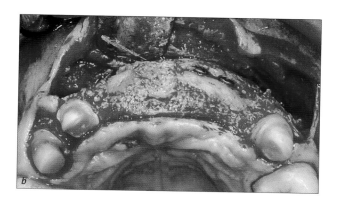

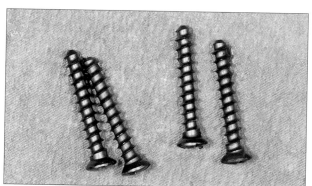

Fig 17   Fixation screws.

A surgical guide was used to facilitate ideal three-dimensional implant placement in accordance with the planned position of the future implant-supported restoration. This guide ensured correct both orofacial and coronoapical positioning of the implants (Figs 18a-d).

A thick bone wall was present around the ideally positioned implants (Figs 19a-b).

Due to the cortical nature of the autologous grafts, however, a low-substitution bone filler was additionally used for buccal overcontouring, followed by coverage with a resorbable collagen barrier membrane (Figs 20a-b).

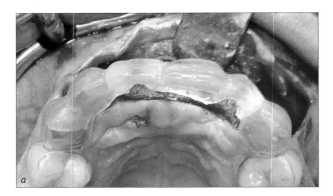
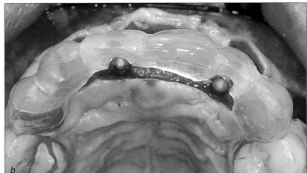
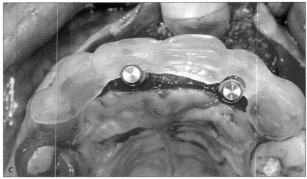
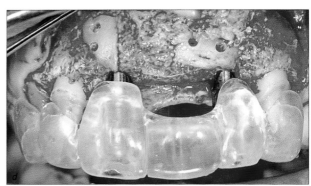

Figs 18a-d   Placement of implants using a surgical guide derived from the temporary restoration.

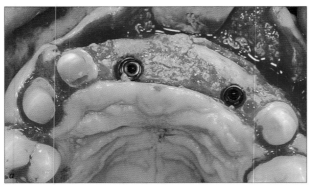
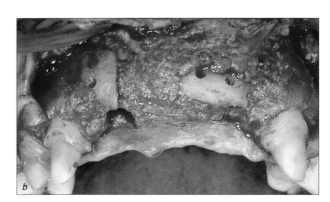

Figs 19a-b   Implants in place.

The soft-tissue wound was sealed using the same technique as described above.

Primary wound closure was achieved, and the postoperative period was uneventful (Figs 21a-b).

Eight weeks after implant placement, the soft tissue had matured under the temporary fixed restoration (Fig 22). Even though a significant horizontal gain in hard tissue was noted, soft tissue was still lacking buccal to the cervical margins of the temporary crowns (Fig 23a).

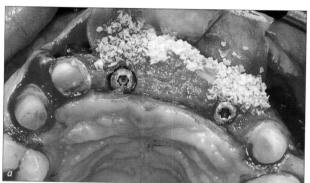 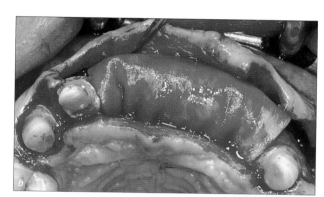

Figs 20a-b   Adjunctive bone grafting.

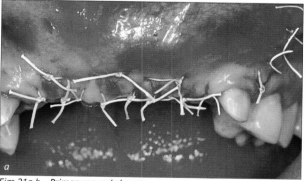 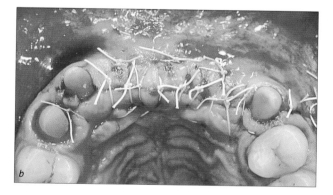

Figs 21a-b   Primary wound closure.

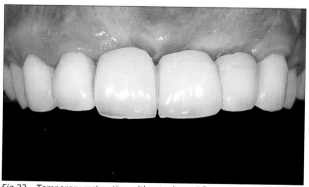

Fig 22   Temporary restoration without a buccal flange.

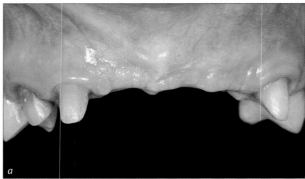
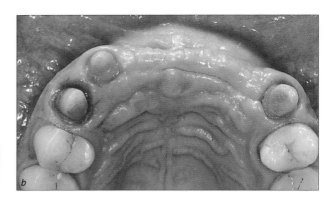

Figs 23a-b   Anatomy of the alveolar ridge following tissue maturation.

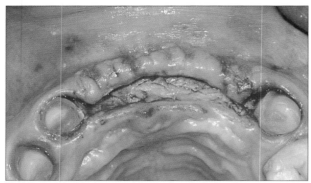

Fig 24   Recipient bed prepared for the free gingival graft.

The various coronal flap advancements performed to achieve soft-tissue closure of the graft had also reduced the depth of the vestibulum and had displaced the band of keratinized mucosa in a palatal direction (Fig 23b). A spindle-shaped, free gingival graft was planned to increase the horizontal soft-tissue volume and width of the keratinized buccal mucosa.

A partial-thickness horizontal incision was performed over the alveolar ridge connecting the distopalatal angles of the two teeth adjacent to the edentulous area, followed by a partial-thickness dissection undermining the buccal flap and extending beyond the mucogingival junction (Fig 24).

The free gingival graft was harvested from the premolar/molar region of the palate, remaining at a safe distance of 4 mm from the gingival margin. The graft had a spindle shape on an axial section and a wedge shape in the sagittal area. The wedge allowed for harvesting a considerable amount of connective tissue under the epithelial layer (Figs 25a-b).

The connective-tissue segment was slipped into the pocket created under the buccal flap. The epithelial segment was sutured to the wound margins with single interrupted 6-0 non-resorbable sutures (Figs 26a-d).

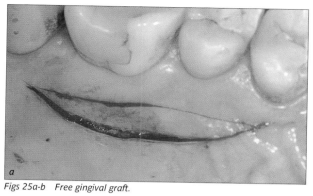
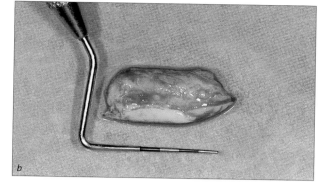

Figs 25a-b   Free gingival graft.

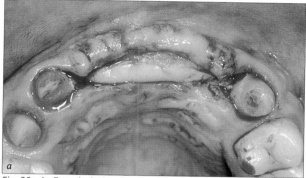
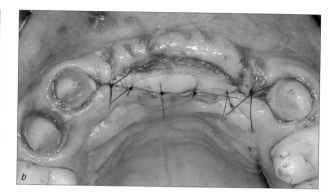

Figs 26a-d   Free gingival-graft suture technique.

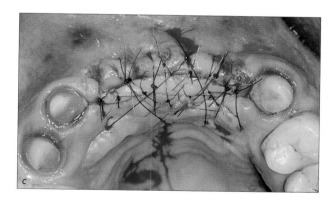
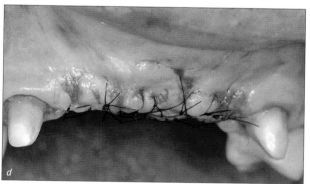

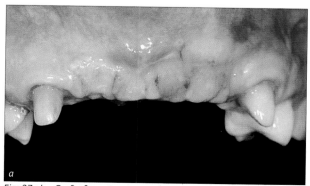
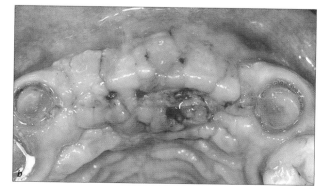

Figs 27a-b   Graft after suture removal on postoperative day 7.

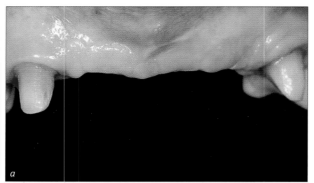

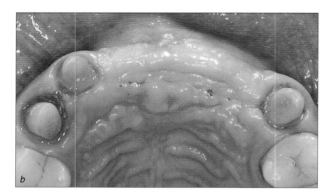

Figs 28a-b   Postoperative view 4 weeks after soft-tissue grafting.

The reason for the spindle-shaped graft design was to facilitate primary closure of the wound margin at the level of the mesial papilla of the teeth adjacent to the edentulous area. If the graft had been rectangular, the tissue excess in the papilla area would have created an unsightly depression at the host-graft connection.

At the 1-week follow-up, the sutures were removed. Good revascularization of the graft was confirmed (Figs 27a-b).

After tissue maturation, no unsightly scars or invaginations were present on the buccal and occlusal tissue surfaces. In the presence of ideal vertical and horizontal contours, the phase of tissue conditioning could be initiated (Figs 28a-b).

Second-stage surgery began with a horizontal incision to access the implant cover screws, leaving the tissues adjacent to the teeth intact. After removing the cover screws, 5-mm healing caps were inserted whose volume displaced the tissue in a buccal direction for contour enhancement. Single interrupted sutures were used to close the wound margins (Figs 29a-b).

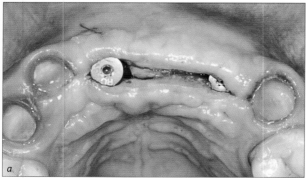

Figs 29a-b   Second-stage surgery.

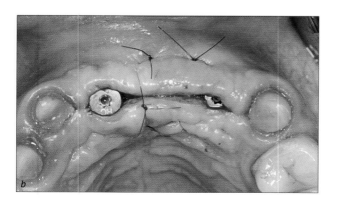

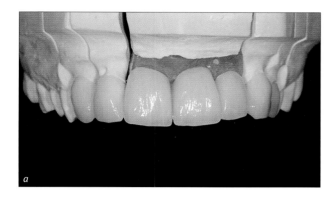

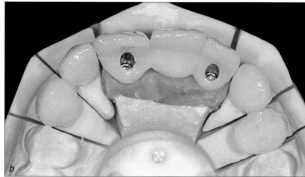

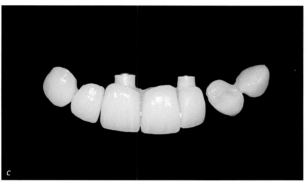

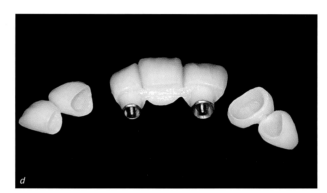

Figs 30a-d   Second set of temporary restorations.

Soft-tissue conditioning and provisionalization

Four weeks after connecting the implant abutments, an impression of the tooth and implant abutments was taken and a new set of temporary restorations fabricated.

Single-unit restorations and a screw-retained three-unit fixed partial denture were fabricated for the tooth and implant abutments, respectively (Figs 30a-d).

The transocclusally screw-retained, temporary fixed partial denture was fabricated on a titanium post for temporary restorations. Its cervical portion was kept slim on the labial surface for chairside optimization of the cervical shape. The pontic area was also conditioned chairside.

Step by step, a flowable composite material was added where the mucosa needed modeling (Fig 31).

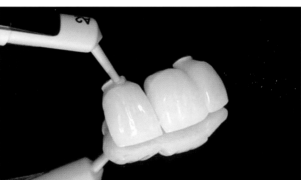

Fig 31   Chairside conditioning of temporary restoration.

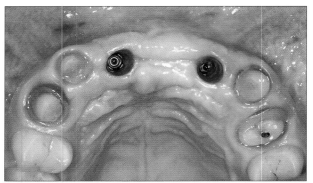

Fig 32   Soft-tissue structures prior to conditioning of the emergence profile with the temporary restorations.

The desired emergence profile was created by the cervical portion of the temporary crown exerting pressure to the mucosa.

After 2 to 4 weeks, additional soft-tissue conditioning was initiated to improve the emergence profile and marginal mucosa line. Soft-tissue maturation takes place within 3 to 6 months of second-stage surgery. During this time, changes to the peri-implant soft tissue may occur.

To avoid any tissue recessions following delivery of the definitive crown, the temporary restoration was kept in place during these 3 to 6 months.

Once this period had elapsed, the final soft-tissue shape was considered established and stable (Figs 32 and 33a-b).

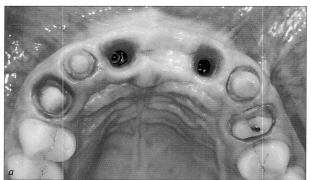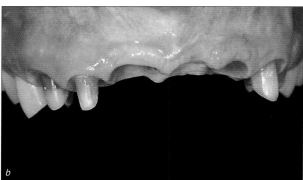

Figs 33a-b   View of the soft-tissue structures 4 months into wearing the conditioned temporary restorations.

Taking the impression for the final restorations

To capture and transfer the final tissue shape, an individual impression cap was fabricated by connecting the temporary restoration to an implant analog and pressing both into silicone (Figs 34a-b).

Once the silicone had set, the temporary restoration was unscrewed from the implant analog, with the emergence profiles remaining sculpted in the impression material just above the level of the implants (Fig 35).

After screwing two impression transfer copings to the analogs (Fig 36), the spaces created by the emergence profiles were filled with a flowable composite and polymerized (Figs 37a-b).

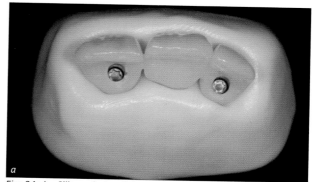

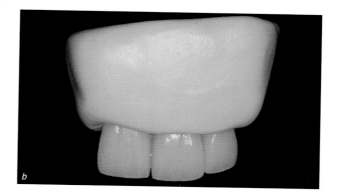

Figs 34a-b   Silicone index of the cervical area of the temporary restoration.

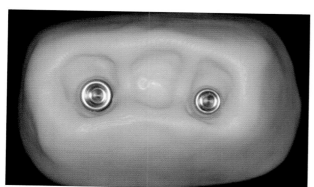

Fig 35   Silicone index with the emergence imprints.

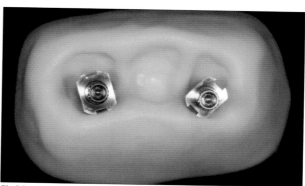

Fig 36   Impression transfer copings screwed to the implant analogs.

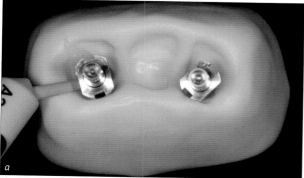

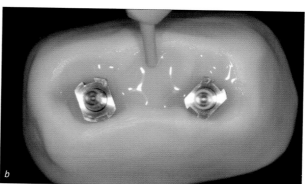

Figs 37a-b   Application of a flowable composite to fill the emergence imprints.

The contour created by the pontic was also included in the customized composite transfer, such that a three-unit complex was obtained for transfer (Fig 38).

This customized impression coping not only prevented the conditioned peri-implant mucosa from collapsing after temporary removal, but it also offered ideal support for the mucosa during impression-taking and accurately captured the emergence profile in the impression. An open-tray technique with polyether material was selected to record the tooth preparations and implant positions.

Final restoration

To diagnose the contours and proportions of the final restoration, the dental technician fabricated a wax-up (Figs 39a-b).

When the patient showed a slight smile, the incisal edges of the restoration harmoniously followed the line of the lower lip (Figs 40a-d).

Once the decision had been reached on how the final restoration should be fabricated, the laboratory technician was able to accurately design the metal framework (Figs 41a-b).

The framework was checked for accuracy of fit and passive seating.

A light-body polyether material was used to record the soft-tissue anatomy under the implant-supported restoration (Fig 42). In this way, the technician was able to adjust the cervical contour of the final restoration.

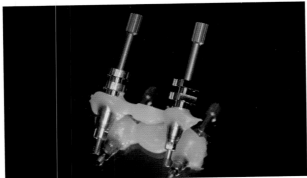

Fig 38   Customized impression transfer.

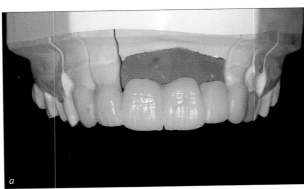
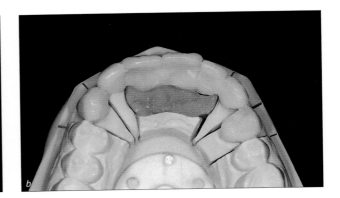

Figs 39a-b   Wax try-in of the final restoration.

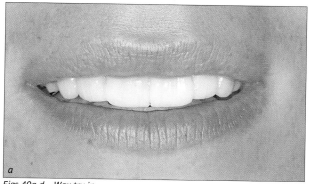
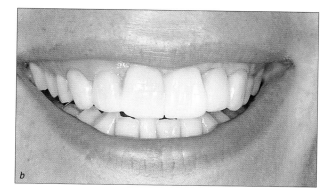

Figs 40a-d   Wax try-in.

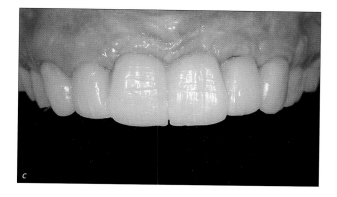
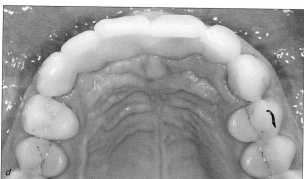

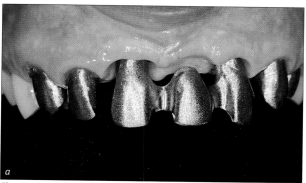

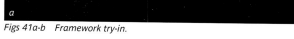
Figs 41a-b   Framework try-in.

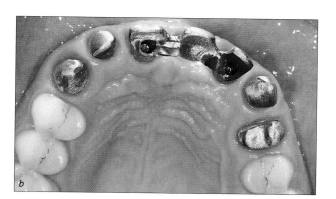

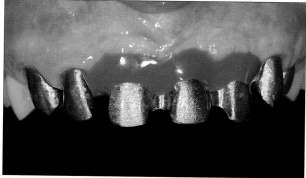

Fig 42   Polyether impression of the marginal soft-tissue anatomy.

The final crown parameters (shape, size, color, surface texture) were checked during a bake try-in (Figs 43a-b).

Slight modifications in tooth length were performed. A black permanent marker was used to "erase" the incisal surfaces of teeth 13, 22, 23. On removing the light from the chair lamp, the black markings merged with the black background of the oral cavity to change the shape of the teeth (Figs 44a-b).

Once recontouring of the incisal edges was completed and the dental technician had glassed the ceramic crowns, the restorations were ready for delivery (Figs 45a-b to 48a-d).

Metallic occlusal contacts were left on the palatal aspect of the implant-supported restoration due to the deep overbite presented by the patient.

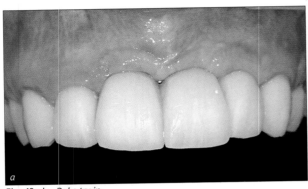
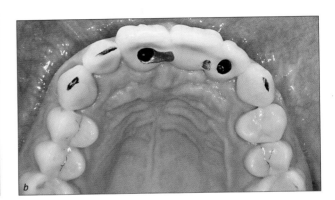

Figs 43a-b   Bake try-in.

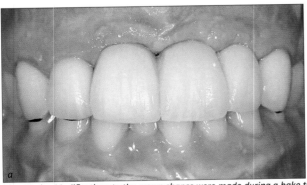
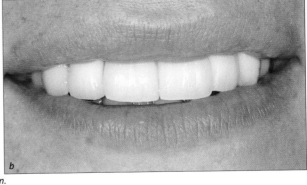

Figs 44a-b   Modifications to the crown shapes were made during a bake try-in.

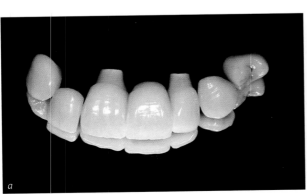
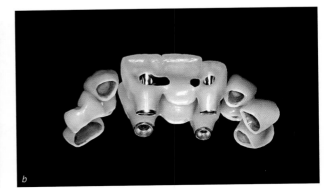

Figs 45a-b   Final restoration.

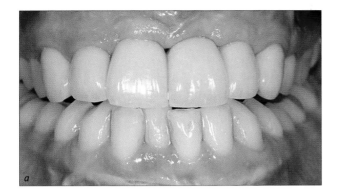
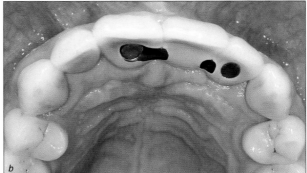
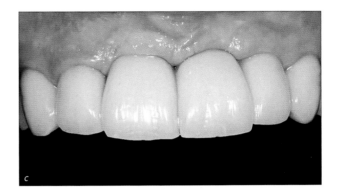

Figs 46a-c   Delivery of the final restoration.

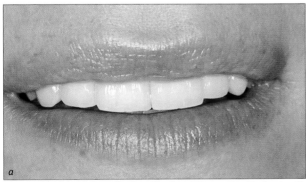

Figs 47a-b   View of the patient's smile after delivery of the final restoration.

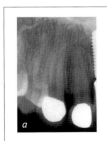
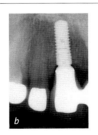
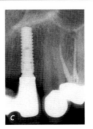
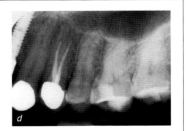

Figs 48a-d   Radiographic verification following delivery.

Post-treatment follow-up and maintenance
At the 1-year follow-up, no mechanical or biological complications were noted (Figs 49a-c and 50a-b). The patient was perfectly satisfied with the stability of her restoration. There was no evidence of tissue complications around any of the abutments, which confirms the excellent plaque control maintained by the patient and facilitated by the prosthetic design.

Excellent integration of the grafted bone blocks is also supported by the stability of the peri-implant marginal bone levels 1 year after loading (Figs 51a-d).

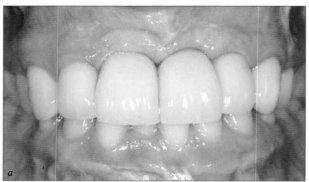

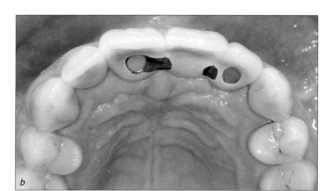

Figs 49a-c   Views of the restoration at the 1-year follow-up.

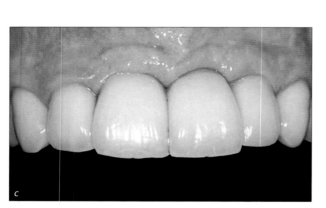

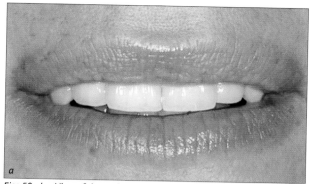

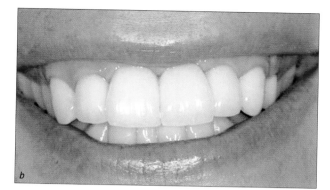

Figs 50a-b   View of the patient's smile 1 year after prosthetic delivery.

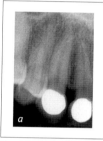
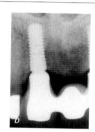
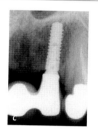
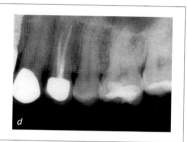

Figs 51a-d   Radiographic verification 1 year after prosthetic delivery.

Acknowledgments

The author is indebted to Dr. Manual Sancho Puchades for his support in preparing the manuscript and pictures. He also wishes to thank dental technician Walter Gebhard for excellent collaboration.

6.5   Replacement of Two Central Incisors and One Lateral Incisor with a Fixed Dental Prosthesis on Two Tissue-Level Implants

D. Buser, C. Hart

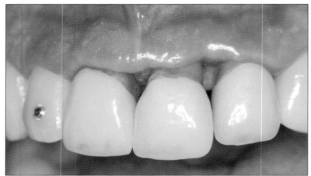

Fig 1   Initial clinical situation with three tooth-supported crowns following a major car accident more than 10 years previously. The patient's main concern was about the interproximal black triangles and the gingival recession.

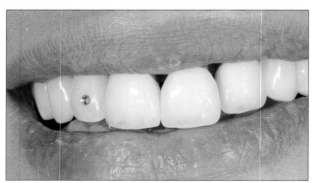

Fig 2   Due to the medium smile line, the black triangles were not covered by the lips.

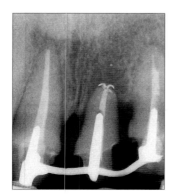

Fig 3   Periapical   radiograph demonstrating severe vertical bone loss around teeth 11 to 22.

A 29-year-old woman was referred to our department for implant therapy. At the day of examination, a detailed Esthetic Risk Assessment (ERA) was performed (Martin and coworkers 2006). The patient was in good general health, but a heavy smoker (more than 20 cigarettes per day). When her midface had been injured in a severe car accident 10 years earlier, the dentition in the anterior maxilla was also affected. The injured anterior teeth (11, 21, 22) required endodontic treatment and were restored with crowns.

Within a few years of the accident, the patient developed a considerable esthetic problem due to progressive recession of the gingiva in the area of the restored teeth. The local status demonstrated severe exposure of the root surfaces, especially of root 21, and black triangles between the three teeth (Fig 1). Thanks to her medium smile line, the patient was able to conceal the exposed root surfaces, but not the black triangles (Fig 2). A periapical radiograph was obtained and revealed extensive loss of the vertical bone height around tooth 21 (Fig 3). No periapical lesions were seen on the three teeth with root canal fillings.

Table 1 Esthetic Risk Assessment (ERA)

Esthetic Risk Factor	Low	Moderate	High
Medical status	Healthy, co-operative patient with an intact immune system		Reduced immune system
Smoking habit	Non-smoker	Light smoker (< 10 cigs/day)	Heavy smoker (≥ 10 cigs/day)
Patient's esthetic expectations	Low	Medium	High
Lip line	Low	Medium	High
Gingival biotype	Low-scalloped, thick	Medium-scalloped, medium thick	High-scalloped, thin
Shape of tooth crowns	Rectangular		Triangular
Infection at implant site	None	Chronic	Acute
Bone level at adjacent teeth	≤ 5 mm to contact point	5.5 to 6.5 mm to contact point	≥ 7 mm to contact point
Restorative status of neighboring teeth	Virgin		Restored
Width of edentulous span	1 tooth (≥ 7 mm)	1 tooth (< 7 mm)	2 teeth or more
Soft-tissue anatomy	Intact soft tissue		Soft-tissue defects
Bone anatomy of alveolar crest	Alveolar crest without bone deficiency	Horizontal bone deficiency	Vertical bone deficiency

Clearly, the three teeth had to be removed, which was going to create an extended edentulous space. Based on the ERA summary of clinical parameters, the case was classified as complex, with 7 of the 12 examined parameters falling into the high-risk category (Table 1).

After thoroughly discussing the situation with the patient, an agreement was reached to pursue the following treatment plan:

- Cutting nicotine use below 10 cigarettes per day
- Forced orthodontic eruption of teeth 11 to 22 to minimize the vertical tissue deficiency
- After 3 months of retention, extraction of teeth 11 to 22 and temporary insertion of a removable partial denture
- After 8 weeks of healing, early implant placement with simultaneous contour augmentation using guided bone regeneration (GBR)
- Following surgical re-entry, initiation of soft-tissue conditioning using an implant-supported temporary fixed partial denture
- Final restoration with a three-unit metal-ceramic prosthesis 4 to 6 months later.

This surgical protocol was in accordance with the concept of "early implant placement with soft-tissue healing." After obtaining the patient's informed consent, treatment was initiated by orthodontic treatment for forced eruption, which resulted in correction of the vertical tissue deficiency 3 months later (Fig 4). Following a retention phase of roughly 3 months, the three teeth were extract-ed without elevating a flap (Fig 5). Debridement of the extraction sockets was followed by insertion of collagen plugs to stabilize the blood clot, and the patient was provided with a removable partial denture (Fig 6). The extraction sites were allowed to heal for an increased width of keratinized mucosa (Figs 7 and 8).

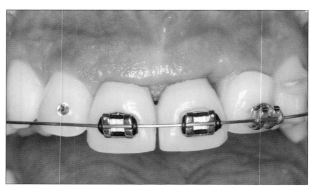

Fig 4   A course of orthodontic treatment for forced eruption of the three teeth (11, 21, 22) was applied to improve the soft-tissue situation in this area.

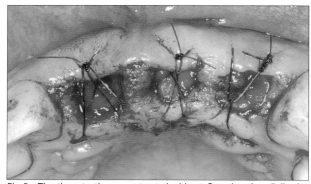

Fig 5   The three teeth were extracted without flap elevation. Following debridement, collagen plugs were inserted to stabilize the blood clot and sutures applied to keep the collagen plugs in place.

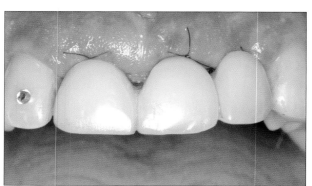

Fig 6   Clinical situation after flapless tooth extraction and delivery of a removable partial denture.

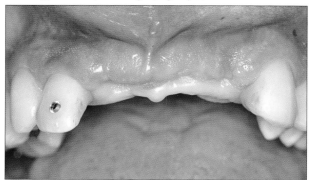

Fig 7   Clinical situation of the healed sites 8 weeks after extracting the teeth. The plan was to conduct the implant procedure with simultaneous contour augmentation, utilizing the concept of early implant placement.

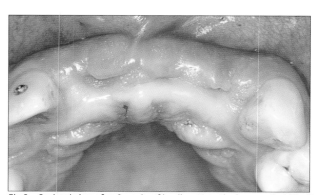

Fig 8   Occlusal view after 8 weeks of healing. Note the increased width of keratinized mucosa in the edentulous area.

After 8 weeks of healing, implant surgery was performed under local anesthesia, combined with sedative premedication and perioperative antibiotic prophylaxis (Augmentin 2 g orally 1 hour prior to surgery). The procedure was initiated with a trapezoidal flap design, using a midcrestal incision in the edentulous area and two vertical releasing incisions at the distal line angles of teeth 12 and 23. After elevation of a full-thickness flap, the full extent of the local bone defect became apparent in the edentulous area (Fig 9). The bone defect was most significant at the future pontic site 21 (Fig 10). Luckily, the vertical dimension of the palatal bone wall was adequate.

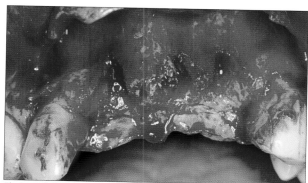

Fig 9   A full-thickness flap was raised to expose the edentulous area. As usual, the extraction sockets were still visible 8 weeks after removal of the teeth. Note the bone defect at the future pontic site 21.

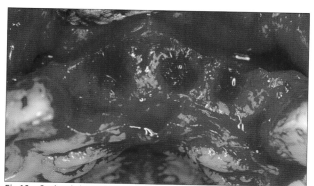

Fig 10   Occlusal view confirming a crest width adequate for implant placement at sites 11 and 22. Again, the most significant bone defect can be seen at the site of the future pontic.

Following debridement, the two implants were inserted in correct three-dimensional positions at sites 11 and 22 with the help of a translucent surgical stent (Fig 11). Care was taken to position each implant shoulder or platform within the mesiodistal, orofacial, and corono-apical "comfort zones" (Buser and coworkers 2004). In the coronoapical direction, the implant shoulders were positioned roughly 2 mm apical to the future mucosal margins, using the outline of the surgical stent as reference (Fig 12). Tissue-level implants were utilized in this specific patient. A TE implant with a Regular Neck (RN) configuration was inserted at site 11, whereas a Narrow Neck (NN) implant was used at site 22 (Straumann AG, Basel, Switzerland).

As expected, both implants exhibited good primary stability and were associated with medium-sized, crater-like dehiscence defects in the crestal area (Fig 13). Both bone defects had a two-wall morphology, with the exposed implant surfaces located inside the alveolar crest, which is favorable for a highly predictable outcome of the regeneration.

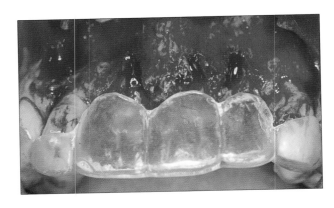

Fig 11   At extended edentulous sites with multiple missing teeth, a translucent surgical stent is mandatory for correct three-dimensional implant placement. This stent includes the outline of the future crowns and the incisal edge, thereby allowing the surgeon to select a correct implant axis.

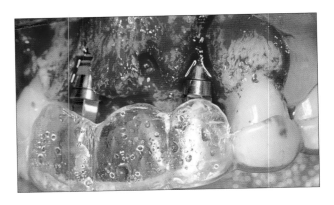

Fig 12   Correct positioning of the implant shoulder (or platform) in the coronoapical direction is paramount. For tissue-level implants, a distance of 2 mm apical to the future mucosal margin is normally selected. In addition, the platform is placed in a slightly palatal position of the alveolar crest, approximately 1.0–1.5 mm palatal to the future point of emergence.

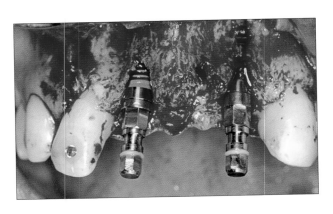

Fig 13   Status after correct three-dimensional positioning of both implants. As expected, both implants presented a crater-like defect in the crestal area. Two-wall defects were present, with the exposed implant surfaces located inside the alveolar crest. The most significant vertical defect was noted at the pontic site, requiring both horizontal and vertical contour augmentation.

The next step was to harvest autologous bone chips from the same surgical site, using a flat chisel on the nasal spine and a bone scraper on the perinasal facial bone surface (HuFriedy, Chicago, IL, USA). These bone chips were applied onto the exposed surfaces of both implants (Fig 14). An additional bone filler was used as a second, superficial layer for local contour augmentation. Since 1998, deproteinized bovine bone mineral (Bio-Oss; Geistlich, Wolhusen, Switzerland) has been the preferred material for contour augmentation at our department. Given its low substitution rate, this filler is important for long-term maintenance of the bone volume created. Bio-Oss particles embedded in a collagen matrix (Bio-Oss Collagen; Geistlich) were used at the pontic site 21 because of the enhanced mechanical stability it offers following application (Fig 15) and in the initial phase of wound healing.

The graft was covered with a non-crosslinked porcine-derived resorbable collagen membrane (Bio-Gide; Geistlich) as a temporary barrier (Fig 16) during initial bone healing in accordance with the principle of guided bone

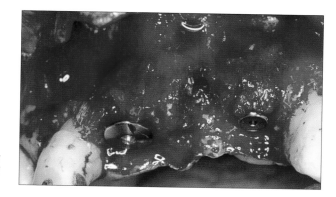

Fig 14   Contour augmentation was initiated by applying locally harvested autologous bone chips to the exposed implant surfaces to stimulate rapid new bone formation in the defect areas.

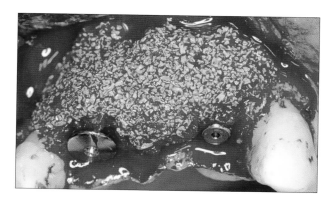

Fig 15   Contour augmentation is completed with a second layer of deproteinized bovine bone mineral (DBBM) particles as a low-substitution bone filler. In the pontic area, collagen-embedded DBBM is used, since this bone filler offers better mechanical stability in the initial phase of wound healing.

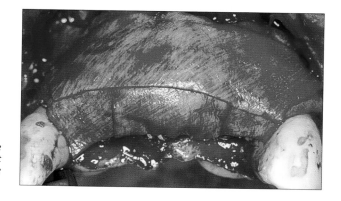

Fig 16   Using the GBR principle, the graft was covered with a resorbable collagen membrane as temporary barrier – a user-friendly material that carries a low risk of complications in the event of a postsurgical soft-tissue dehiscence.

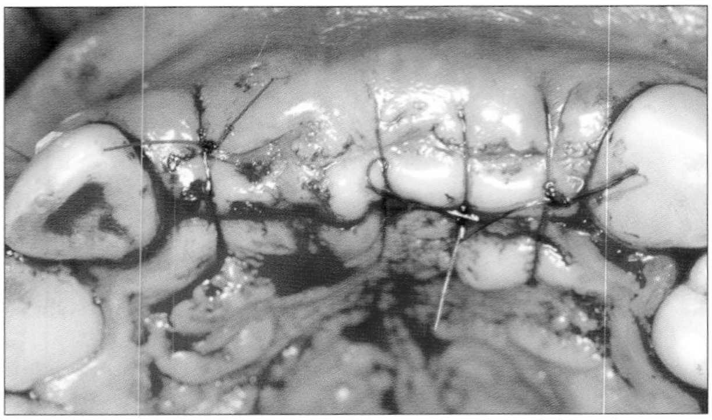

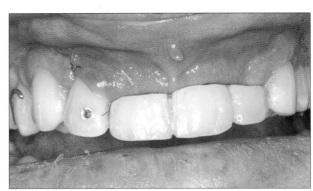

Fig 17   *Following extensive relief of the mucoperiosteal flap, the surgery was completed by tension-free primary wound closure using interrupted single sutures. In the crestal area, 4-0 sutures were used for 2 weeks of healing.*

Fig 18   *After surgery, the existing removable partial denture was reduced in length in the edentulous area to avoid direct contact with the wound surface.*

regeneration (GBR). Surgery was completed by primary wound closure to allow submerged healing of the applied biomaterials (Fig 17). Extended periosteal relief was needed to achieve tension-free adaptation of the wound margins. After surgery, the existing removable partial denture was reduced in the edentulous area to avoid direct contact with the wound surface (Fig 18).

Both implants were exposed following an uneventful healing period of 8 weeks (Fig 19), using a minor punch technique without flap elevation to minimize morbidity in the surgical area (Fig 20). Within 1 week, a temporary

fixed partial denture with titanium copings and acrylic (Fig 21) was inserted to initiate the phase of soft-tissue conditioning (Fig 22). After good adaptation of the peri-implant soft tissue was seen within a few weeks, the esthetic outcome was quite pleasing (Fig 23). The periapical radiograph obtained at the same time confirmed stable levels of the bone crest following the typical phase of remodeling (Fig 24). The contour enhancement achieved in the pontic area was quite significant. The final restoration with a metal-ceramic fixed partial denture was inserted and treatment completed (Figs 25 to 27).

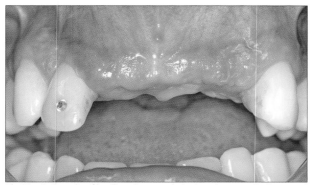

Fig 19   *At 8 weeks of healing, the extended edentulous area had matured well and uneventfully.*

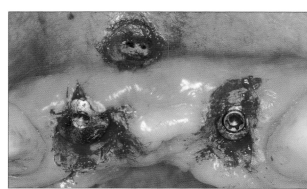

Fig 20   *A reopening procedure using a punch technique was performed to establish access to both implants. The healing caps were replaced, and the prominent frenulum was cut using a CO_2 laser.*

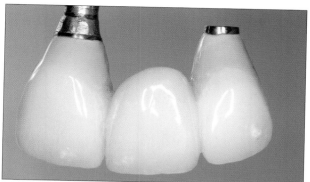

Fig 21 Three-unit temporary prosthesis for soft-tissue conditioning. Temporary restorations of this type always have a screw-retained design.

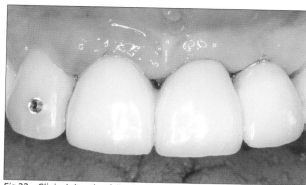

Fig 22 Clinical situation following insertion of the temporary prosthesis to initiate the essential phase of soft-tissue conditioning.

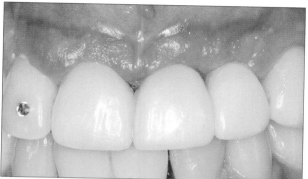

Fig 23 Within a few weeks, good adaptation of the soft tissue to the outline of the temporary prosthesis was noted.

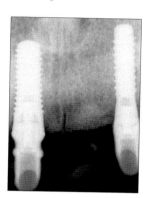

Fig 24 Periapical radiograph showing good integration of both implants. Note the excellent bone level with radiopaque particles of deproteinized bovine bone mineral (DBBM) at the pontic site.

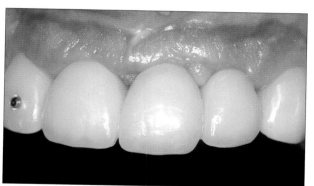

Fig 25 Clinical situation with the definitive metal-ceramic fixed partial denture. Both the three-unit restoration and the course of the soft-tissue margin are harmonious and esthetically acceptable.

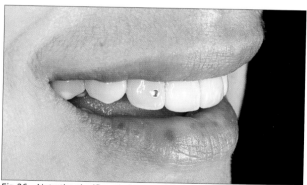

Fig 26 Note the significantly improved facial esthetics compared to the initial situation.

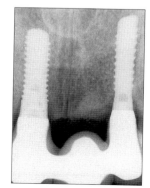

Fig 27 Periapical radiograph obtained at the same time, demonstrating stable levels of the crestal bone.

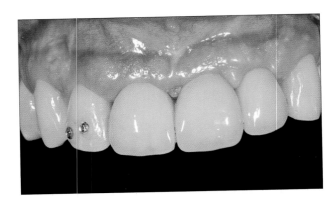

Fig 28 Intraoral view at the 5-year follow-up, confirming stability of the peri-implant soft tissue. Also note the stable outcome of contour augmentation with good convexity of the alveolar crest at the implants and the pontic site.

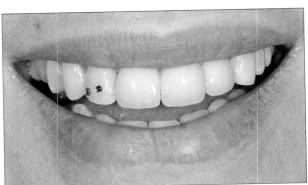

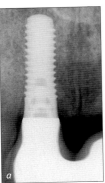 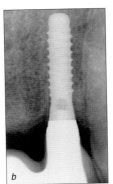

Fig 29 Perioral view of the patient's smile at the 5-year follow-up. A pleasing esthetic outcome had been achieved.

Figs 30a-b This radiograph, obtained after 5 years, confirms good stability of the crestal bone levels at both implant sites and the pontic site.

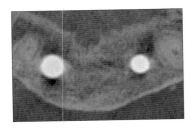

Fig 31 Horizontal section of three-dimensional CBCT scan, demonstrating an excellent bone volume in the grafted area at the 5-year follow-up.

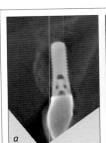 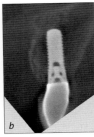 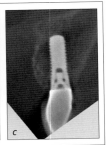

Figs 32a-c Orofacial sections of the CBCT scan, confirming good thickness of the facial bone wall at both implants and at the pontic site at the 5-year follow-up.

At the 5-year follow-up, the clinical situation was characterized by pleasing esthetics and good stability of the peri-implant soft tissues (Figs 28 and 29). The radiographic examination confirmed that the peri-implant crestal bone levels were stable and without indications of bone resorption (Figs 30a-b). The cone-beam computed tomography (CBCT) scan demonstrated an excellent dimensional stability overall on the facial aspects of both implants and at the pontic sites (Figs 31 and 32a-c).

Discussion

Treatment of the present case resulted in a pleasing esthetic outcome even though the initial clinical situation had been highly demanding. The Esthetic Risk Assessment (ERA) described previously by Martin and coworkers (2006) revealed a high risk for 7 of the 12 parameters examined. The most significant problem was a vertical bone and soft-tissue defect around tooth 21, which was a long-term complication of a car accident that the patient had experience around 10 years previously. The risk situation was greatly compounded by the patient's smoking habit of more than 20 cigarettes per day. Being unwilling to quit, she finally agreed to cut her nicotine use to approximately five cigarettes per a day (two packs a week).

Extracting only one tooth (the left central incisor) was not an option because an implant-supported single crown would clearly have compromised the esthetics of the outcome, given two short papillae proximal to the implant-supported crown following vertical bone loss at both adjacent roots. Extracting two teeth (21 and 22) was not an option either, since edentulous spaces with two adjacent teeth missing remain the most difficult clinical indication for implant therapy, particularly if one site was previously occupied by a lateral incisor. The most appropriate treatment plan in this patient included extraction of all three teeth. Edentulous spaces extending over three missing teeth are today routinely managed by placing only two implants, thereby avoiding the risks of inserting adjacent implants in the esthetic zone. Horizontal and vertical contour augmentation at the pontic site offers an opportunity to optimize the esthetic outcome with this approach.

In the present case, an attempt was made to reduce the soft-tissue defect by forced eruption using orthodontic therapy before performing the extractions. This treatment strategy dates back to the 1990s, when it was first recommended to address vertical bone defects on teeth to be extracted with the objective of regaining vertical bone volume at future implant sites (Salama and Salama 1993). Today it must be questioned if the time and cost going into this pretreatment strategy was justified, considering that bone grafting was still required during implant placement.

The teeth were extracted without elevating a flap, minimizing morbidity to the patient and postsurgical bone resorption. Any bone resorption following this extraction technique will largely remain confined to the bundle bone of the extraction sockets during soft-tissue healing (Araújo and coworkers 2005). A period of 4 to 8 weeks is respected to achieve soft-tissue healing and an increased width of keratinized mucosa at future implant sites. As the local crest width will not be reduced within this short healing period, the implants can be placed with simultaneous guided bone regeneration (GBR). Two ITI Consensus Conferences in 2003 and 2008 have established the terminology for this approach as "early implant placement with soft-tissue healing" (Hämmerle and coworkers 2004; Chen and coworkers 2009c). Furthermore, the approach has been described in a methodology paper and in a textbook (Buser and coworkers 2008; Buser and Chen 2009).

After correct three-dimensional placement of the implants at sites 11 and 22, a GBR technique was performed for contour augmentation in the same session. Ever since 1998, we have preferred bioabsorbable non-crosslinked collagen membranes (Bio-Gide; Geistlich, Wolhusen, Switzerland) for GBR procedures in our clinic, since these are easy to handle and do not require a second open flap surgery for removal. Also, they minimize the risk of complications in the event of a soft-tissue dehiscence after guided bone regeneration (GBR) (von Arx and Buser 2006). These collagen membranes are routinely combined with autologous bone chips and with deproteinized bovine bone mineral (DBBM) particles, which offer synergistic properties for optimized regenerative outcomes with the GBR technique. Autologous bone grafts are used to accelerate new bone formation not only for rapid osseointegration at the implant surface but also for ingrowth into the surface layer of bone substitutes to result in DBBM particles embedded in bone. Superiority of autologous bone chips to bone substitutes has been confirmed in several histomorphometric experimental studies (Buser and coworkers 1998; Jensen and coworkers 2006; Jensen and coworkers 2007; Jensen and coworkers 2009). It is believed that the osteogenic properties of autologous bone chips are due to non-collagenous proteins and growth factors being entrapped in bone matrix (Bosshardt and Schenk 2009). It has also been hypothesized that entrapped osteocytes might have a positive impact on osteogenic cells (Bonewald 2011). Recent in-vitro studies using osteoblast cell cultures have demonstrated that the harvesting technique also influences the osteogenic potential of autologous chips (Miron and coworkers 2011; Miron and coworkers 2012). Of four harvesting techniques tested, the use of a bone mill or bone scraper clearly yielded the most favorable bone grafts in terms of osteogenic potential.

Deproteinized bovine bone mineral (DBBM) particles are routinely used as a secondary bone filler to cover the applied layer of autologous bone chips, enhancing the contour of the alveolar crest around dental implants. This technique of "contour augmentation" is intended to optimize esthetic outcomes around dental implants (Buser and coworkers 2008; Buser and Chen 2009). It can also be applied, as in the present case, both horizontally and vertically in pontic areas of implant-supported prostheses. Although the low substitution rate of DBBM particles has been demonstrated in several preclinical studies (Jensen and coworkers 1996, 2006, 2007, 2009), evidence has since been growing that only DBBM particles embedded in bone will offer this property. A recent preclinical study has demonstrated that, in fibrous tissue, these fillers exhibit severe resorption (Busenlechner and coworkers 2012). The cellular mechanism of this resorption is currently not understood and requires further investigation. These findings emphasize the importance of the first layer of autologous bone grafts to stimulate ingrowth of bone into the surface layer of DBBM particles.

The cone-beam computed tomography (CBCT) scan obtained at the 5-years follow-up demonstrated that a very favorable graft volume had been attained in the present patient. This finding is consistent with stable and favorable esthetic outcomes in a prospective case series study of single-tooth replacements following early implant placement with simultaneous GBR for contour augmentation (Buser and coworkers 2009; Buser and coworkers 2011). However, clinical long-term studies of contour augmentation with 5 to 10 years of follow-up are needed to better document the long-term stability of this grafting technique.

6.6 Replacement of Four Incisors with a Fixed Dental Prosthesis on Two Bone-Level Implants

H. Katsuyama, M. Hojo, M. Ogawa

In November 2007, a 52-year-old woman presented with a failing restoration of the anterior maxilla in the form of a four-unit metal-ceramic fixed partial denture (Fig 1). As secondary caries had led to fracture of the abutment teeth bilaterally, the existing restoration could not be preserved. The patient was in good systemic health, and her medical history was without significant findings. Nor did the ensuing intra- and extraoral examination yield any significant findings. The patient had both a high lip line and high esthetic expectations (Fig 2). The pre-extraction findings suggested that no hard-tissue augmentation would be required before implant placement (Figs 3 to 5). After discussing the higher risk of immediate placement with the patient, she agreed to undergo "early implant placement after soft-tissue healing" simultaneously with guided bone regeneration (GBR) for hard-tissue augmentation.

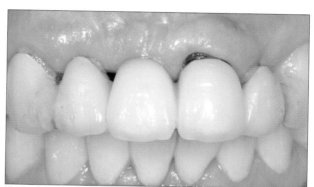

Fig 1   Buccal view of the failing metal-ceramic prosthesis. The prosthesis was mobile and had been temporarily bonded to the adjacent teeth.

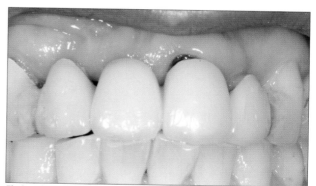

Fig 2   Close-up view of the high lip line.

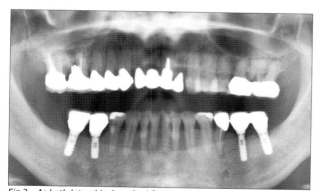

Fig 3   As both lateral incisors had fractured, the metal-ceramic prosthesis was supported by the left central incisor only.

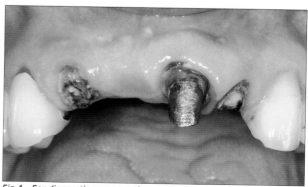

Fig 4   For diagnostic purposes, the prosthesis was removed prior to finalizing the treatment plan. Both lateral incisors were horizontally fractured and revealed decay. The surrounding tissues seemed reasonably healthy.

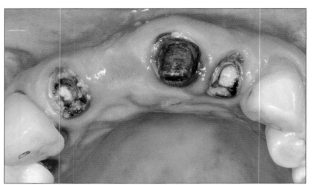

Fig 5   The right central incisor had been extracted more than 10 years previously. Slight resorption at was noted on the labial aspect of the site.

To optimize the chance for an esthetic treatment outcome, a protocol of early implant placement following tooth extraction and completion of soft-tissue healing was selected (Figs 6 to 8). Tissue resorption after tooth extraction was moderate both horizontally and vertically, being ideal for implant placement. After various treatment options had been discussed with the patient, she expressed her preference for an implant-supported fixed restoration. The final treatment plan was to extract the two lateral incisors and place the implants there, using the concept of early placement. The central incisor was to be extracted also but, for the time being, was preserved to serve as an abutment for the temporary fixed restoration. After the phase of provisionalization, delivery of an implant-supported four-unit fixed partial denture was planned (Fig 9).

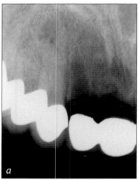
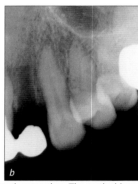

Figs 6a-b   Periapical radiograph after tooth extraction. The vertical bone height was adequate for implant placement.

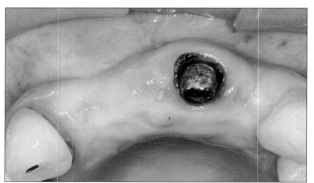

Fig 7   Situation 8 weeks after tooth extraction. Note the excellent healing progress, including an adequate amount of keratinized mucosa.

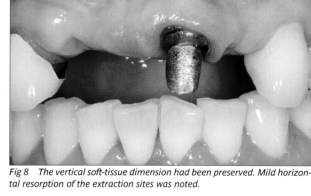

Fig 8   The vertical soft-tissue dimension had been preserved. Mild horizontal resorption of the extraction sites was noted.

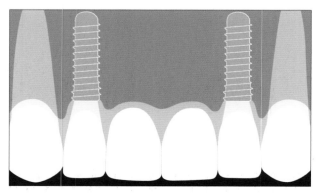

Fig 9   To minimize the esthetic risk, only two implants were placed at the sites previously occupied by the lateral incisors to support a four-unit fixed dental prosthesis. Current recommendations are to place fewer implants in areas with multiple missing teeth with a view to optimizing esthetic results, as pontics will often facilitate the task of creating esthetically ideal soft-tissue contours at adjacent sites compared to implants placed next to each other.

Clinical examination (Figs 10 and 11) and a cone-beam computed tomography (CBCT) scan demonstrated that the vertical and horizontal bone quantity was adequate, with slight resorption of the crestal area. A GBR procedure was indicated, to be performed simultaneously with implant placement (Fig 12).

Under local anesthesia and a mild tranquilizer (Cercine 5 mg; Takeda Pharmaceutical, Osaka, Japan), two bone-level implants (Straumann Bone Level, diameter 4,1 mm, length 10 mm) were placed and a GBR procedure simultaneously performed. Autologous bone chips from the ramus and grafting material (HA particles; Zimmer Dental, CA, USA) were applied. Additional grafting material was applied over the autologous bone graft to reduce horizontal resorption of the augmented site and was covered by a resorbable collagen membrane (Collatape; Zimmer Dental, CA, USA). Complete primary flap closure was obtained over the surgical sites. Healing was uneventful. Postsurgical medications included Flomox (Shionogi, Osaka, Japan; 3×100 mg/d for 7 days), Voltaren (Novartis, Basel, Switzerland, 3×25 mg/d for 7 days), and Neosterine Green (oral rinse agent; Nippon Shika Yakuhin, Yamaguchi, Japan).

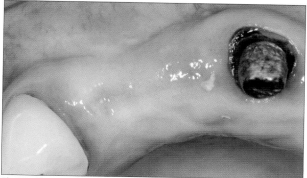

Fig 10   Close-up view of the site previously occupied by the right lateral incisor. The clinical examination revealed adequate bone width and healthy soft tissue.

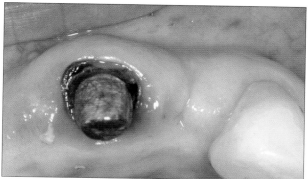

Fig 11   Close-up view of the site previously occupied by the right lateral incisor. Note the limited mesiodistal dimension associated with a minimal degree of tissue resorption since the tooth had been extracted.

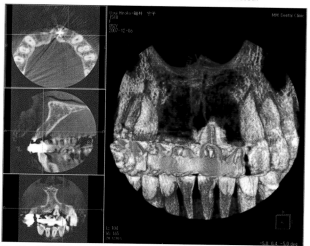

Fig 12   A CBCT scan with a radiographic template was performed 8 weeks after extracting both teeth, confirming the vertical and horizontal dimensions were sufficient for implant placement. However, the alveolar crest was compromised in the crestal areas of both proposed implant sites, suggesting that implant placement should be combined with a GBR procedure.

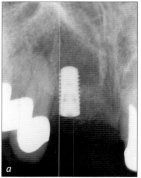
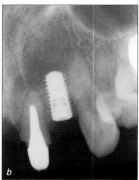

Figs 13a-b Periapical radiographs obtained after implant placement bone-level implants (Straumann Bone Level, Regular CrossFit).

Immediately after surgery, periapical radiographs and a cone-beam computed tomography (CBCT) scan were obtained. The implants were ideally positioned and aligned for the planned restoration (Figs 13a-b to 15a-b).

Postsurgical healing was uneventful. A 12-week healing period was respected before the second-stage surgery for impression-taking and soft-tissue management. Slight resorption after augmentation was observed (Figs 16 to 17). The second procedure was performed 12 weeks after implant placement under local anesthesia (Fig 18) and by using a minimized incision line above the implants to avoid damage to surrounding tissue. A periapical radiograph was taken to confirm the precise fit of the impression posts (Figs 19a-b).

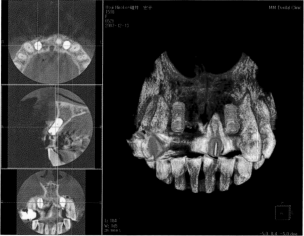

Fig 14   CBCT scan obtained after implant placement. The three-dimensional implant positions and the results of bone augmentation were favorable.

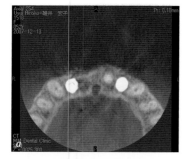

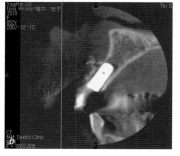

Figs 15a-b Close-up CBCT views showing good alignment of the implants in all three dimensions.

After the impression, master casts for the provisional restoration were fabricated (Fig 20). This restoration was designed prior to extraction of the central incisor and was to be delivered immediately after the extraction. Indicated by the implant positions, a cemented temporary restoration on customized temporary abutments was selected (Figs 21 to 22). Insertion of this first temporary restoration marked the initiation of soft-tissue management.

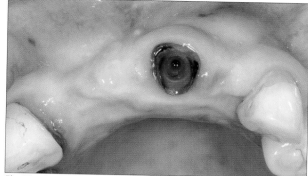

Fig 16   Situation 12 weeks after implant placement. Soft-tissue healing seemed to have proceeded smoothly. Note the presence of mild horizontal resorption.

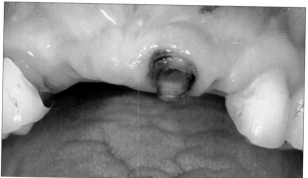

Fig 17   The vertical soft-tissue dimensions were well maintained.

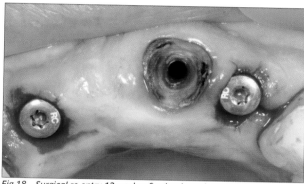

Fig 18   Surgical re-entry 12 weeks after implant placement for impression-taking and soft-tissue management.

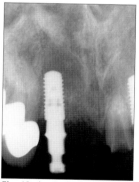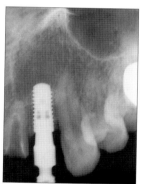

Figs 19a-b   Periapical radiographs obtained to verify that the impression posts were correctly positioned on the bone-level implants.

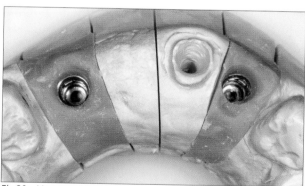

Fig 20   Master cast to fabricate the provisional restoration. The implants were located approximately 3–4 mm below the soft-tissue margin.

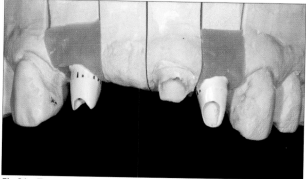

Fig 21   Temporary abutments (Straumann AG, Basel, Switzerland) were selected and prepared as temporary customized abutments for a cemented provisional restoration.

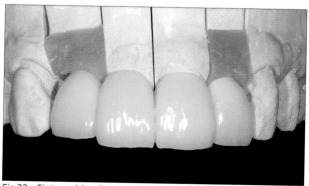

Fig 22   First provisional restoration on the master cast.

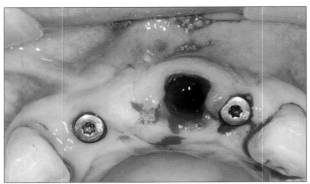

Fig 23 Situation following extraction of the left central incisor before the provisional restoration was inserted.

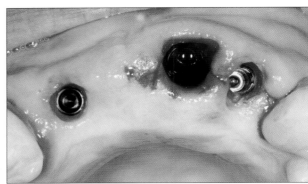

Fig 24 Situation immediately after tooth extraction. The healing caps were removed from the implants.

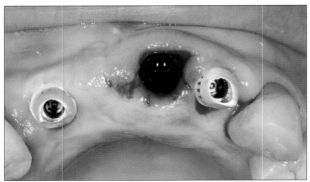

Fig 25 The temporary abutments were inserted with 35 Ncm. The labial margin of the extraction site had a more labial position than the implant sites. Also, the labial shape of the site is disharmonious.

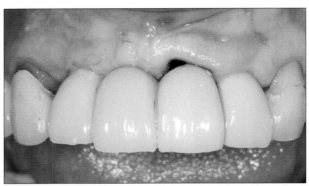

Fig 26 Frontal view of the provisional restoration delivered immediately after extraction.

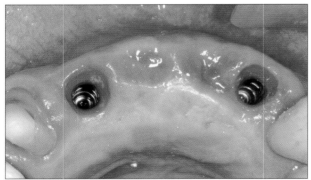

Fig 27 Situation 8 weeks after extraction of the left central incisor. The pontic rest areas in the crestal soft tissue were not sufficiently developed at this point.

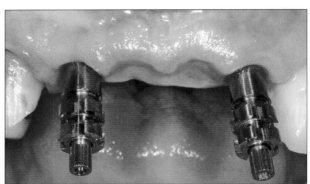

Fig 28 An impression was taken for a second provisional restoration, using open-tray impression posts.

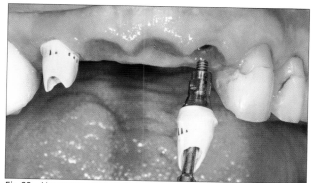

Fig 29   New temporary abutments were installed for the second provisional restoration.

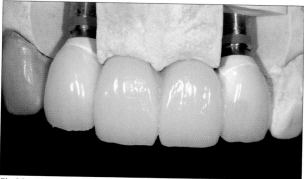

Fig 30   The margins of the temporary custom abutments were prepared at a level 1 mm below the soft-tissue margin. The shapes of the retainer crowns and pontics were carefully designed.

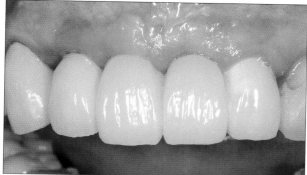

Fig 31   Second provisional restoration immediately after insertion.

Under local anesthesia, the central incisor was carefully extracted to minimize any damage to the extraction socket (Figs 23 and 24). Then the temporary abutments were screwed in place and the provisional restoration delivered, using a water-resorbable temporary cement (Shofu, Kyoto, Japan) to avoid complications with any cement remnants in the adjacent soft tissue (Figs 25 and 26).

The soft-tissue situation was revisited 8 weeks after extraction (Fig 27). While the extraction socket had completely healed by that time, the peri-implant soft-tissue framework and the soft tissue in the pontic area were still developing. The healing period was extended for the tissue to mature. At 12 weeks after extraction, soft-tissue maturation had improved, but the site was not considered ready for the final restoration. After consultation with the patient, it was decided to fabricate a second provisional restoration for further tissue management. A new impression was taken with open-tray impression posts (Fig 28) and a second provisional restoration fabricated (Figs 29 to 32).

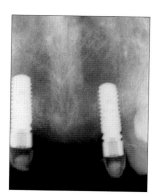

Fig 32   Periapical radiograph after delivery of the second provisional restoration. The peri-implant bone levels were well maintained.

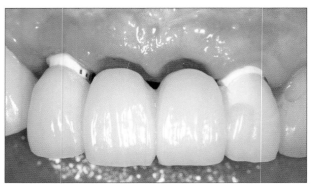

Fig 33   Verification of soft-tissue maturation 4 weeks after insertion of the second provisional restoration.

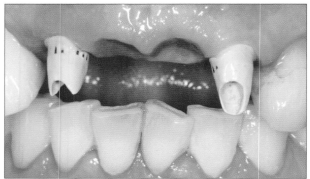

Fig 34   Verification of the restorative space. Note the harmonic relations with the opposing mandibular teeth.

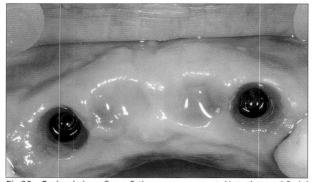

Fig 35   Occlusal view after soft-tissue management. Note the good facial harmony of the sites previously occupied by the left and right central incisors.

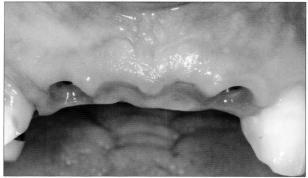

Fig 36   Situation prior to the final impression.

An additional period of 8 weeks was considered to further enhance the soft tissue by means of a second provisional restoration. Only 4 weeks later, appropriate soft-tissue maturation was confirmed in all three dimensions (Figs 33 to 35). The treatment steps required for the permanent prosthesis were initiated.

Prior to the final impression, the soft-tissue situation was reevaluated (Figs 36 to 38). The patient exhibited well-matured and stable soft tissue, consistent with a medium biotype. While CAD/CAM-generated ceramic abutments were initially considered for the final prosthesis, space and biomechanical considerations prompted a change of mind in favor of titanium anatomical abutments (Figs 39 to 41) and a CAD/CAM-generated zirconia framework (Figs 42 and 43). The periapical radiograph disclosed stable peri-implant bone levels (Fig 44). Cone-beam computed tomography (CBCT) scanning also confirmed the stability of hard tissues around both implants in all three dimensions, and particularly on the facial aspect (Fig 45). The patient was instructed to use various cleaning tools to maintain healthy conditions around the implants. A 3-month recall and aftercare schedule was proposed. Conditions remained stable throughout the follow-up period, yielding an esthetically satisfactory outcome after 3 years (Fig 46). To summarize, careful soft-tissue handling was essential to achieving a predictable and stable esthetic outcome in this moderate esthetic risk patient (Fig 47).

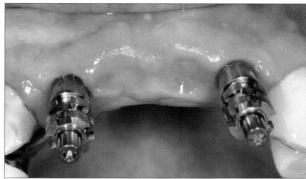

Fig 37   Final impression with open-tray impression posts.

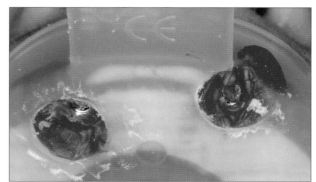

Fig 38   An open tray was utilized for the final impression.

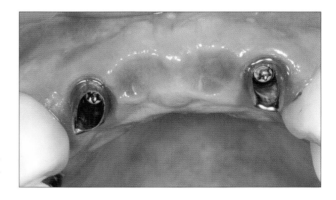

Fig 39   Thanks to a favorable thickness of the peri-implant soft tissue, standard titanium anatomical abutments were selected and modified. The tip of the abutment was very thin; biomechanical aspects should be carefully considered in these situations.

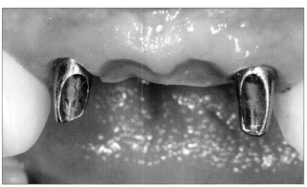

Fig 40   The soft tissue was adequately thick to conceal the metallic color of the titanium custom abutments.

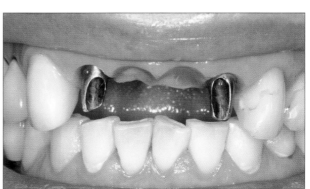

Fig 41   Final soft-tissue frame prior to delivering the fixed prosthesis.

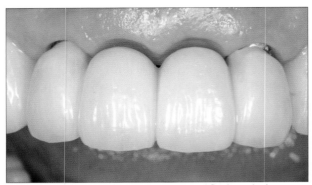

Fig 42   First try-in of the final implant-supported fixed prosthesis.

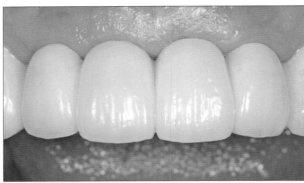

Fig 43   Final implant-supported prosthesis upon delivery.

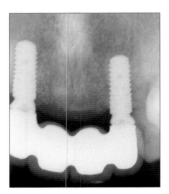

Fig 44 Radiograph obtained at the 3-year follow-up. Note the well-preserved bone level around both implants.

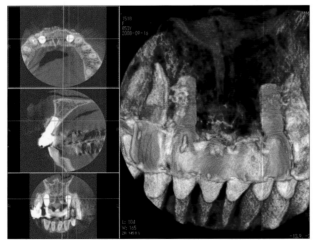

Fig 45   CBCT scan obtained after delivery of final restoration. The hard tissue surrounding both implants is well maintained in all three dimensions.

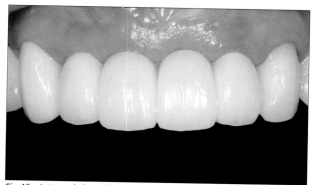

Fig 46 Intraoral view of the treated area at the 3-year follow-up.

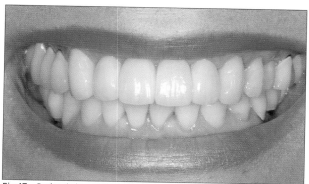

Fig 47 Perioral view of the patient's smile line, which shows good integration of the prosthesis wth the surrounding tissues and neighboring teeth.

Acknowledgments

The authors wish to thank Mr. Isamu Saitoh for his excellent technical work and contributions for superstructure. In addition, we feel indebted to all members of the team at Center of Implant Dentistry (CID), Yokohama, Japan.

6.7 Replacement of Five Teeth with a Fixed Dental Prosthesis on Bone-Level Implants

D. Dragisic

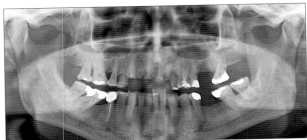

Fig 1   Orthopantomograph of the initial situation.

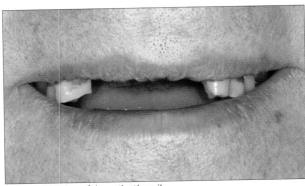

Fig 2   Initial view of the patient's smile.

A 52-year-old male patient presented at our clinic, his concern being that most of his maxillary anterior dentition (teeth 13 to 22) was missing. This extensive tooth loss was due to trauma, which had occurred several years previously, after which the patient had been wearing a removable partial denture. He stated that the residual roots were asymptomatic, did not express any other concerns, and reported not having a routine dental history with regular dental examinations. His medical history was uneventful, and he did not smoke.

A clinical and radiographic examination (Fig 1) revealed the presence of generalized periodontal disease associated with fair to poor oral hygiene, moderate plaque, subgingival fracture of teeth 13 to 22 with a poor prognosis, defective restorations on several teeth (18, 17, 14, 24, 25, 27, 37, 45, 47, 48), periapical radiolucencies around several teeth (38, 35, 33, 43, 47), and erosive/abrasive lesions on most teeth (notably in the fifth sextant).

The patient's gingival tissue was characterized by a moderately scalloped, medium to thick biotype with an adequate band of keratinized mucosa. Evaluation of his smile revealed a low lip line (Fig 2). It should be noted that despite the aforementioned indications of periapical periodontitis, vitality testing of teeth 38, 33, 43, 47 (ethyl-chloride test, electric pulp test, cavity test on tooth 38) yielded normal pulp reactions. Tooth 35 did not respond to these tests. The patient asked for a fixed rehabilitation with a "natural" appearance matching his existing dentition.

Treatment Planning

The patent's existing occlusion was correct in the transverse and vertical planes. There was evidence of structural loss on the teeth, possibly due to chemical erosion and abrasion.

Based on the clinical and radiographic examination, a preoperative surgical and restorative analysis was conducted to assess the complexity of the case (Table 1).

Based on a comprehensive evaluation of clinical and radiographic parameters using a risk assessment table (see Volume 1 of this ITI Treatment Guide), it was concluded that the case posed a medium esthetic risk and offered a good prognosis for implant therapy.

Proposed treatment plan:

- Extraction of the non-restorable roots (13 to 22 and 26) and replacement with implant-supported restorations
- Comprehensive periodontal assessment and treatment
- Endodontic retreatment of tooth 14 and endodontic treatment of tooth 35
- Replacement of defective direct restorations (teeth 18, 17, 14, 24, 25, 27, 37, 45, 47, 48)
- Replacement of full-coverage restoration on tooth 45
- Provision of a night guard

The main objectives of the proposed final treatment plan were to accomplish implant-supported fixed rehabilitation of a number of teeth (13 to 22, 26 and 36) once periodontal treatment to re-establish stability and hygiene would have been completed. An additional requirement was to replace all defective restorations for optimal function and esthetics. To achieve these goals, the treatment protocol included not only extraction of teeth 13 to 22 with early implant placement, simultaneous bone grafting, and subsequent delivery of definitive restorations, but also soft-tissue conditioning with screw-retained temporary prostheses.

Definitive restorations for the anterior maxilla included one screw-retained single crown at site 13 and two separate restorations at sites 11 and 21 region with distal cantilever units for the adjacent sites 12 and 22. The proposed design would enable the patient to optimally meet his oral hygiene requirements and had no mechanical or technical disadvantages as long as the cantilever extensions did not exceed 15 mm (Salvi and Bragger 2009). Also, there is no evidence that splinting of implant-supported restorations might be biomechanically advantageous, while non-splinted units offer the added benefit that they can be repaired in the event of ceramic failure.

Table 1   SAC assessment.

Standard SAC criteria			
Esthetic Risk Factor	**Low**	**Moderate**	**High**
Medical status	Healthy, cooperative patient with an intact immune system		Reduced immune system
Smoking habit	Non-smoker	Light smoker (< 10 cigs/day)	Heavy smoker (≥ 10 cigs/day)
Patient's esthetic expectations	Low	Medium	High
Lip line	Low	Medium	High
Gingival biotype	Low-scalloped thick	Medium-scalloped, medium thick	High-scalloped, thin
Shape of tooth crowns	Rectangular		Triangular
Infection at implant site	None	Chronic	Acute
Bone level at adjacent teeth	≤ 5 mm to contact point	5.5 to 6.5 mm to contact point	≥ 7 mm to contact point
Restorative status of neighboring teeth	Virgin		Restored
Width of edentulous span	1 tooth (≥ 7 mm)	1 tooth (< 7 mm)	2 teeth or more
Soft-tissue anatomy	Intact soft tissue		Soft-tissue defects
Bone anatomy of alveolar crest	Alveolar crest without bone deficiency	Horizontal bone deficiency	Vertical bone deficiency

White: not assessed

Supplementary criteria			
Oral hygiene and compliance	Good	Sufficient	Insufficient
Craniofacial/skeletal growth	Completed		In Progress
Visibility of treatment area upon smiling	No		Yes
Zone selection	Posterior		Anterior
Loading protocol	Conventional	Early	Immediate
Soft-tissue contour and volume	Ideal	Slightly compromised	Significantly deficient
Intermaxillary relationship	Angle Class I and III	Angle Class II Div. 1 and 2	Severe malocclusion
Occlusion	Harmonious	Irregular	Occlusal modifications necessary
Interim restoration	Non required	Removable	Fixed
Bruxism	Absent		Present
Retention	Cemented		Screw-retained

Assessment	
Esthetic risk	Medium
Normative SAC classification	Complex

Surgical procedures

The patient was referred to a periodontologist for comprehensive evaluation and treatment. Advanced periodontitis was diagnosed and treated by non-surgical full-mouth debridement, followed by monthly recalls. During periodontal treatment, the residual roots of teeth 13 to 22 and tooth 26 were extracted. Tooth 35 was removed elsewhere as an emergency measure while the patient was on vacation.

Nine months after periodontal pre-treatment and following a strict 3-month maintenance program, the patient was referred back to our clinic for further treatment.

Our reassessment showed that all prospective implant sites had healed satisfactorily (Figs 3 and 4). Based on a radiographic examination, inspection of the post-extraction sockets, and measurements performed on study casts, implants with regular dimensions (enossal diameter 4.1 mm) could be inserted within the area between sites 14 and 23.

A palatocrestal incision was performed at sites 13 to 22 and a full-thickness flap reflected, also using two distal vertical release incisions at sites 14 and 23. After removing granulation tissue from the surgical site, initial osteotomies were prepared at sites 13, 12, 21, and the proposed implant positions were radiographically assessed using radiopaque depth and direction indicators (Fig 5).

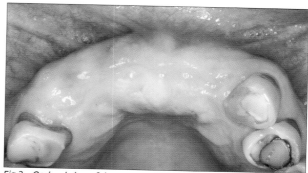

Fig 3   Occlusal view of the maxillary anterior ridge.

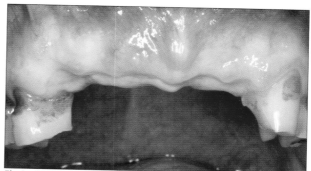

Fig 4   Frontal view of the maxillary anterior ridge.

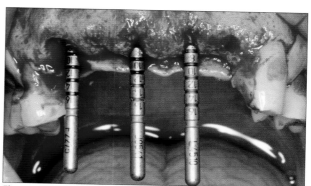

Fig 5   Verification of implant beds using depth gauges.

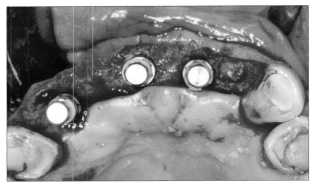

Fig 6   Occlusal view of the implants with the insertion mounts still attached.

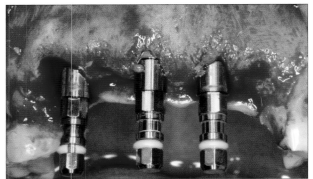

Fig 7   Frontal view of the implants with the insertion mounts still attached.

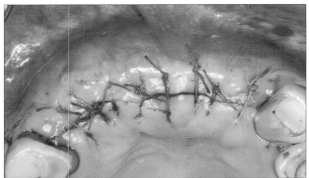

Fig 8   Frontal view after tension-free closure with resorbable sutures.

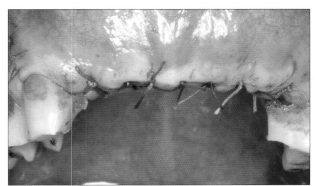

Fig 9   Occlusal view after tension-free closure with resorbable sutures.

Three bone-level implants (Straumann Bone Level, SLActive, Regular CrossFit, diameter 4.1 mm, length 10 mm) were inserted and closed with Regular CrossFit (RC) cover screws (Figs 6 and 7). Cancellous bone that had been collected during preparation was mixed with deproteinized bovine bone mineral (DBBM) particles (Bio-Oss; Geistlich, Wolhusen, Switzerland), packed to the vestibular area, and covered with a resorbable collagen membrane (Bio-Gide; Geistlich). After extended relief of the periosteum, full closure with resorbable interrupted sutures (Vicryl 4-0 and 6-0; Ethicon, Somerville, NJ, USA) was obtained (Figs 8 and 9). The patient was prescribed antibiotics and a chlorhexidine mouth rinse.

After the soft tissue had been allowed to mature under a removable temporary restoration for 2 months, the implants were surgically exposed and all three cover screws replaced with tapered healing abutments to create the initial emergence profile.

Soft-tissue conditioning and provisionalization

Two weeks later, an impression was taken at implant level, followed by the provision of a set of implant-supported screw-retained provisional restorations, including one single-unit restoration on tooth 13 and two double-unit (crown plus cantilever) restorations at sites 11/12 and 21/22 (Fig 10). These provisional restorations were designed to reflect the contours and proportions of the final restorations. The double-unit provisional restorations had a transocclusally screw-retained design and were fabricated on meso-abutments for temporary restorations. The main reason for designing three separate restorations rather than a one that would connect all implants was to optimize conditions for oral hygiene. The temporary restorations restored the incisal guidance, and lateral excursion on the right side was mainly supported by the premolars to keep the articulation with full proprioception.

Over the following 4 weeks, flowable composite was gradually added to the pontics, conditioning the soft tissue and improving the emergence profiles (Figs 11 and 12). After achieving a satisfactory outcome, the provisional restorations were kept in place to achieve a predictable outcome with the final restorations in terms of soft-tissue volume. Another important function of this period was to evaluate the patient's esthetic expectations and to identify any parafunctional habits.

Fitting the final restorations was preceded by revising the defective restorations (direct composite filling of two or three surfaces on teeth 18, 17, 14, 23, 24, 25, 38, 37, 47, 48; indirect composite filling of four surfaces on tooth 27; metal-ceramic crown on tooth 45). Tooth 35 had been extracted elsewhere due to acute apical periodontitis while the patient was vacationing. For restoration of structural loss—possibly by chemical erosion and abrasion—ceramic veneers or direct composite restorations were recommended. The latter were selected by the patient for budget reasons and were executed after fitting the final implant-supported crowns in the maxilla. Three implants were placed at sites 26, 35, 36.

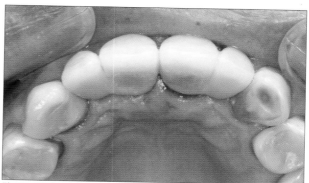

Fig 10   Occlusal view of the inserted provisional restorations.

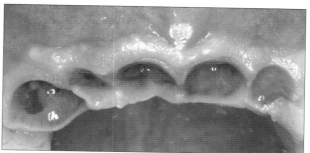

Fig 11   Frontal view of the tissue contours 6 months after delivery of the provisional restorations.

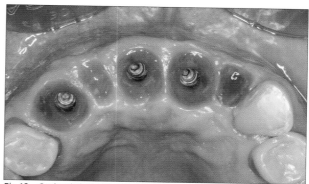

Fig 12   Occlusal view of the tissue contours 6 months after delivery of the provisional restorations.

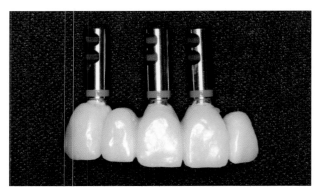

Fig 13   Provisional restorations with implant analogs attached.

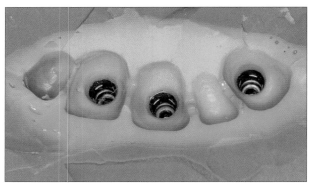

Fig 14   Implant analogs in silicone reflecting the gingival contour.

Impression

For precision in capturing and transferring the shaped soft tissue, customized impression copings were fabricated. This was accomplished by fitting the temporary restorations on implant analogs and submerging them in putty silicone. Once the material had set, the restorations were unscrewed, leaving the contour of the emergence profile replicated in the silicone. The next step was to place the impression copings on the analogs and fill the concavities with flowable composite. This resulted in customized impression copings suitable for transferring not only the position of the implants but also the shape of the soft tissue to the cast, ensuring a predictable outcome at the mucosa level (Figs 13 to 17).

An open-tray technique was selected to record the tooth preparations and implant positions, using an addition-type silicone as impression material (Fig 18).

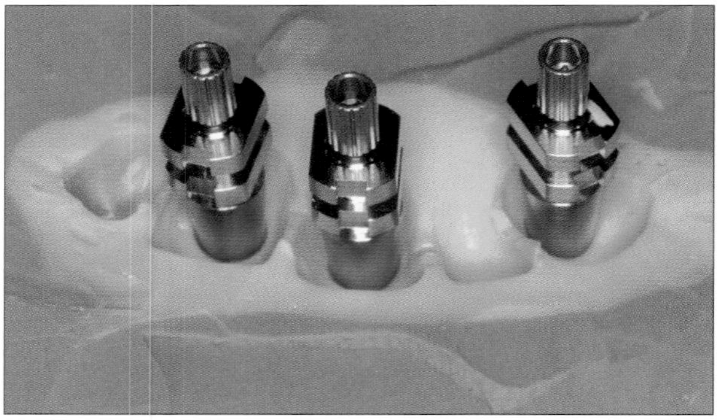

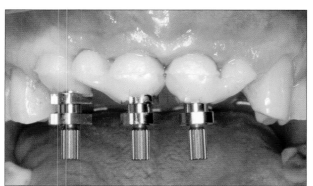

Fig 15   Impression copings on implant analogs for customization.

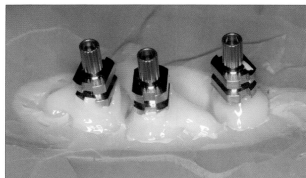

Fig 16   Customized impression copings.

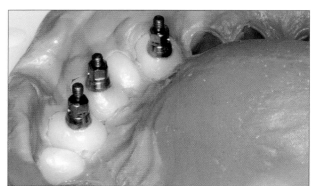

Fig 17   Taking the impression with the customized copings in place.

Fig 18   Customized copings after the impression.

Final restoration

Before entering into this phase of treatment, the patient's current satisfaction was evaluated from an esthetic and functional viewpoint. No significant abrasion was noted, and no episodes of acrylic fracture had occurred. The patient was already happy with the temporary restorations as they were. An alginate impression was taken with the temporary restorations in situ to guide the laboratory technician in designing the metal frameworks and the ceramic veneer (Figs 19 and 20).

The framework try-in confirmed adequate fit and correct metal support. Minor final adjustments were made during a subsequent bisque try-in. Following glazing of the ceramic crowns by the dental technician, the restorations were ready for delivery (Figs 21 to 25).

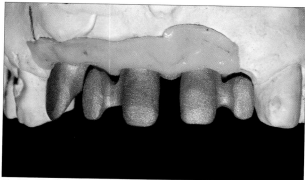

Fig 19   Metal frameworks.

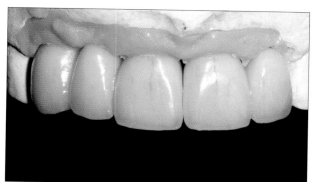

Fig 20   Final restorations on the master cast.

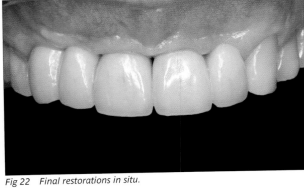

Fig 21   Final restorations ready for delivery.

Fig 22   Final restorations in situ.

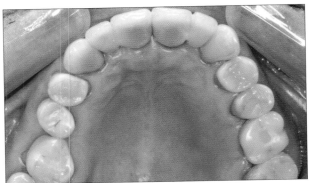

Fig 23   Palatal view of final restorations.

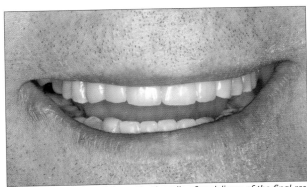

Fig 24   Perioral view of the patient's smile after delivery of the final restorations.

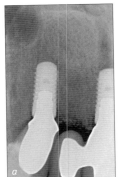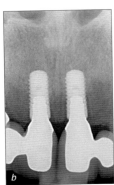

Figs 25a-b   Radiographic verification after delivery of the restorations.

Post-treatment follow-up and maintenance

At the 12-month follow-up, no mechanical or biological complications had occurred (Figs 26 to 27a-c).

The patient was perfectly satisfied with the stability of his restoration. No signs of peri-implant complications were noticed around any of the implant abutments, which confirmed that the patient had performed adequate plaque control, favored by a restorative design that offered good access to hygiene instruments.

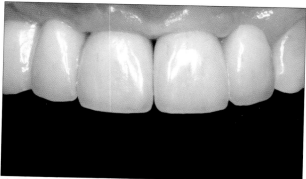

Fig 26   Intraoral view of the restorations at the 12-month follow-up.

Acknowledgments

Restorative procedures
Raul Costa and Dejan Dragisic

Laboratory procedures
Somanu Luang Phaxay and Nilou Sotouhi

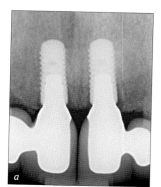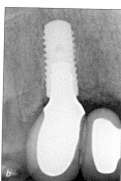

Figs 27a-c   Radiographic images obtained at the 12-month follow-up.

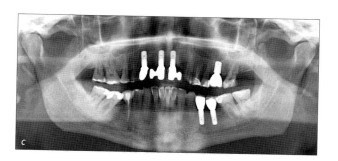

6.8 Replacement of Six Teeth with a Fixed Dental Prosthesis on Four Bone-Level Implants

M. Mokti, G. Gallucci

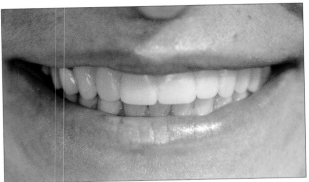

Fig 1   Perioral view of the patient's smile line.

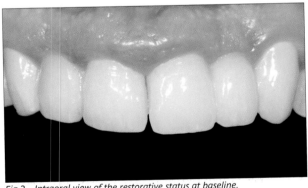

Fig 2   Intraoral view of the restorative status at baseline.

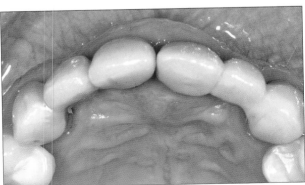

Fig 3   Occlusal view the existing metal-ceramic restorations.

In November 2010, a 44-year-old woman presented to the Harvard School of Dental Medicine seeking options to replace her failing six-unit conventional prosthesis. Having served for approximately 10 years, the fixed partial denture had repeatedly needed recementation after chronic dislodgement over the past few months. Following these episodes, the patient requested further evaluation of her current prosthesis and showed interest in exploring other options for a fixed solution.

The patient was in good overall health, presenting with no systemic contraindications to implant therapy or any history of allergies; she did not smoke and was on no medications. Being a well-motivated individual, she regularly saw her general dental practitioner and effectively complied with oral hygiene requirements.

During an extraoral examination, the patient's facial contour and lip support was found to be within normal limits. Her full smile was associated with a medium lip line displaying more than two-thirds of the tooth crowns while concealing the gingival margins and interproximal papillae of the maxillary anterior segment (Fig 1).

The intraoral examination revealed a prosthesis supported by four abutment teeth (sites 13, 11, 21, 23) and replacing tooth 12 and 22 (Figs 2 and 3). Radiographs were obtained which showed that the abutment teeth were non-vital, had been restored with inadequate obturation of the root canals, featured short metal posts, and exhibited periapical pathology (Figs 4 to 6). A detailed clinical examination with the prosthesis removed showed recurrent carious lesions and potential root fractures affecting the abutment teeth.

Based on these findings, the abutment teeth were deemed non-restorable, and the patient was informed that extraction of teeth was inevitable and possibly would have to be followed by replacement with an implant-supported fixed partial denture after 2 months of healing.

After discussing treatment options and sequencing with the patient, she agreed to the proposed treatment plan. An appointment was scheduled to extract the non-restorable teeth under local anesthesia, followed by immediate delivery of a removable partial denture.

After 6 weeks of healing, the patient was recalled for further soft-tissue evaluation and a diagnostic mock-up of the future prosthesis. The soft tissue had healed well, showing minor dehiscences at the extractions sites. The coronal third of the alveolar ridges was well preserved buccolingually, while apically a buccal concavity seemed to be present. The diagnostic mock-up was also used to assess the patient's esthetic demands and phonetics, and she expressed her satisfaction with the parameters concerned.

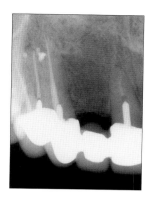

Fig 4   Radiographic status at baseline.

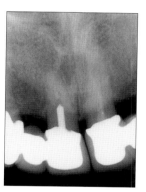

Fig 5   Radiographic status at baseline.

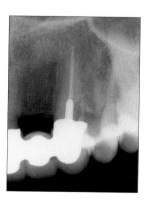

Fig 6   Radiographic status at baseline.

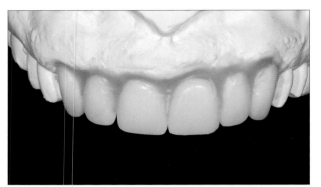

Fig 7   Diagnostic wax-up with consideration of the soft-tissue defect and dental rehabilitation.

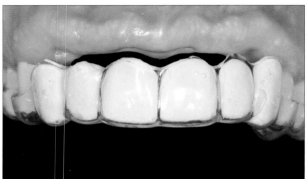

Fig 8   Radiographic template.

Based on the diagnostic set-up, the evaluated size of the six anterior teeth was used to guide fabrication of the radiographic and surgical template (Fig 7). A cone-beam computed tomography (CBCT) scan was taken with the patient wearing a custom radiographic stent for computer-assisted treatment planning (Fig 8). Simplant software (Materialise Dental, Glen Burnie, MD, USA) was used for reformatted cross-sectional images to determine the number, location and axial orientation of implants. The treatment plan was to place four bone-level implants (Straumann Bone Level, Regular CrossFit, diameter 4.1 mm, length 10 mm) at sites 13, 11, 21, 23 (Figs 9 to 14).

A surgical appointment to place four implants (sites 13, 11, 21, 23) under local anesthesia was scheduled for 1 week after the cone-beam computed tomography (CBCT) scan. The procedure started with a crestal incision in a slightly palatal position and extending to the distal aspect of the line angles of 14 and 24, followed by divergent incisions apically to the labial vestibule. A full-thickness flap was raised and reflected with black-silk sutures both in labial and palatal directions. All granulation tissue was excavated and the ridge continuously rinsed with saline to avoid drying of the implant sites (Figs 15 to 18).

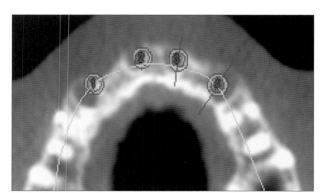

Fig 9   Computer-assisted implant planning: occlusal view

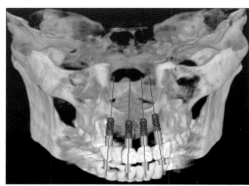

Fig 10   Computer-assisted implant planning: frontal view.

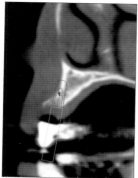

Fig 11 Computer-assisted implant planning: maxillary right canine.

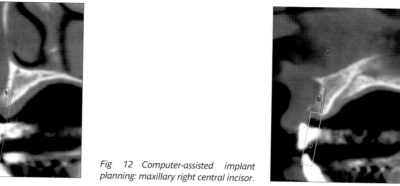

Fig 12 Computer-assisted implant planning: maxillary right central incisor.

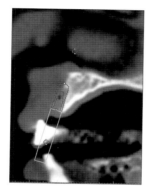

Fig 13 Computer-assisted implant planning: maxillary left central incisor.

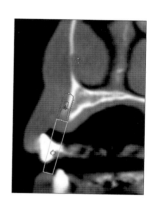

Fig 14 Computer-assisted implant planning: maxillary left canine.

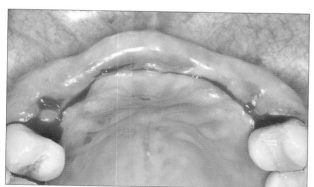

Fig 15 Occlusal view of the midcrestal incision.

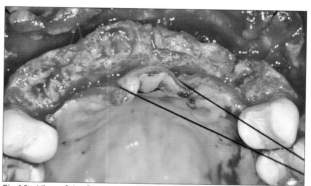

Fig 16 View of the flap procedure.

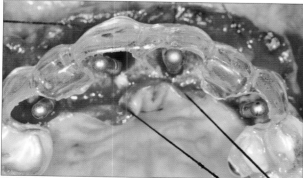

Fig 17 View of the surgical template and guide pins in place.

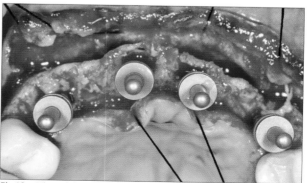

Fig 18 View of the 2.8 mm paralleling pins.

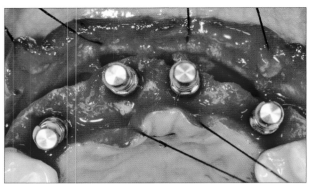

Fig 19   View of the inserted implants with the mounting devices.

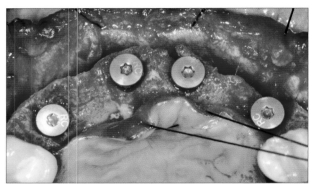

Fig 20   View of the healing abutments connected to the implants before suturing.

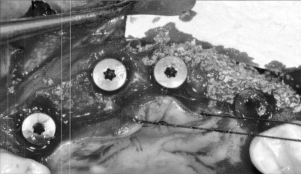

Fig 21   View of the buccal bone graft, including the collagen membrane.

Surgical templates were used to create the entry points of all implant sites and to establish parallelism, using the first pilot drill to a depth of 6 mm. Upon achieving parallelism of the implant sites, the pilot drill was continued and the subsequent drill sequence carried out to the established planned implant positions. Four bone-level implants (Straumann Bone Level, SLActive, Regular CrossFit, diameter 4.1 mm, length 10 mm) were placed (sites 13, 11, 21, 23) in their correct three-dimensional positions as previously defined in the planning phase. Each implant was then fitted with a 2-mm Regular Cross-Fit (RC) healing abutment (Figs 19 to 20).

Buccal dehiscences were noted at implant sites 11, 21, 23. A guided bone regeneration (GBR) procedure was performed using a xenograft of demineralized bovine bone matrix (Bio-Oss; Geistlich, Wolhusen, Switzerland) followed by coverage with a double layer of collagen membrane (Bio-Gide; Geistlich). A mucoperiosteal releasing incision was performed to achieve complete closure of the implants and xenograft. The flaps were then repositioned and sutured using Gore-Tex sutures (WL Gore and Associates, Flagstaff, AZ, USA) to submerge the implants and the graft (Figs 21 and 22). After the procedure, a panoramic radiograph was obtained to verify the implant positions (Fig 23).

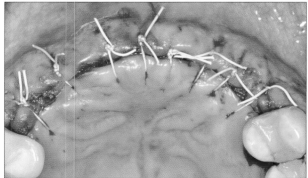

Fig 22   View of the tension-free primary wound closure.

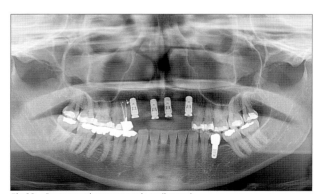

Fig 23   Postoperative panoramic radiograph.

After 4 weeks of postsurgical healing, the patient was recalled for a review visit. The soft tissue was healing well, and some of the healing abutments were partially or completely exposed. The implants did not show any clinical signs of mobility or infection (Fig 24).

Regular CrossFit (RC) impression posts for open trays were connected to the implants and utilized for a pickup impression in a medium-body polyether material (Impregum Penta; 3M ESPE, St. Paul, MN, USA), which was used to fabricate a temporary acrylic fixed partial denture (Figs 25 and 26).

A six-unit, one-piece, screw-retained, temporary prosthesis had been fabricated and was ready for loading the implants 2 weeks after the impression. Good seating was obtained on torqueing the prosthesis to the implants. Also, care was taken to ensure that the restoration did not impinge on the soft tissue in an excessive way. The patient was satisfied with the overall esthetic and functional outcome of this prosthesis (Figs 27 to 29).

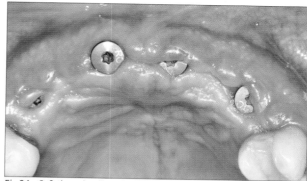
Fig 24   Soft-tissue healing after 4 weeks.

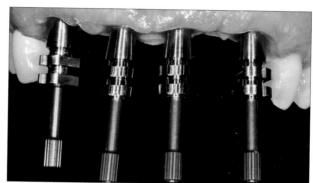
Fig 25   Preliminary implant-level impressions.

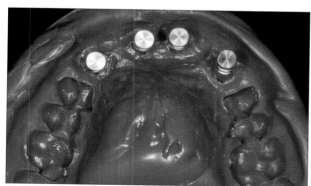
Fig 26   Implant analogs repositioned into the impression.

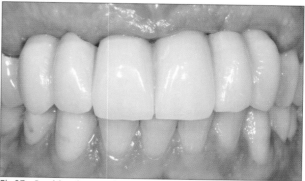
Fig 27   Provisional restoration.

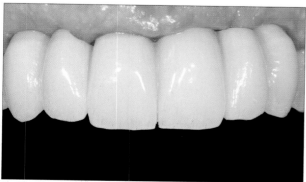
Fig 28   Close-up view of the provisional restoration.

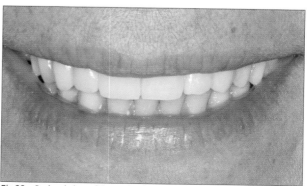
Fig 29   Perioral view of the patient's smile with the provisional restoration.

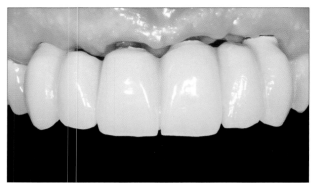
Fig 30 Soft-tissue contour after 3 months of loading.

Six weeks after tissue conditioning and 3 months after implant placement, the final impression of the implants and soft tissue was taken using the splinted technique. Regular CrossFit (RC) impression posts for open trays were connected to the implants, followed by the use of dental floss and a light-curing colorless gel (Triad; Dentsply International, York, PA, USA) material to splint the impression posts together such that they formed a single complex. Impressions were taken with a heavy-body polyvinyl siloxane (PVS) material (3M ESPE, MN, USA) together with a light-body PVS material to capture the soft-tissue contours (Figs 30 to 36).

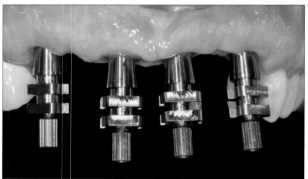
Fig 31 Final impression using an open-tray technique.

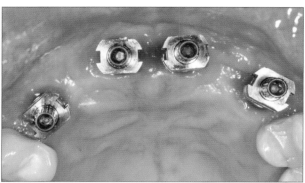
Fig 32 Final impression using an open-tray technique.

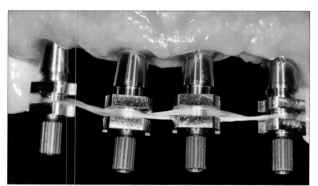
Fig 33 Splinting of the impression copings.

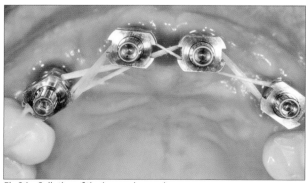
Fig 34 Splinting of the impression copings.

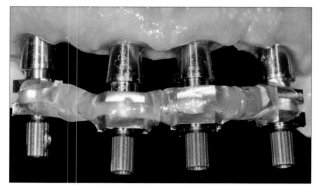
Fig 35 Impression copings splinted with dental floss and a light-cured colorless gel.

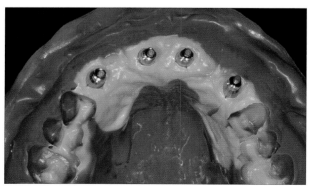
Fig 36 View of the final impression.

After the final impression appointment, abutments were waxed up and subjected to an intraoral try-in with full seating and evaluation of the margins to ensure that these were submucosal (Figs 37 and 38). The waxed abutments were scanned (Etkon; Straumann AG, Basel, Switzerland) for the final CAD/CAM-generated zirconia abutments (Figs 39 and 40).

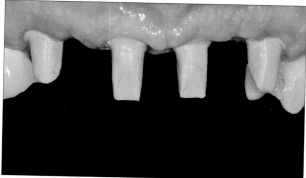

Fig 37   Try-in of waxed abutments to verify the location of their margins.

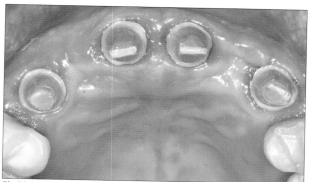

Fig 38   Try-in of waxed abutments to verify the location of their margins.

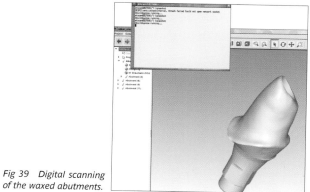

Fig 39   Digital scanning of the waxed abutments.

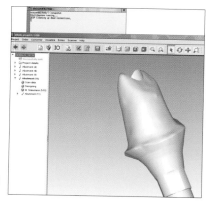

Fig 40   Digital scanning of the waxed abutments.

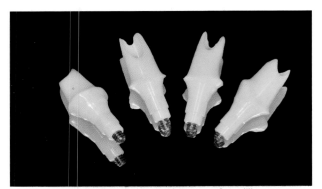

Fig 41   CAD/CAM-generated zirconia abutments after milling.

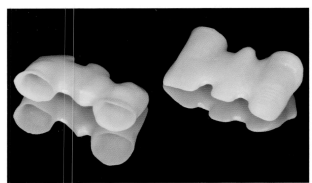

Fig 42   CAD/CAM-generated zirconia copings after milling.

The next appointment was scheduled to try in the final CAD/CAM-generated zirconia abutments and zirconia frameworks for verification before the final prosthesis was going to be processed. This try-in again included full seating of the abutments, and the frameworks were evaluated for their passivity upon insertion and for marginal adaptation (Figs 41 to 46).

By the final visit, two three-unit fixed partial dentures with zirconia frameworks and ceramic veneering had been fabricated and were ready for delivery to the patient. Parameters that were evaluated prior to their cementation included marginal adaptation, contact points and occlusion. Once the final prostheses were cemented, the patient expressed her satisfaction with the esthetic and functional outcome and with the treatment rendered (Figs 47 to 49). Delivery of the rehabilitation was followed by obtaining radiographs for assessment (Fig 50).

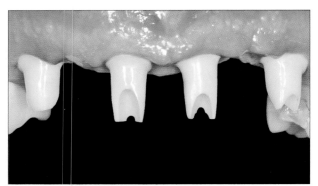

Fig 43   Try-in of the CAD/CAM-generated zirconia abutments.

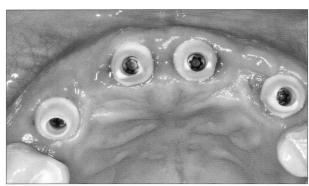

Fig 44   Try-in of the CAD/CAM-generated zirconia abutments.

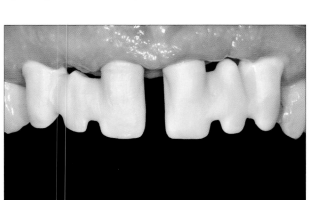

Fig 45   Try-in of the CAD/CAM-generated zirconia copings.

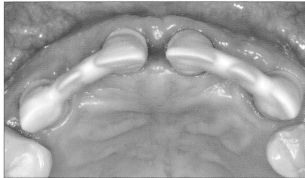

Fig 46   Try-in of the CAD/CAM-generated zirconia copings.

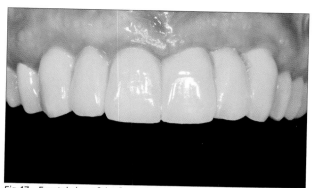

Fig 47   Frontal view of the final rehabilitation.

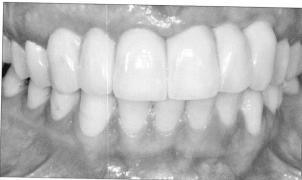

Fig 48   Final rehabilitation in occlusion.

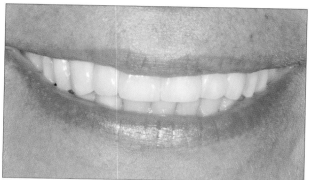

Fig 49   Perioral view of the patient's smile with the final rehabilitation in place.

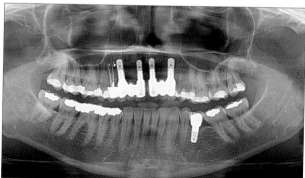

Fig 50   Final panoramic radiograph.

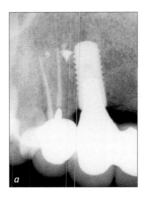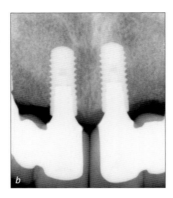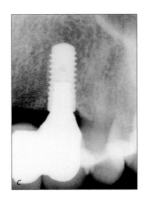

Figs 51a-c   Periapical radiographs at 1-year follow-up.

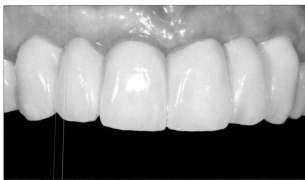

Fig 52   Intraoral situation at the 1-year follow-up.

A recall program was instituted and a radiographic review conducted at the 1-year follow-up (Figs 51 and 52).

7 Complications: Causes, Prevention, and Treatment Options

H. P. Weber, J.-G. Wittneben

7.1   Causes of Complications

7.1.1   Introduction

Along with the growing popularity of dental implants to replace missing teeth, the incidence of related complications of various etiologies has dramatically increased (Froum 2010). This observation also applies to treatments performed in the maxillary anterior segment. In addition, the likelihood of complications related to implants, components, and superstructures is increasing as more and more years of intraoral service are accumulating. Reasons for this growing incidence of complications include:

- A substantial growth in the number of implants placed and restored over the past 10 to 15 years
- An increasing number of dentists placing or restoring dental implants, involving varying levels of knowledge, experience and skills
- Dentists with informal or inadequate education and training are undertaking treatment that is beyond their capabilities
- Implants placed at compromised sites (insufficient bone volume or space)
- Increasing aggressiveness of implant placement and loading protocols
- Non evidence-based information is presented at meetings that may be misleading
- Poor risk assessment or understanding of risks
- Lack of experience in how to handle problems during implant surgery

Malposition of implants is a major cause of complications. In the esthetic zone, the consequences are especially severe. The only modifying factor that may temper patient dissatisfaction with the resultant outcomes is the presence of a low smile line (Figs 1a-d).

Implant malposition may occur for a variety of reasons (Table 1).

7.1.2   Risk Factors for Complications Reported in the Literature

The available evidence for potential risk factors in implant therapy has been assessed as part of the 4th ITI Consensus Conference in 2008 in Stuttgart, Germany. Systematic reviews were prepared on four issues:

- Systemic conditions and treatments as risks for implant therapy
- History of treated periodontitis and smoking as risks for implant therapy
- Mechanical and technical risks in implant therapy
- Local risk factors for implant therapy

Summarizing the findings of these reviews, we must accept that, given the limited volume and quality of published data, true evidence has been provided on a sporadic basis at best. In the context of discussing complications, it is nevertheless relevant to summarize the findings of the 4th ITI Consensus Conference.

Systemic conditions and treatments as risks for implant therapy
Certain systemic conditions may represent biological risk factors in implant therapy. Patients who could benefit from implant treatment in the esthetic zone may present with concomitant systemic diseases. No information pertaining to the use of dental implants is available for many of those systemic conditions. The most substantial body of reports on systemic risks is available for diabetes mellitus, osteoporosis, and radiotherapy (Bornstein and coworkers 2009; Cochran and coworkers 2009). While none of the studies indicate that dental implants should be withheld from patients with diabetes mellitus or osteoporosis, cases involving recent irradiation therapy may require at least a treatment delay. There is also a risk of publication bias and overestimation of success, since numerous articles are based on clinical cases or case series. Furthermore, some patients may present with multiple interrelated risks, making it

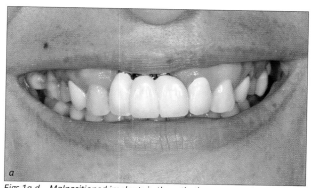
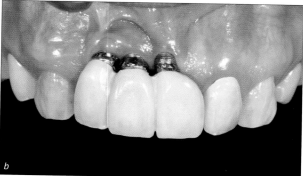

Figs 1a-d   Malpositioned implants in the esthetic zone, associated with severe labial tissue dehiscences, in patients with a high (a-b) or low (c-d) smile line.

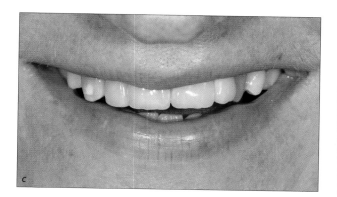
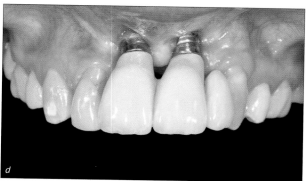

difficult to single out the effects of individual factors. It is therefore important to distinguish between risks of implant failure and risks of medical complications (e.g. bisphosphonate treatment, radiotherapy). Whenever the risk of either is potentially increased, dental implants should be used restrictively and only if specific requirements of patient information have been satisfied.

History of treated periodontitis and smoking as risks for implant therapy

In a review by Heitz-Mayfield and coworkers (2009), cigarette smoking and histories of treated periodontitis were evaluated, both alone and in combination, as risk factors for adverse implant outcomes. Pertinent studies available in the literature were found to be so heterogeneous that their outcomes could not be readily compared. Different definitions as to what constituted presence or absence of periodontitis were used. Where the type of periodontitis was specified at all, it was usually referred to as chronic periodontitis. While all reports stated that periodontal patients had been treated—most of them also indicating that periodic supportive periodontal therapy had been provided—details about the periodontal status were rarely given. A range of definitions for smokers, nonsmokers, and former smokers were used, and few studies reported and adjusted for confounding

Table 1   Potential causes of implant malposition

Inadequate diagnostic information or interpretation
Inadequate treatment planning and communication
Inadequate bone volume
Inadequate horizontal or vertical space
Inadequate template or position of template
Inadequate template
Inadequate implant selection
Inadequate knowledge or experience
Inadequate care, negligence

Table 2   Risk factors for mechanical/technical complications.

• Cantilever extension(s) on fixed dental prostheses	NO
• Cemented versus screw-retained fixed dental prostheses	NO
• Angled abutments	NO
• Bruxism	YES
• Crown-to-implant ratio	NO
• Length (span) of superstructure	YES
• Prosthetic materials	YES

factors. The outcomes that the review could address included implant survival, implant success (as defined by the authors), longitudinal radiographic bone levels, and occurrence of peri-implantitis.

- *History of treated periodontitis.* There is evidence in the literature that patients with a history of periodontitis are at greater risk for peri-implantitis than are patients without a history of periodontitis (reported odds ratios ranged from 3.1 to 4.7). It is important that periodontal disease be treated prior to implant placement.
- *Smoking.* There is strong evidence that smoking is a risk factor for adverse implant outcomes. Smokers have an increased risk of peri-implantitis (reported odds ratios ranged from 3.6 to 4.6) and radiographic marginal bone loss (reported odds ratios ranged from 2.2 to 10) compared to nonsmokers. There is some evidence for a dose effect of cigarette smoking. Nevertheless, smoking is not a contraindication for dental implants. Heavy smokers in particular need to be informed about their increased risk, and every attempt should be made to motivate these patients to quit smoking.
- *History of treated periodontitis and smoking* combined. Few studies have evaluated the effect of smoking combined with histories of periodontitis. There is some evidence for an increased risk of implant failure and bone loss in smokers compared to nonsmokers with a history of treated periodontitis. Again, this condition is not considered an absolute contraindication, but patients need to be informed about the increased risk of implant failure.

Mechanical and technical risks

Certain mechanical and technical risks, as they have been reported in the literature, also apply to the indication of multiple missing teeth in the anterior maxilla. A review by Salvi and Brägger (2009) addressed mechanical/technical risks in implant therapy at large. Some of their findings have implications for the clinical situations discussed in this book. Their review is particularly interesting because it included controlled studies. In other words, the individuals evaluated in those studies were either exposed not exposed to the assessed mechanical or technical risks. Outcome variables included (a) implant-related mechanical and technical risk factors; (b) abutment-related mechanical and technical risk factors; and (c) superstructure-related mechanical and technical risk factors. Depending on the presence or absence of a specific mechanical or technical risk factor, survival and success rates of implants, abutments, and related superstructures were extracted from the publications. Survival was defined as presence of the implant, abutment, or superstructure in its original and extended position with or without complications at any of the follow-up examinations. Success was defined as presence of the implant, abutment, or superstructure without any mechanical or technical complications during the entire follow-up period. Data were grouped in accordance with ten risk factors identified after literature screening. While one risk factor applied only to overdentures, the remaining nine deserve consideration in context with the replacement of multiple missing teeth in the anterior maxilla. Those nine potential risk factors are listed in Table 1 and marked "YES" in the presence of a potentially increased risk or "NO" in its absence (Table 2).

Local risk factors

While the clinical evidence for complications due to local risk factors during replacement of multiple adjacent teeth in the esthetic zone seems obvious and has been reported in case reports and case series (see Chapter 2), the systematic review by Martin and coworkers (2009) revealed that there is little scientific evidence to facilitate clinical decision-making. As mentioned earlier, implant malposition is presumably the greatest risk factor for unfavorable (esthetic) treatment outcomes in the anterior maxilla. The impact of implant malposition on implant or prosthetic survival and success has not been adequately studied even though it is a serious problem for esthetic treatment outcomes.

7.2 Prevention of Complications

Clinicians need to be well aware of potential pitfalls on the road to successful treatment outcomes, notably in the presence of advanced or complex indications for implant treatment, one example being extended edentulism in the anterior maxilla. By identifying the risks and addressing them appropriately in the diagnostic and planning phase, including consultations with or referral to specialist colleagues, numerous esthetic short- or long-term complications may be prevented. It is considerably easier to prevent complications than to treat them.

General and esthetic modifying factors that may influence treatment outcomes in positive or negative ways have been outlined in the book "SAC Classification in Implant Dentistry" by Chen and Dawson (Chen and Dawson 2009 a, Chen and Dawson 2009 b, Chen and coworkers 2009 b). These general and esthetic modifiers—the latter specifically relating to the esthetic zone—form the basis of the SAC Assessment Tool, which is freely accessible on the ITI website (www.iti.org).

Refer to Table 3 for details on general modifiers, which include:

- Clinician's competence and experience
- Compromised patient health
- Growth considerations in children and young adults
- Iatrogenic factors

Table 3   General risk factors for candidates for implant therapy (Buser and coworkers 2004)

Risk Factor	Remarks
Medical	• Severe bone disease causing impaired bone healing • Immunological disease • Medication with steroids • Uncontrolled diabetes mellitus • Irradiated bone • Others
Periodontal	• Active periodontal disease • History of refractive periodontitis • Genetic predisposition
Oral Hygiene/ Compliance	• Home care measured by gingival indices • Personality, intellectual aspects
Occlusion	• Bruxism

Table 4   *Esthetic Risk Assessment (ERA).*

Esthetic Risk Factor	Level of Risk		
	Low	**Moderate**	**High**
Medical status	Healthy, cooperative patient with an intact immune system		Reduced immune system
Smoking habit	Non-smoker	Light smoker (< 10 cigs/day)	Heavy smoker (≥ 10 cigs/day)
Patient's esthetic expectations	Low	Medium	High
Lip line	Low	Medium	High
Gingival biotype	Low-scalloped, thick	Medium-scalloped, medium thick	High-scalloped, thin
Shape of tooth crowns	Rectangular		Triangular
Infection at implant site	None	Chronic	Acute
Bone level at adjacent teeth	≤ 5 mm to contact point	5.5 to 6.5 mm to contact point	≥ 7 mm to contact point
Restorative status of neighboring teeth	Virgin		Restored
Width of edentulous span	1 tooth (≥ 7 mm)	1 tooth (≤ 7 mm)	2 teeth or more
Soft-tissue anatomy	Intact soft tissue		Soft-tissue defects
Bone anatomy of alveolar crest	Alveolar crest without bone deficiency	Horizontal bone deficiency	Vertical bone deficiency

A detailed discussion of esthetic modifiers can also be found in Volume 1 (Implant Therapy in the Esthetic Zone) of the ITI Treatment Guide (Martin and coworkers 2007). The "Esthetic Risk Assessment" (ERA) presented is an extremely useful tool to evaluate the risk of undesirable outcomes in specific treatment situations in the diagnostic and planning stage (Table 4).

Other modifying factors defined in the book "SAC Classification in Implant Dentistry" include surgical modifiers (Chen and coworkers 2009b; Table 5) and restorative modifiers (Dawson and Martin 2009; Tables 6a-b). These considerations further elaborate on the potentially increased risk of (esthetic) complications from the surgical and prosthodontic perspectives.

Table 5   Surgical modifiers.

Site Factors	Risk or Degree of Difficulty		
	Low	**Moderate**	**High**
Bone Volume			
Horizontal	Adequate	Deficient, but allowing simultaneous augmentation	Deficient, requiring prior augmentation
Vertical	Adequate	Small deficiency crestally, requiring slightly deeper corono-apical implant position. Small deficiency apically due to proximity to anatomical structures, requiring shorter than standard implant lengths.	Deficient, requiring prior augmentation
Anatomic Risk			
Proximity to vital anatomic structures	Minimal risk of involvement	Moderate risk of involvement	High risk of involvement
Esthetic Risk			
Esthetic zone	No		Yes
Biotype	Thick		Thin
Thickness of facial bone wall	Sufficient ≥ 1 mm		Insufficient < 1 mm
Complexity			
Number of prior or simultaneous procedures	Implant placement without adjunctive procedures	Implant placement with simultaneous procedures	Implant placement with staged procedures
Complications			
Risk of surgical complications	Minimal	Moderate	High
Consequences of complications	No adverse effect	Suboptimal outcome	Severely compromised outcome

Table 6a   Restorative modifiers (A).

Issue	Notes	Degree of Difficulty		
		Low	Moderate	High
Oral Environment				
General oral health		No active disease		Active disease
Condition of adjacent teeth		Restored teeth		Virgin teeth
Reason for tooth loss		Caries/Trauma		Periodontal disease or occlusal parafunction
Restorative Volume				
Inter-arch distance	Refers to the distance from the proposed implant restorative margin to the opposing occlusion	Adequate for planned restoration	Restricted space, but can be managed	Adjunctive therapy will be necessary to gain sufficient space for the planned restoration
Mesiodistal space	The arch length available to fit tooth replacements	Sufficient to fit replacements for missing teeth	Some reduction in size or number of teeth will be necessary	Adjunctive therapy will be needed to achieve a satisfactory result
Span of restoration		Single tooth	Extended edentulous space	Full arch
Volume and characteristics of the edentulous saddle	Refers to whether there is sufficient tissue volume to support the final restoration, or some prosthetic replacement of soft tissues will be necessary.	No prosthetic soft-tissue replacement will be necessary		Prosthetic replacement of soft tissue will be needed for esthetics or phonetics

Table 6b   Restorative modifiers (B).

Issue	Notes	Degree of Difficulty		
		Low	Moderate	High
Occlusion				
Occlusal scheme		Anterior guidance		No guidance
Involvement in occlusion	The degree to which the implant prosthesis is involved in the patient's occlusal scheme	Minimal involvement		Implant restoration is involved in guidance
Occlusal parafunction	Risk of complication to the restoration, but not to implant survival	Absent		Present
Provisional Restorations				
During implant healing		None required	Removable	Fixed
Implant-supported provisionals needed	Provisional restorations will be needed to develop esthetics and soft tissue transition zones	Not required	Restorative margin < 3 mm apical to mucosal crest	Restorative margin ≥ 3 mm apical to mucosal crest
Loading protocol	To date immediate restoration and loading procedures are lacking scientific documentation	Conventional or early loading		Immediate loading
Materials/manufacture	Materials and techniques used in the manufacture of definitive prostheses	Resin-based materials ± metal reinforcement	Porcelain fused to metal	
Maintenance needs	Anticipated maintenance needs based on patient presentation and the planned prosthesis	Low	Moderate	High

7.3 Management of Complications— Clinical Case Presentations

Given the multifaceted etiology of complications, it would be beyond the scope of this ITI Treatment Guide to address comprehensively the treatment options available for any type of complication. What follows is a sequence of clinical case presentations that will illustrate a number of different complications and their treatment, imparting to clinicians an understanding of some of the associated "troubleshooting" concepts.

7.3.1 The Consequences of Non-Retrievability in Implant-Supported Fixed Prosthodontics

S. Scheuber, U. Braegger

Introduction
Technical failures and complications may occur when implant-supported restorations are exposed to function in the oral cavity. In a recent review (Salvi and Braegger 2009), the conclusion has been drawn that long-term studies on the survival and success of implant-supported restorations should report any observed events separately depending on whether they affect mechanical devices such as implants and components on the one hand, or laboratory-fabricated restorations on the other.

Several systematic reviews combined data from original articles to calculate the estimated events per 100 objects and per year of exposure to risk (Pjetursson and coworkers 2007). On this basis, meaningful statistical evaluations can be performed and evidence-based conclusions drawn for clinical decision-making (Pjetursson and Lang 2008). Some cohorts that included restorations of a specific de-

sign showed increased rates of adverse events compared to other designs (Lang and coworkers 2004; Aglietta and coworkers 2009; Stafford 2010). Identifying risk factors, however, would require direct prospective comparison of cases exposed to a certain condition versus cases not exposed to that condition (Salvi and Braegger 2009).

Numerous essential aspects in the cascade of events leading to technical and mechanical failures or complications, however, remain obscure and were neither controlled for nor reported in the clinical long-term studies mentioned. This includes the role of process standardization related to the equipment and materials used in dental laboratories. Human error, too, may lead to incorrect clinical handling of components or materials.

Given the growing number of cases treated daily and the different levels of expertise on the part of users, a number of errors and misguided decisions are bound to occur in the fabrication of implant-supported restorations. This phenomenon has already been addressed in some reports on the learning curve experienced by centers starting to offer implant surgery.

From a practical point of view, it seems reasonable to prefer retrievable implant-supported restorations, as these will facilitate the clinical procedures needed to initiate repair or refabrication, in addition to being less stressful for the patient. This logic will, of course, only apply if the retrievability itself does not subject the restoration to increased risk.

The purpose of this case report is to present the remake of an implant-supported restoration and to discuss and propose ways to reduce risks and improve quality control in implant-based fixed prosthodontics.

Case presentation

A 39-year-old woman was in need of replacing teeth 11, 21, and 22, which had been lost due to trauma. She also exhibited chronic periodontitis.

The patient consented to being treated as part of an undergraduate dental medicine class (University of Bern, Switzerland). As an incentive for participation, she received treatment at a reduced cost. The expenses for the instructors' contributions (i.e. implant placement, materials, laboratory steps) were covered by an accident insurance company. Tutors and senior clinical instructors were present to supervise treatment planning and all steps executed by the undergraduates.

After initial periodontal and restorative treatment, the patient received two 12-mm bone-level implants (Straumann Bone Level, SLActive, diameter 4.1 mm, length 12 mm) at sites 11 and 22. The surgical procedure was performed by a senior instructor for oral surgery, using a surgical splint indicating the ideal implant positions for a transocclusally screw-retained prosthesis. However, the actual positions at which the implant ended up after healing precluded the use of transocclusal screws for retention of the fixed partial denture.

The treatment plan was changed to a cemented ceramic prosthesis retained by two customized Regular CrossFit (RC) zirconia abutments. The final impression was taken with customized impression posts using an open-tray technique. Customized abutments were shaped with CAD software and milled in a CAD/CAM center (CARES; Straumann, Basel, Switzerland). For use on top of the abutments, a separate zirconia framework was designed and milled by CAD/CAM. The veneering was accomplished by manual layering of a feldspathic ceramic.

Several try-ins were performed. Following active participation by and information given to the patient, it was decided to proceed with cementation of the ceramic restoration (Figs 1 and 2). The zirconia abutments were torqued to 35 Ncm and the access holes for the abutment screws closed. Despite the use of a zirconia framework, the instructors were concerned about delivering the fixed partial denture with a temporary cement. The crucial error committed at this point was to use an adhesive cement (Panavia 21; Kuraray Medical, Frankfurt, Germany). Residual cement was eliminated, the patient given instructions for home care, and a radiograph taken for post-delivery verification (Fig 3).

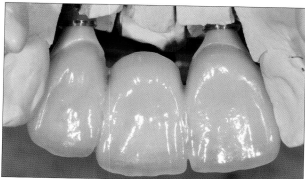

Fig 1 The laboratory work included two CARES zirconia abutments on bone-level implants at sites 11 and 22 and a fixed partial denture with a CAD/CAM zirconia framework. Veneering was accomplished by manual layering of feldspathic ceramics.

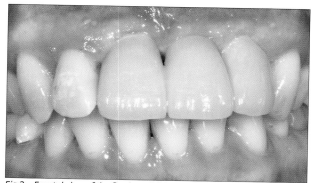

Fig 2 Frontal view of the fixed partial denture during try-in. Both the prosthesis (color, shape, contour) and the mucosal conditions were considered acceptable by the instructors. The patient also accepted the prosthesis.

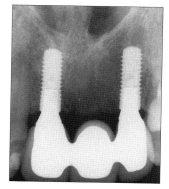

Fig 3 Radiograph obtained after delivery of the final prosthesis. Precise marginal fit and ideal peri-implant bone levels.

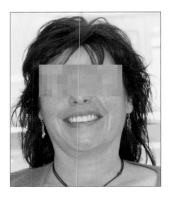

Fig 4 Smile line with the final prosthesis. Unfortunately, the fixed partial denture had already been cemented with Panavia (Kuraray Medical, Frankfurt, Germany) after torqueing the abutments to 35 Ncm and covering the access hole for the abutment screw. The restoration appeared bulky, artificial, and unsightly.

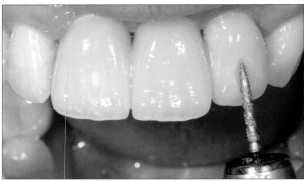

Fig 5 Special-purpose diamond cutters for application to high-density ceramics were used to find the access holes to the CARES abutment screws.

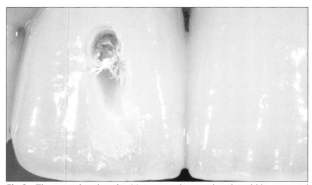

Fig 6 The screw head at site 11 was not damaged and could be removed with the screwdriver.

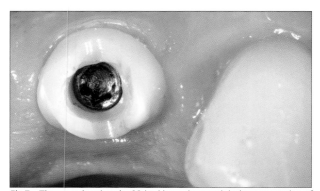

Fig 7 The screw head at site 22 had been damaged during preparation of the abutment and could not be handled with a regular screwdriver.

When the patient returned for the follow-up 1 week later, she was extremely dissatisfied and insisted that the restoration should be removed. In particular, she demanded a different shade. A second opinion was also requested by the course director.

On reassessing the situation using objective esthetic parameters, the fixed partial denture was considered unacceptable. There was a need for better adaptation of color, shape, and contour to the clinical situation (Fig 4).

At this juncture, retrieving the prosthesis turned out to be a challenge. It was necessary to inform the patient about the consequences of this dilemma, about the procedures and time requirements, and about the worst-case scenario of having to remake the superstructure from scratch. However, it was made clear from the outset that none of this would have financial implications for the patient.

After scheduling the patient for a special open-ended session, all necessary equipment was prepared. A special service set (Straumann, Basel, Switzerland) was ordered well ahead of time.

In a first attempt, the fixed partial denture was gripped with rubber-protected forceps and tapped. However, the superstructure would not move. The second attempt was to attach the slings of a Coronaflex system (CORONAflex; KaVo Dental, Brugg, Switzerland) underneath the pontic. Even at maximum intensity, the shocks of the instrument had no effect at all.

The third attempt was to use special-purpose diamond cutters from a service kit (Jota, Rüthi, Switzerland) to separate the zirconia framework and to find the access holes for the abutment screws. The access hole at implant site 11 was uncovered and could be removed with a screwdriver. At implant site 22, however, the screw head was damaged and could not be handled with a regular screwdriver (Figs 5 to 7).

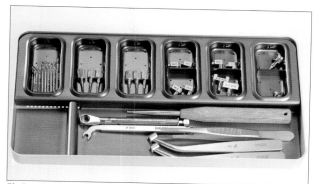

Fig 8a   Service set basic kit.

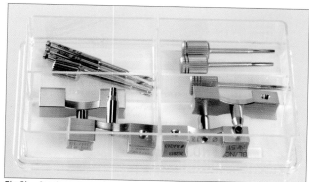

Fig 8b   Service set supplement for bone-level prosthetics.

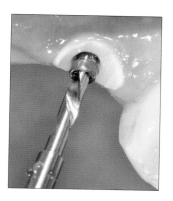

After cutting the zirconia abutment almost entirely down to the mucosa, a special stainless-steel drill from the service kit (Fig 8a-b) was applied to cut an access directly into the head of the abutment screw.

Fig 9   A stainless-steel drill was applied counterclockwise at low speed. Liberal cooling was used to avoid propagation of heat.

The Straumann Service Set is comprised of a basic kit and four supplemental kits, which are provided upon request to retrieve any damaged prosthetic components. It comes with a brochure giving step-by-step instructions. It is also recommended to request service support by an instructor from the manufacturer of the implant system.

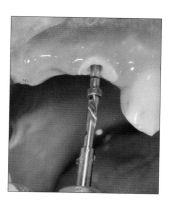

As the preparations had been made counterclockwise, it was assumed that the vibration could lead to the loosening of the abutment screw. Drilling under continuous cooling with a spray is mandatory to avoid heat development in the implant body (Brägger and coworkers 1995). The drilling speed needs to be controlled and should not exceed 600 rpm. Otherwise the sharp edges of the drills are not capable of effectively cutting into titanium (Figs 9 to 11). In the case described here, the screw became mobile and could be easily removed.

Fig 10   The abutment screw was mobilized by the drilling process and was unscrewed by counterclockwise rotation from the implant.

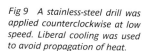

Fig 11   The torque applied was sufficient to mobilize the component.

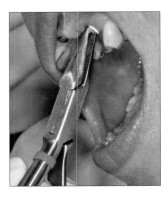

Fig 12   The residual base of the CARES (Straumann, Basel, Switzerland) abutment was removed with forceps.

Had the screw still persisted in the inserted abutment, "extraction bolts" contained in the Straumann Service Set would have been used to apply reverse torque undoing the abutment screw via a ratchet.

Due to the tight friction of the CrossFit connection (Straumann, Basel, Switzerland), the residual fragment had to be removed with a forceps (Fig 12).

Now that the patient was able to wear a screw-retained provisional prosthesis, she was scheduled for a complete remake of the CARES abutments (Straumann, Basel, Switzerland) and provision with a new implant-supported fixed partial denture. As the 3D data of the abutments and CAD/CAM framework were still available, the technician could reorder the same components and the framework. This time, however, retrievability was ensured by the use of temporary cement (Temp Bond; Kerr Scafati, Italy). This choice was prompted by the biomechanical stability of both the zirconia abutments and the prosthetic framework. The patient was pleased by the new restoration, which significantly improved the situation (Figs 13 to 16).

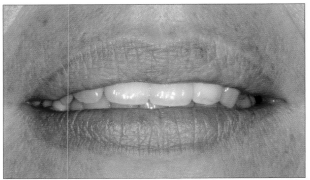

Fig 13   Perioral view of the patient's smile. Pleasing appearance of the new prosthesis.

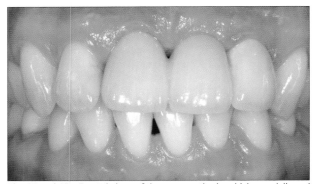

Figs 14 and 15   Frontal views of the new prosthesis, which was delivered with temporary cement and can be retrieved if required.

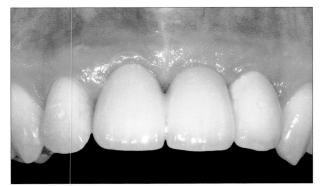

Fig 15

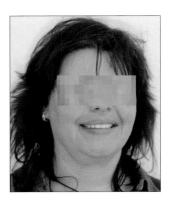

Fig 16   Portrait of the patient with her new retrievable prosthesis replacing teeth 11, 21, 22.

Discussion

Mechanical/technical complications and failures may occur at the level of the implant, the abutment, the occlusal screw or cement line, or the superstructure. Events should be expected to occur more frequently in the presence of specific reconstructive designs, abutment distributions, anatomical conditions, and functional disturbances.

The consequences of these events may be minor in some cases, being confined to requiring additional service time, and may be catastrophic in others.

Over the past decade, cases of abutment/screw loosening and fracture have declined in number due to progress made in implant manufacturing and design (Theoharidou and coworkers 2008).

Veneer fractures are clearly the most common events observed with metal-ceramic and ceramic structures, and they occur more frequently on implant-supported than tooth-supported restorations (Pjetursson and coworkers 2007). Areas damaged by cohesive chipping can often be polished, while areas damaged by adhesive chipping may expose the framework and create an esthetic problem requiring a remake.

Retrieving a single-tooth restoration or a fixed partial denture that has been delivered with a definitive cement may not be possible without damaging the structure. Retrieving a blocked or fractured abutment/screw without damaging the implant is a truly challenging task, particularly if the screwdriver can no longer engage the screw head.

Luterbacher and coworkers (2000) reported on how a Service Set was used to retrieve two broken synOcta abutments (Straumann Dental Implant System). Their step-by-step approach consisted of assembling the guide devices to locate the center of the implant, guided drilling through the fractured part of the component remaining in the implant, and removal of residual metal particles in the implant by means of taps.

Only one drill was needed to handle this complication by removing the damaged component. Ever since bone-level implants were first introduced, the service set has been supplemented to include special-purpose drills and guide devices to fit onto and into the CrossFit connection (Straumann, Basel, Switzerland). The main purpose of these precision instruments is to avoid damaging the threads in the internal connection of both bone-level and tissue-level implants. It is very important to follow the instructions in the manuals supplied with the Service Set. None of the steps must be omitted.

Any chain of events resulting in failure of a non-retrievable restoration can have enormous financial implications. In the case described here, at least the remakes of the abutments and the framework were accomplished with relative ease, as the same 3D designs could be reordered from the production center. It should be emphasized, however, that this may be not always be possible, notably if the soft-tissue contour has changed in the meantime. Also, some fine adjustments will need to be performed on the abutments supplied by the production center. In other cases, the abutments will have to be designed from scratch, requiring initiation of a wholly new CAD/CAM process for the framework.

The availability of the service set customized for a particular implant system helps to mitigate worst-case scenarios. By following the step-by-step instructions in removing any blocked or fractured components, it will be possible to solve almost any problem that may conceivably occur in clinical practice.

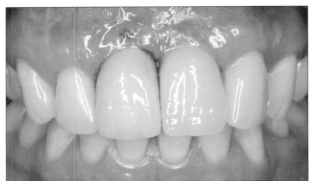

Fig 1   Draining sinus associated with implant 11.

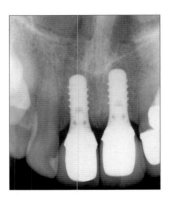

Fig 2   Periapical radiograph obtained after cementation of the crowns in 2005. Radiopaque material (cement) at the crown margin on implant 11.

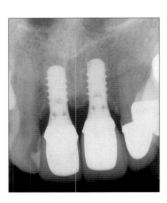

Fig 3   Periapical radiograph taken in 2009. Crestal bone loss.

7.3.2   Treatment of Peri-Implant Infection at Adjacent Implant-Supported Single Crowns

L. Heitz-Mayfield

A 45-year-old woman was referred for management of an infection associated with two implant-supported crowns replacing the maxillary central incisors. Two tissue-level implants had been placed and restored with cemented single metal-ceramic crowns in those sites 4 years previously.

The patient presented with a draining sinus (i.e. a pathological duct from an abscess cavity to a surface) 3 mm from the midfacial peri-implant mucosal margin of the maxillary right implant crown (Fig 1). She was in good general health, did not smoke, showed a good oral hygiene status, and had no history of periodontal disease. The implants were well positioned. While the patient was very satisfied with the appearance of her crowns, she had noted that the peri-implant soft tissue had receded since their insertion and was concerned about the possibility of further recession.

A clinical examination revealed probing depths of 4 – 5 mm with bleeding on gentle probing. The patient had a thin gingival biotype. A radiograph showed crestal bone levels apical to the rough-smooth interface of the implants approximating the first thread of the implant. In comparison with a radiograph taken after cementation of the crowns in 2005 (Fig 2), it was apparent that there had been bone loss over the past 4 years.

While the radiograph obtained upon presentation of the patient in 2009 (Fig 3) did not show any cement remnants at the crown margins, some remnants were visible in the 2005 radiograph taken immediately after cementation of the crowns. This residual cement may have initiated the peri-implant infection.

The patient was informed that treatment would likely be associated with recession of the peri-implant mucosa and that some titanium may be visible after treatment, the plan being to provide non-surgical management with adjunctive antimicrobial therapy. She was informed that surgical access for assessment and decontamination of the implant surface may be required if a conservative approach to resolving the infection would fail. The patient was also informed of potential side effects of systemic antibiotics. The treatment provided included oral hygiene instructions using floss and a soft manual toothbrush. Following local anesthesia, submucosal debridement with titanium-coated curettes was performed, and the patient was prescribed systemic antibiotics (metronidazole 3×400 mg/d and amoxicillin 3×500 mg/d for 7 days). She was instructed to apply chlorhexidine digluconate 0.2% to the affected region with an ultra-soft toothbrush for 2 weeks.

Four weeks after treatment, the draining sinus had resolved with reductions in probing depth and no more bleeding on probing. While some mucosal recession had occurred, there was no exposure of the titanium margin (Fig 4).

The patient was reviewed at 3-month intervals. At the 9-month follow-up, additional recession was noted, this time involving exposure of the titanium margin (Figs 5 and 6).

The patient was informed that an attempt at soft-tissue grafting could be made to cover the exposed metal margin. Another possibility would be to replace the implant-supported crown after preparation of the implant shoulder to below the level of the peri-implant mucosa. She opted against these treatment modalities, as the metal margin did not show in her smile.

The patient has maintained good oral hygiene and has been seen every 6 months for monitoring and maintenance.

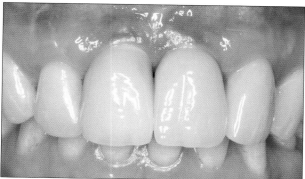

Fig 4   Close-up view 4 weeks after treatment. The peri-implant tissue was healthy, as the inflammation and the draining sinus had resolved.

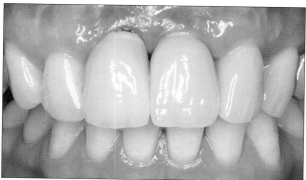

Fig 5   Close-up view 9 months after non-surgical treatment. The peri-implant tissue was healthy. Exposed titanium margin.

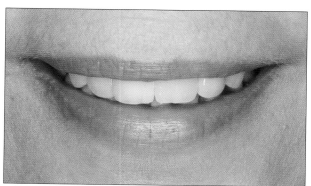

Fig 6   View of the patient's smile line.

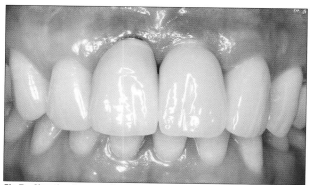

Fig 7   Situation 2 years after treatment. Healthy peri-implant tissues and stable mucosal margin.

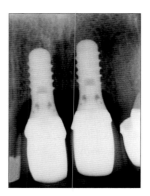

Fig 8   Radiograph taken 1 year after non-surgical treatment.

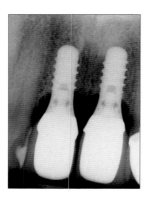

Fig 9   Radiograph taken 2 years after non-surgical treatment.

Two years after treatment, the peri-implant mucosal margin was stable, and there was continued peri-implant health (Fig 7). Radiographs taken 1 and 2 years after treatment indicated stable crestal bone levels (Figs 8 and 9).

7.3.3 Replacement of Failing Hydroxyapatite-Coated Cylinder-Type Implants with Bone-Level Implants and a Screw-Retained Fixed Partial Denture in the Anterior Maxilla

S. Keith, G. Conte

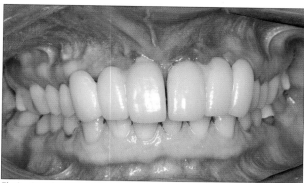

Fig 1   Anterior view of the existing implant-supported three-unit prostheses.

This 49-year-old woman was referred for treatment by her general dentist with the request that she be evaluated for her "failing implants." This very cooperative patient presented for care with no significant medical conditions, no known drug allergies, and was not taking any prescription medications. She did report a history of mild insomnia in the previous 7 years and was taking a multi-vitamin supplement in addition to over-the-counter vitamin D and calcium supplements. She complained of mild discomfort and swelling around her dental implants and occasional foul taste and unpleasant aroma in her mouth. A thorough history and examination revealed no evidence of parafunctional habits or temporomandibular joint disorder.

A complete oral examination and full mouth radiographic series revealed four press-fit type, cylinder-shaped dental implants in the maxillary canine (sites 13 and 23) and central incisor (sites 11 and 21) positions. The implants were supporting two three-unit fixed partial dentures, each extending from canine to central incisor (Fig 1). The patient reported that the implants had been placed about 20 years before. The radiographic presentation and timing of placement seemed consistent with typical hydroxyapatite- (HA-) coated press-fit cylinder-type implants (Figs 2a-d). All four implants showed radiographic evidence of extensive bone loss, with periapical radiolucency surrounding most of the two anterior implants (sites 11 and 21). There was slight mobility of the two implant-retained fixed partial dentures, gingival edema, and absence of attached keratinized tissue. Apical palpation of the area elicited discomfort and produced a purulent exudate from the peri-implant sulcus (Fig 1).

The patient's existing metal-ceramic restorations were overcontoured and protruded facially. She had never been completely satisfied with the appearance of the prostheses. Her chief complaint was general discomfort around the implants and a more recent sensation that the teeth had shifted position. The patient suspected that the chronic, low-grade inflammatory process around her implants might have contributed to the development of insomnia over the previous few years.

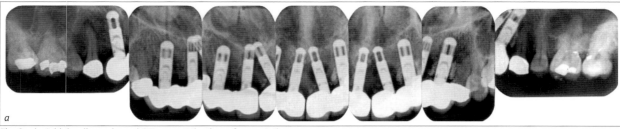

Figs 2a-d   Initial radiographs and CT scans at the time of presentation.

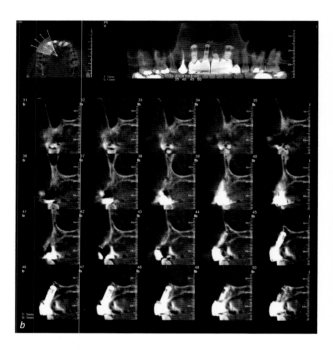

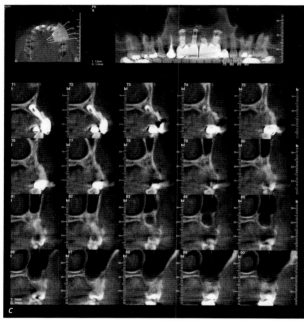

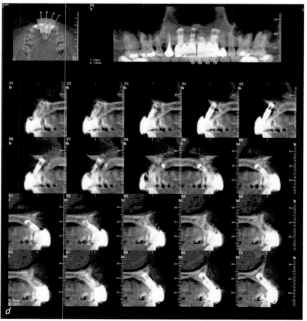

Following a complete clinical examination and an evaluation of mounted study casts, the patient was advised of the various treatment options available. She fully understood that the existing implants and fixed partial dentures would need to be removed and that the area would require a multi-stage approach to the eventual fixed restoration. Once all of her questions regarding the phases of treatment and overall treatment duration had been answered, she agreed to the following treatment plan.

The existing HA cylinder implants were to be surgically removed and the residual structures of the alveolar ridge to be reconstructed by guided bone regeneration (GBR). A transitional removable prosthesis would be fabricated for delivery at the time of implant removal and bone grafting. Upon completion of preliminary soft-tissue healing, a secondary transitional removable partial denture would be fabricated for use throughout the remainder of the healing period. Two standard-diameter, bone-level implants would be placed in the maxillary canine positions (sites 13 and 23). After an appropriate healing interval, soft tissue maturation and gingival emergence would be achieved using an acrylic-resin, six-unit, provisional fixed partial denture on temporary implant abutments. Finally, the definitive metal-ceramic prosthesis would be fabricated, adjusted, and delivered to satisfy the patient's functional and esthetic demands and to return her to a state of oral health.

Treatment was started by surgery to remove the existing failing implants, to reconstruct the damaged alveolar process, and to prepare the site for future implant placement. The patient began a course of preoperative amoxicillin (3 × 500 mg/d) starting on the day before the procedure. After removal of the palatal fixation screws, the existing fixed partial dentures were unseated (Fig 3). This exposed the underlying mesostructures connected to the failing implants (Fig 4). Under local anesthesia, a crestal incision was performed and a full-thickness mucoperiosteal flap elevated to expose the implants and osseous defects (Fig 5). The existing implants were carefully removed using a trephine and luxation to separate the last few millimeters of apical bone-implant contact. The various legacy implants, abutment screws, and components used in this dental restoration from 1989 demonstrated what had been state of the art in implant dentistry at that early stage (Fig 6). The site was thoroughly debrided of residual granulation tissue and irrigated with copious amounts of sterile saline solution (Fig 7).

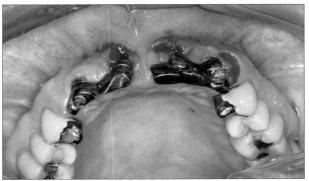
Fig 3 Removal of fixed partial dentures revealing underlying mesostructures.

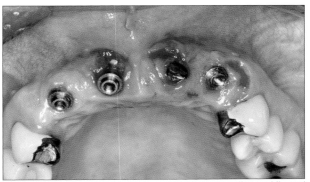
Fig 4 Removal of screw-retained mesostructures revealing mobile and infected legacy implants.

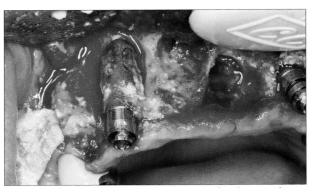
Fig 5 Elevation of a full-thickness flap demonstrating the expansive nature of osseous defects around the remaining implants.

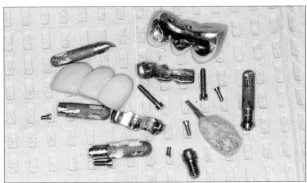
Fig 6 Hardware from failing implant-supported prostheses.

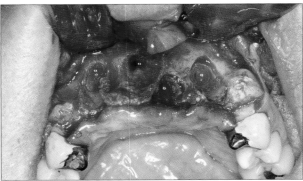
Fig 7 Situation after implant removal and site degranulation.

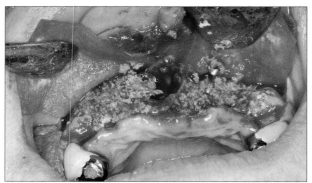

Fig 8 Titanium bone-tenting screws in place with defect grafted using human cancellous allograft and platelet derived growth factor.

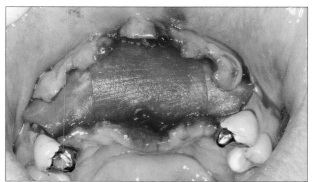

Fig 9 Double layers of a resorbable collagen barrier membrane in place over the graft material.

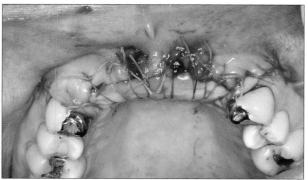

Fig 10 Primary closure of site with multiple interrupted sutures.

The site was prepared for guided bone regeneration (GBR) with three titanium tenting screws 1.5 × 8 mm (Ace Surgical, Brockton, MA, USA). The residual defect was grafted with a combination of large-particle, human cancellous bone allograft (Puros, Zimmer, Carlsbad, CA, USA) that had been saturated with platelet-derived growth factor-β (Gem-21; Osteohealth, Shirley, NY, USA) (Fig 8). The graft material was covered with a double layer of slowly resorbing collagen barrier membrane (BioMend Extend; Zimmer, Carlsbad, CA, USA) (Fig 9). A high periosteal release of the mobilized soft-tissue flap allowed for tension-free closure of the site with multiple interrupted sutures (Fig 10).

A tooth-supported transitional Essix-type removable partial denture was adjusted and delivered for esthetic replacement of the missing maxillary anterior teeth in the early healing phase of treatment (Fig 11). This allowed healing to proceed without loading on the grafted site. After about 6 weeks of initial healing, new impressions were made, followed by delivery of a more traditional tissue-supported removable partial denture for better comfort and esthetics (Fig 12).

Following 6 months of healing (Fig 13), a new impression of the maxillary arch allowed the fabrication of a radiographic guide. A diagnostic wax-up of the extended edentulous area from site 13 to site 23 revealed limited space in a mesiodistal dimension. An attempt to place four implants would yield the same difficulties encountered with the original failed restoration. It was decided that only two implants would be placed in the canine positions to restore the six missing teeth with a single implant-supported fixed partial denture (Fig 14). A CT scan was taken to evaluate the volume and quality of bone in the anterior maxilla and to confirm the location and angulation of the proposed implant sites in the canine positions (Figs 15a-c).

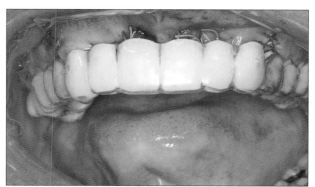

Fig 11 Removable (tooth-supported, clear, vacuform-type) partial denture for temporary use.

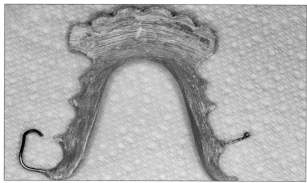

Fig 12 Transitional removable partial denture (subsequent version).

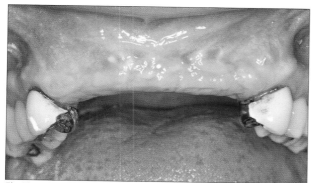

Fig 13 Edentulous anterior maxilla 6 months following implant removal and guided bone regeneration.

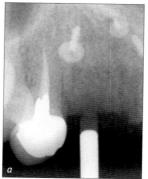
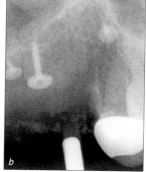

Fig 14 Periapical radiographs showing the planned implant positions with radiographic markers in place.

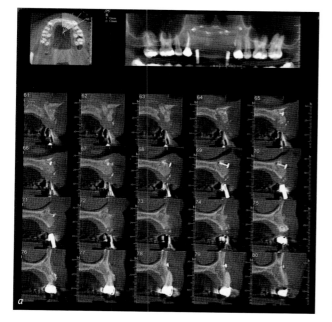

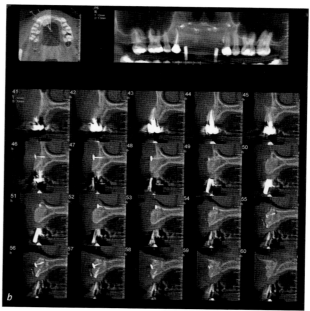

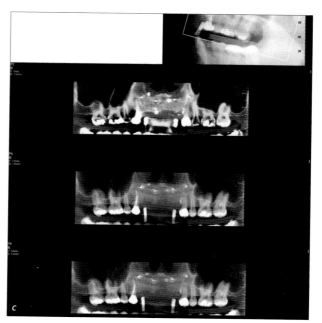

Figs 15a-c CT scan to evaluate three-dimensional anatomy in areas of planned implant placement.

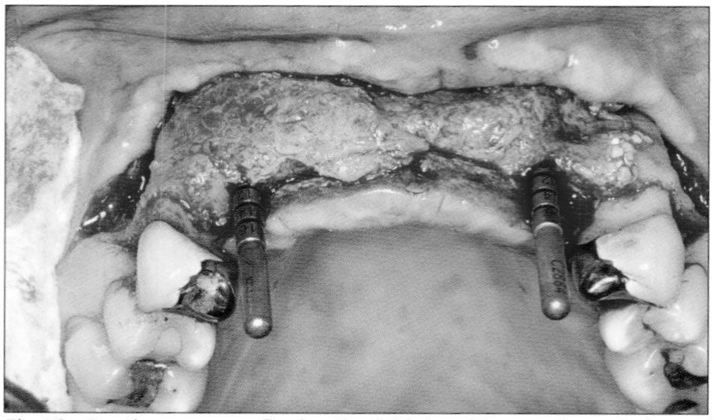

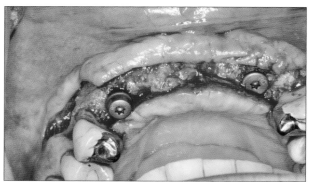

Fig 16   Depth gauges confirming the initial positions and angulations of the osteotomies.

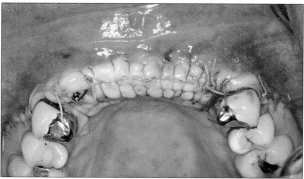

Fig 17   Implants and 4.3-mm "bottle-shaped" healing abutments in place.

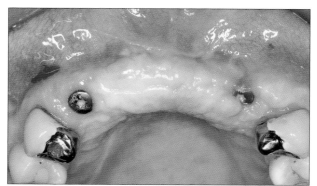

Fig 18   Semi-submerged closure after implant placement.

A surgical template assisted in locating the desired implant sites (Fig 16). Osteotomies were prepared at 650 RPM drilling speed with a surgical motor (Nouvag, Lake Hughes, CA, USA) and chilled sterile saline irrigation. The two implants (Straumann Bone Level, SLActive, Regular CrossFit, diameter 4.1 mm, length 12 mm) were placed using a hand ratchet to assess and confirm primary stability (Fig 17). The implant mounts were used to confirm the positions and were then replaced by healing abutments. The tissue was then re-approximated in a semi-submerged approach (Fig 18).

The patient's existing transitional prosthesis was adjusted to relieve the areas over the implant sites. She was given postoperative instructions and completed another course of amoxicillin (3 × 500 mg/d for 7 days), followed by rinsing with chlorhexidine digluconate (2 × 0.12%).

The patient was recalled for suture removal at 10 days and for periapical radiographs to assess healing of the implant sites at 6 weeks. After 10 weeks of undisturbed healing, the prosthetic restoration phase was initiated (Fig 19). Following limited infiltration of a local anesthetic, the healing abutments were removed without incident and replaced with Regular CrossFit (RC) provisional mesoabutments (Straumann, Basel, Switzerland) (Fig 20). The implants were deemed well healed and osseointegrated with the delivery of a 35-Ncm seating torque on the mesoabutments. The mesoabutments were prepared in situ using a high-speed handpiece and diamond burs under air-water spray to create a finish line that was only slightly (0.5 mm) subgingival on the facial aspect (Fig 21). A laboratory-processed, metal-wire-reinforced, acrylic-resin, provisional fixed partial denture was relined to fit over the mesoabutments. The screw access holes in the provisional mesoabutments were closed with a cotton pellet and soft-setting composite resin. The provisional restoration was delivered with a temporary luting agent. During this time, the patient was able to evaluate the provisional restoration for esthetic and functional parameters of tooth shape and arrangement, incisal edge position, and phonetics (Fig 22).

Fig 19   Healing status 10 weeks after implant placement.

After a 6-week period, a mature soft-tissue architecture had developed around the implant sites (Fig 23), and a master impression was made using a polyvinyl siloxane material (Take-1; Kerr Dental, Orange, CA, USA) in a custom tray. Using a new soft-tissue cast (Resin Rock, Whip Mix Corporation, Louisville, KY) and a cast of the temporary restoration, the laboratory technician started fabricating the final prosthesis. It was determined from the master cast that a six-unit fixed partial denture could be supported on two non-engaging UCLA-type gold abutments (RC gold abutments, non-engaging, Straumann; Straumann, Basel, Switzerland). The framework was waxed up in two separate units, then invested and cast using a traditional method. The metal was finished and reassembled on the solid master cast with pattern resin and delivered to the office for clinical verification.

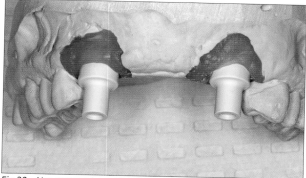

Fig 20   Non-prepared provisional mesoabutments for RC Bone Level implants.

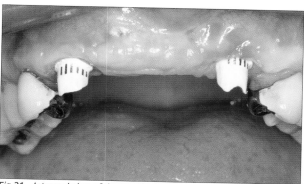

Fig 21   Intraoral view of the modified mesoabutments for RC Bone Level implants.

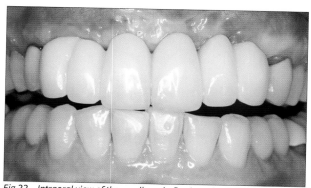

Fig 22   Intraoral view of the acrylic-resin fixed provisional restoration over temporary mesoabutments.

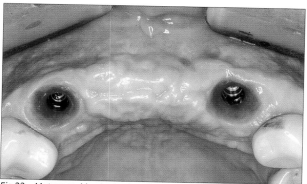

Fig 23   Mature peri-implant sulcus formation following 6 weeks under the temporary restoration.

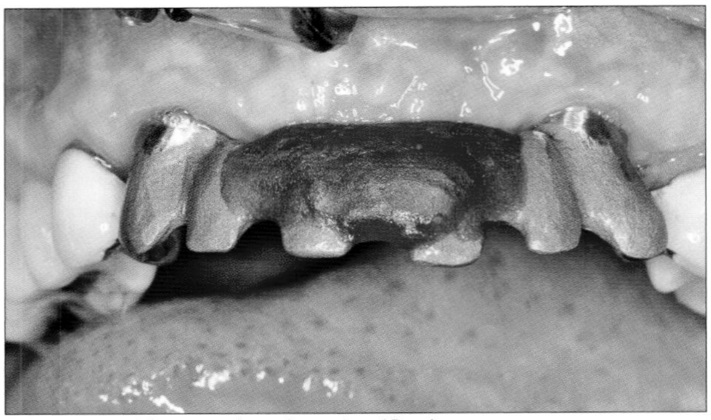

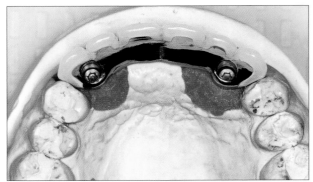

Fig 24   Metal framework try-in and verification.

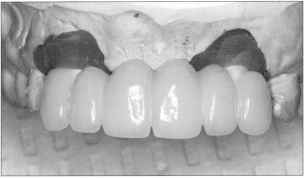

Fig 25   Screw-retained metal-ceramic fixed partial denture.

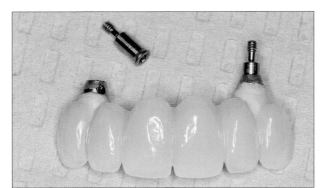

Fig 26   Six-unit fixed partial denture.

An appointment was made to try in the metal framework for the screw-retained fixed partial denture (Fig 24). Radiographs were used to confirm passive seating of the metal framework, and a new centric jaw relation record was made as well. The framework was removed and the provisional restoration replaced. Diagnostic photos were recorded for shade verification. The framework was returned to the dental laboratory for soldering and ceramic application (Figs 25 to 27).

Then the final implant-supported metal-ceramic fixed partial denture was prepared for delivery. The provisional restoration and the temporary mesoabutments were removed.

The final prosthesis was tried in and the implant-abutment passive fit confirmed with periapical radiographs (Fig 28). Articulating paper was used to evaluate and adjust the proximal and occlusal contacts. The prosthesis was evaluated for esthetics and phonetics, and the patient approved the result. After finishing and polishing, the prosthesis was returned to the mouth and delivered using 35 Ncm of measured torque on each abutment screw (Figs 29a-b). New impressions were taken with the prosthesis in place to fabricate a maxillary occlusal guard for overnight use. Home care and oral hygiene instructions were reviewed with the patient, including the use of a floss threader for plaque removal under the pontics.

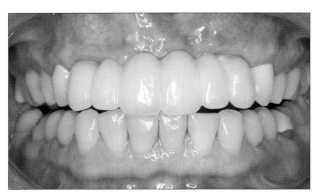

Fig 28   Intraoral view of the implant-supported fixed prosthesis upon delivery.

Fig 27   Construction of prosthesis using non-engaging gold abutments and larger abutment screws that intimately fit into the internal CrossFit prosthetic connection of bone-level implants.

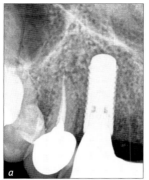
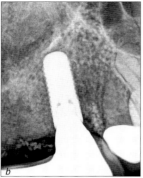

Figs 29a-b   Periapical radiographs of the prosthesis upon delivery.

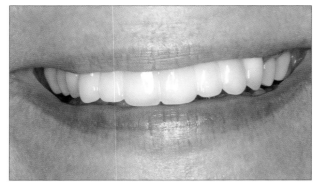

Fig 30   View of the final prosthesis in the patient's full smile.

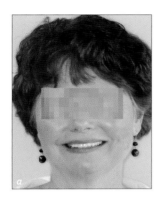

Figs 31a-b   Three-year follow-up.

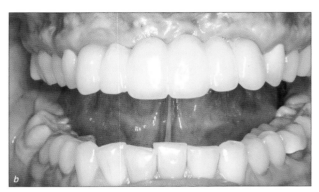

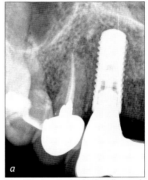
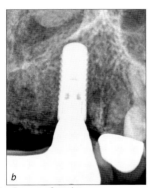

Figs 32a-b   Periapical radiographs after 3 years of service.

The patient was recalled at 1 week to re-evaluate gingival response and to check occlusal contacts. The maxillary occlusal guard was adjusted and delivered. Also, a review of oral hygiene procedures was completed. The patient reported her satisfaction with the esthetic and functional outcome of her treatment (Fig 30). After 6 weeks, she was recalled to remove the temporary filling material from the abutment access holes. A torque wrench was used to confirm that the abutment screws remained tightened to 35 Ncm. At this point, cotton pellets were placed over the abutment screws, and the access holes were closed with a more durable composite-resin material.

Further reevaluation appointments took place after 6 and 12 months. No complications or changes in radiographic bone levels were noted. After more than 3 years of service, the patient continues to report satisfaction with her prosthesis (Figs 31a-b and 32a-b).

Acknowledgments

Laboratory procedures
Dental Technician H. Hansen – Parkview Dental Lab, Brisbane, CA, USA

7.3.4   Replacement of Teeth 12 and 13 with Tissue-Level Implants

W. Martin, J. Ruskin

In 2001, a 48-year-old woman presented at a dental clinic with a failing fixed partial denture spanning from teeth 13 to 21. She was experiencing pain upon function, tenderness to palpation facial to tooth 13, and severe mobility of the prosthesis. Radiographic and clinical assessment revealed a subcrestal fracture of tooth 13,

making its restoration unlikely (Fig 1). It was determined by the clinician that the tooth needed to be extracted prior to proceeding any further with dental care. After the extraction, the patient lost confidence in the progression of her treatment and sought consultation at the Center for Implant Dentistry.

At her consultation visit in our clinic, an extra- and intraoral clinical examination revealed a medium lip line at full smile and an edentulous area spanning from 13 to 12 with both vertical and horizontal deficits in hard and soft tissue (Figs 2 to 4).

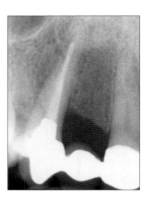

Fig 1   Pretreatment periapical radiograph.

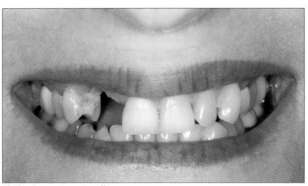

Fig 2   Pretreatment smile.

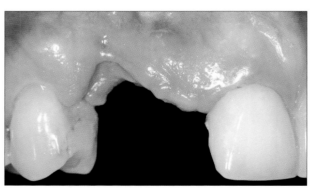

Fig 3   Lateral view of edentulous span 12 and 13.

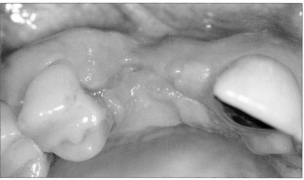

Fig 4   Occlusal view.

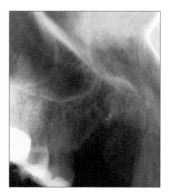

Fig 5   Pretreatment periapical radiograph.

Table 1   Esthetic Risk Assessment (ERA).

Esthetic Risk Factor	Level of Risk		
	Low	Moderate	High
Medical status	Healthy, co-operative patient with an intact immune system.		Reduced immune system
Smoking habit	Non-smoker	Light smoker (< 10 cigs/day)	Heavy smoker ≥ 10 cigs/day)
Patient's esthetic expectations	Low	Medium	High
Lip line	Low	Medium	High
Gingival biotype	Low scalloped, thick	Medium scalloped, medium thick	High scalloped, thin
Shape of tooth crowns	Rectangular		Triangular
Infection at implant site	None	Chronic	Acute
Bone level at adjacent teeth	≤ 5 mm to contact point	5.5 to 6.5 mm to contact point	≥ 7 mm to contact point
Restorative status of neighboring teeth	Virgin		Restored
Width of edentulous span	1 tooth (≥ 7 mm)	1 tooth (≤ 7 mm)	2 teeth or more
Soft-tissue anatomy	Intact soft tissue		Soft-tissue defects
Bone anatomy of alveolar crest	Alveolar crest without bone deficiency	Horizontal bone deficiency	Vertical bone deficiency

The patient exhibited a class I dental relationship with no history of bruxism or parafunctional habits. Radiographic evaluation revealed a recent extraction socket with a retained root tip at site 13 (Fig 5). The patient was highly concerned about the tissue loss and the possibility of an unacceptable esthetic outcome. A review of her medical history revealed no general medical conditions that would prevent routine prosthodontic and surgical procedures.

The patient desired an alternative fixed solution to her previous treatment, wishing to avoid another multi-unit prosthesis in the definitive restoration. In addition, she also wanted a smile makeover with veneering and full-coverage restoration of 14 to 24. She had high esthetic demands and wished to proceed as recommended by our team to maximize the esthetic outcome. A long discussion ensued on treatment options including dental implants. Both pros and cons were discussed, highlighting the difficulty of treating areas with vertical soft and hardtissue defects utilizing dental implants. An Esthetic Risk Assessment (ERA) was generated and reviewed with the patient (see Volume 1 of the ITI Treatment Guide). We felt this was a critical step in the consultation process, setting the tone on the potential esthetic outcome with dental implants. Table 1 highlights the key factors associated with the potential for an esthetic outcome. Based upon these factors, the ERA profile was classified as "high risk."

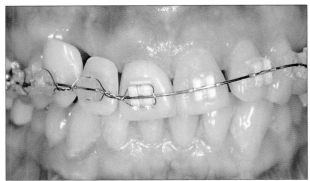

Fig 6   Orthodontic therapy highlighting the inability to move tooth 14 into the edentulous site 13.

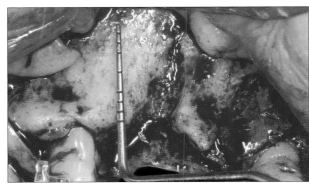

Fig 7   Frontal view of the grafted area as the vertical defect height was being measured.

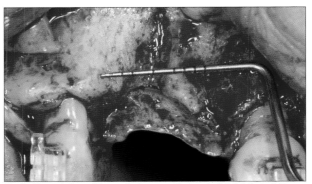

Fig 8   Frontal view of the grafted area as the mesiodistal defect width was being measured.

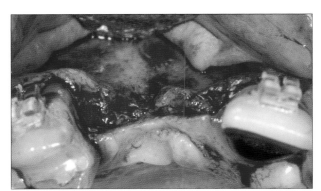

Fig 9   Occlusal view of the defect.

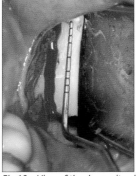

Fig 10   View of the donor site along the ascending ramus.

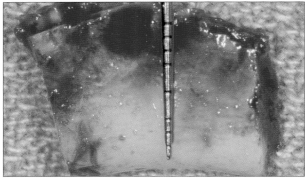

Fig 11   View of the autologous graft.

Based on our planning discussions after reviewing the ERA, we generated a treatment plan for the patient that would utilize orthodontic procedures to move tooth 14 into the canine site, allowing for restoration of a single site with a dental implant. It was the hope of the treatment team that the interproximal bone on tooth 14, once moved into site 13, would allow for more predictable grafting of the edentulous site 12. Orthodontic treatment was initiated, and after 8 months of therapy it was determined that tooth 14 would not move mesially without risking damage to the tooth (Fig 6). The ortho-

dontist then proceeded to level the occlusal plane and create ideal spacing for restoration of sites 13 and 12.

After the attempt at orthodontic movement of tooth 14 had failed, the treatment plan was reevaluated. The alternative plan was to place an autologous block graft in the edentulous sites 13 and 12, followed by implant placement (Straumann Regular Neck and Narrow Neck, respectively) and restoration of the teeth/sites 14 to 24 with all-ceramic single-tooth crowns.

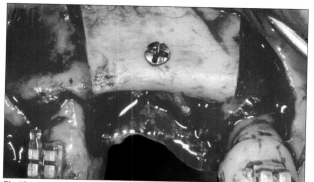

Fig 12   Frontal view of the autologous block fixated in place.

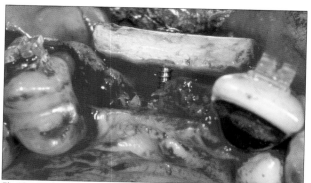

Fig 13   Occlusal view of the autologous block fixated in place.

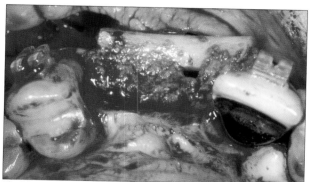

Fig 14   Occlusal view of the autologous block packed with cancellous bone.

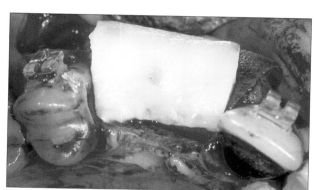

Fig 15   Occlusal view of the acellular tissue graft in place.

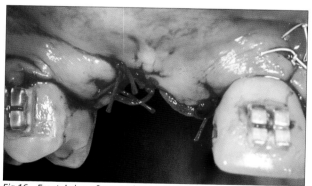

Fig 16   Frontal view after suturing.

Treatment

In the first phase of treatment, grafting of the hard-tissue defect was required. The surgical site was measured and an autologous block graft (12 × 10 mm) harvested from the left lateral ramus (Figs 7 to 11). The graft was then fixated with a 9.0-mm titanium screw, packed with cancellous bone particles, and covered with a resorbable membrane and an acellular tissue graft (Titanium Office System; Lorenz, Jacksonville, FL, USA and Resolut; Gore, Flagstaff, AZ, USA) and Alloderm (LifeCell Corporation, Branchburg, NJ, USA) (Figs 12 to 16).

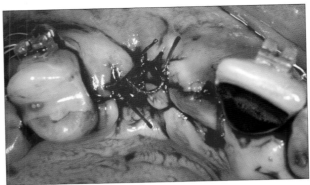

Fig 17   Occlusal view after suturing.

The surgical site was sutured with 4-0 Vicryl (Ethicon Inc, San Angelo, TX, USA) on the crest and the releasing incisions with 5-0 Goretex (WL Gore, Flagstaff, AZ, USA) (Figs 16 and 17). The pontics were modified to relieve the graft of pressure, and the orthodontic archwire was ligated into the brackets (Fig 18).

The graft was allowed to heal for 4 months. The patient returned to the clinic for diagnostic impressions and fabrication of a radiographic template (Figs 19 to 21). A periapical radiograph was obtained and reviewed with the team to confirm proper angulations (Figs 22a-b). Then the surgical template was fabricated and a surgical appointment scheduled.

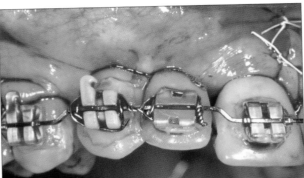

Fig 18   Frontal view with modified pontics on an orthodontic archwire.

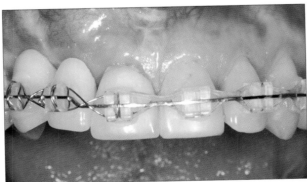

Fig 19   Frontal view of the graft site 4 months after grafting.

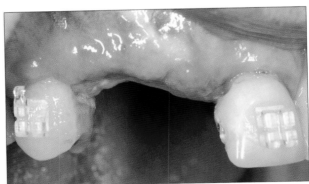

Fig 20   Frontal view after removal of the orthodontic archwire.

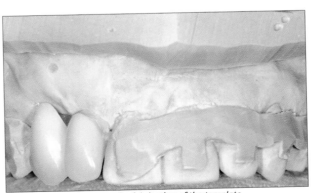

Fig 21   Diagnostic wax-up for fabrication of the template.

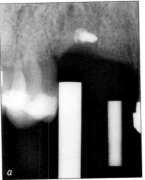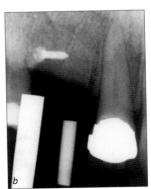

Figs 22a-b   Periapical radiographs with radiographic template in place.

The second phase of treatment was dedicated to placing the implants. First the templates were tried in the patient's mouth to confirm their fit (Figs 23 and 24). The tissue was reflected to expose the healed graft site, and the vertical vacuform template was placed onto the teeth. Using a prosthodontically driven surgical approach, the midfacial position of the planned mucosal margin was isolated on the vacuform template, followed by measuring the distance to the osseous crest. The surgical plan was to place the implant shoulder 1 mm apical to the midfacial mucosal margin so the ridge crest was scalloped to allow for this vertical position (Figs 25 and 26). After preparing the osteotomies in accordance with the manufacturer's instructions, two implants were placed at sites 13 (Straumann SLA, Regular Neck, diameter 4.1 mm, length 10 mm) and 12 (Straumann SLA, Narrow Neck, diameter 3.3 mm, length 10 mm). Figures 27 and 28 show the freshly inserted implants. After tightening the healing caps onto the implants, the tissue was closed by suturing (Fig 29). The pontics were adjusted so they did not contact the tissue, and the archwire was placed onto the brackets (Fig 30). A panoramic radiograph was taken to confirm the implant positions (Figs 31a-b).

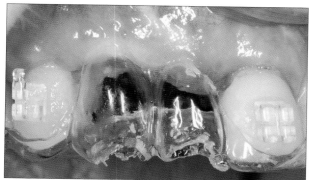

Fig 23   Vacuform surgical template in place.

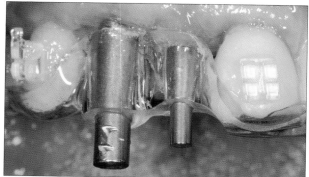

Fig 24   Sleeve template in place, confirming the proposed implant angulations.

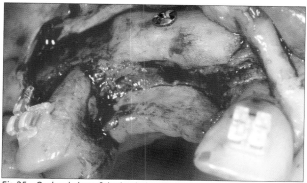

Fig 25   Occlusal view of the healed graft site.

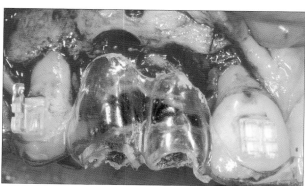

Fig 26   Frontal view of the osseous crest after scalloping.

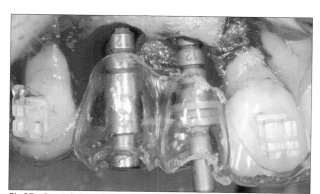

Fig 27   Frontal view of the guide pins in place.

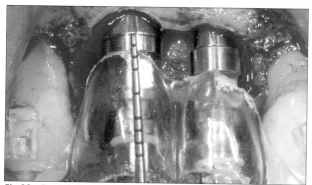

Fig 28   Frontal view of the implants in place, confirming their vertical orientation.

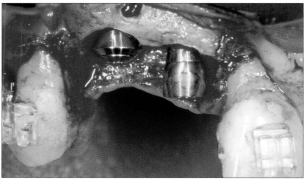

Fig 29 Frontal view of the implants with healing caps in place.

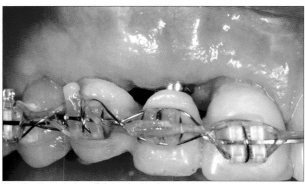

Fig 30 Frontal view of the orthodontic archwire in place.

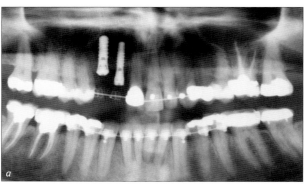

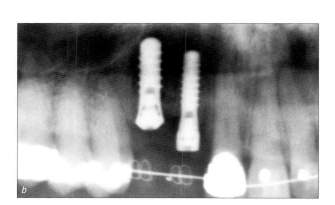

Fig 31a-b Postsurgical panoramic radiograph.

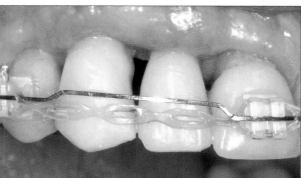

Fig 32 Lateral view of the temporary restorations during loading.

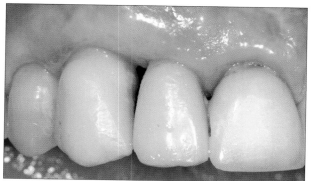

Fig 33 Lateral view at 6 weeks after loading.

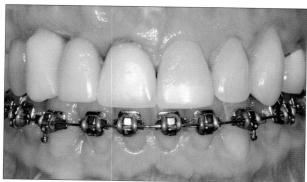

Fig 34 Frontal view at 6 weeks after loading.

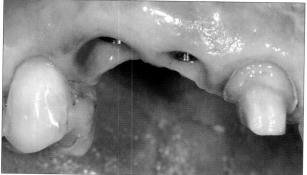

Fig 35 Lateral view of the transition zone after temporary maturation.

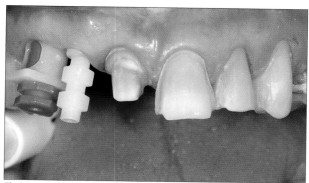

Fig 36 Frontal view prior to final impression-taking.

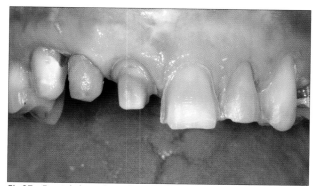

Fig 37 Frontal view prior to fabrication of the second temporary restoration.

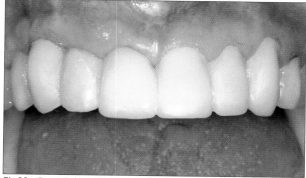

Fig 38 Frontal view with the second temporary restoration in place.

The third phase of treatment was to provide the definitive restorations on the implants. The patient returned to the clinic for loading 6 weeks after placement. Titanium temporary abutments (Straumann, Andover, MA, USA) were placed and restored with a bis-GMA temporary material (Integrity; Dentsply, York, PA, USA). The interproximal contours of the provisional restorations were undercontoured to allow for tissue migration (Fig 32). Six weeks later, the patient returned to the clinic after removal of the braces to follow up on tissue

maturation (Figs 33 and 34). The temporary restorations and abutments were removed and the teeth prepared for all ceramic restorations. As shown in Figures 35 and 36, a polyvinyl siloxane (PVS) impression was made of the teeth and implants (synOcta impression post at site 13 and Narrow Neck impression cap at site 12). After connecting the temporary abutments to the implants, a new interim restoration was fabricated and delivered with temporary cement (Figs 37 and 38).

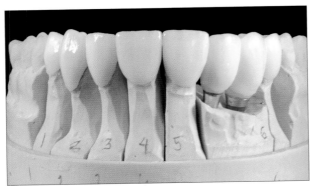

Fig 39   Final all-ceramic restorations.

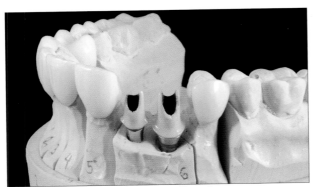

Fig 40   Lateral view of the abutments on the cast.

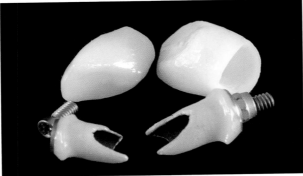

Fig 41   Final abutments and implant restorations.

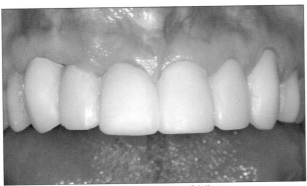

Fig 42   Provisional restorations at the time of delivery.

The restorative plan was to design custom abutments by selecting a 1.5-mm synOcta gold abutment for the implant at site 13 and an oxidizable coping for the implant at site 12 (Straumann, Andover, MA, USA). Once the abutments had been veneered with a thin ceramic layer, all restorations (Finesse, Dentsply, York, PA, USA) were fabricated (Figs 39 to 41). The patient returned to the clinic for delivery of the final restorations (Fig 42). The provisional restorations were removed and the teeth cleaned with pumice, followed by a try-in to verify the fit, contours, and esthetics. After confirmation, the abutments were etched, silanized, tightened to 35 Ncm, and sealed with cotton and Cavit (3M EPSE, St. Paul, MN, USA) (Figs 43 and 44). The teeth were isolated and the restorations delivered with a universal adhesive resin cement (Nexus; Kerr Sybron, Orange, CA, USA). After confirming esthetics and occlusion, the patient was scheduled for a 3-week follow-up visit (Figs 45 to 48a-b). She was placed on a yearly recall schedule and has since continued to report complete satisfaction with the esthetic and functional outcomes of her dental implants and restorations (Figs 49 to 53).

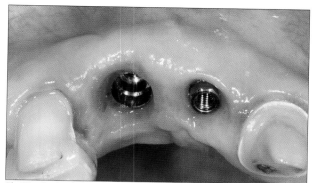

Fig 43   Occlusal view of the transition zone.

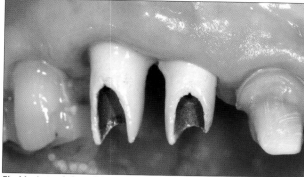

Fig 44   Lateral view of the final abutments prior to sealing with cotton and Cavit (3M EPSE, St. Paul, MN, USA).

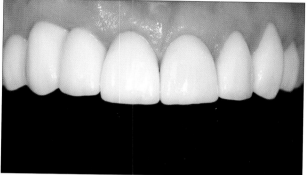

Fig 45   Frontal view of the definitive restorations.

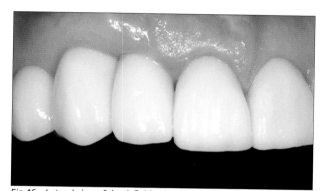

Fig 46   Lateral view of the definitive implant-supported restorations.

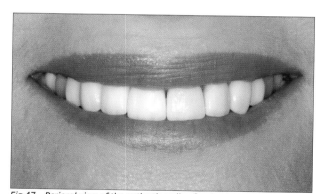

Fig 47   Perioral view of the patient's smile after treatment.

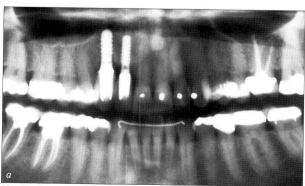

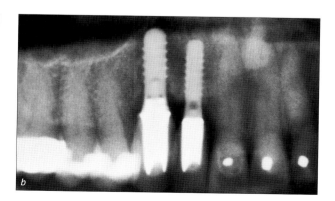

Figs 48a-b   Posttreatment panoramic radiograph.

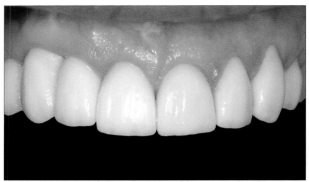

Fig 49   Frontal view at the 4-year follow-up.

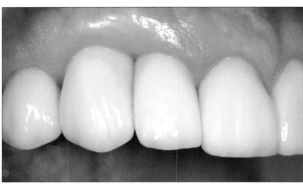

Fig 50   Lateral view at the 4-year follow-up.

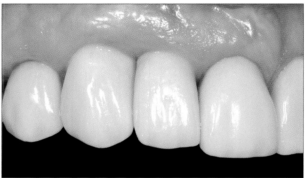

Fig 51   Labial aspect of the restoration at the 8-year follow-up.

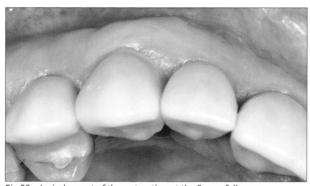

Fig 52   Incisal aspect of the restoration at the 8-year follow-up.

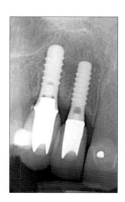

Fig 53   Radiographic control at 8 years.

Acknowledgments

Orthodontic procedures
Dr. Dawn Martin – Gainesville, FL, USA

Laboratory procedures
Dental Technician Lazlo Molnar –
British Columbia, Canada

7.3.5 Replacement of Four Incisors with a Fixed Partial Denture on Two Narrow-Neck Implants after Implant Failure

U.C. Belser, D. Buser

Initial status

A 41-year-old woman was referred to the Clinic of Oral Surgery and Stomatology of the University of Bern due to swelling and acute pain at the site of tooth 11. The patient's history revealed neither medical conditions nor medications incompatible with standard dental treatment. She reported that 4 years previously, due to traumatic loss of teeth 11 and 21, two dental implants had been placed and restored with splinted screw-retained metal-ceramic crowns. Tooth 22 had also been involved in the accident and required endodontic therapy.

Clinical and radiographic examination (Figs 1a-d) confirmed an acute infection at site 11 in the form of marked mucosal swelling on the facial aspect and crevicular suppuration. The patient had a high smile line with display of both the interproximal papillary soft tissue and the cervical alveolar mucosa (Fig 1a). The labial aspect of site 21 exhibited a tissue recession of around 2 mm compared to the mucosal margin of the implant-supported restoration at site 11. This led to the assumption of either buccal malposition of the underlying implant or lack of an adequate labial bone plate at the time of implant placement for which no compensation had been provided by a simultaneous contour augmentation procedure.

The radiographs (Figs 1c-d) documented an active, extended inflammatory peri-implant bone resorption process, involving the coronal 50% of implant 11.

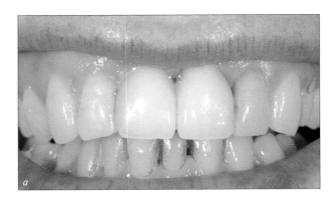

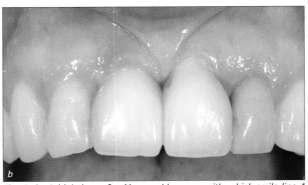

Figs 1a-b Initial views of a 41-year old woman with a high smile line 4 years after implant therapy. The central incisors, lost due to trauma, had been replaced by a two-unit metal-ceramic fixed prosthesis. Soft-tissue swelling and suppuration labial to site 11 and mucosal recession on site 21.

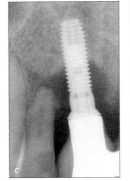
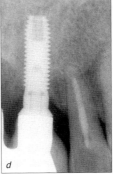

Figs 1c-d Initial radiographs documenting extended peri-implant bone resorption on implant 11, substantial bone loss on the mesial aspects of teeth 12 and 22, and poor marginal fit of the implant-supported two-unit fixed prosthesis.

Furthermore, approximately 60% of bone loss was observed on the mesial aspect of vital tooth 12, whereas about 50% of bone loss was diagnosed on the mesial aspect of non-vital tooth 22. In addition, this tooth presented a noticeable discoloration, which was attributed to its non-vital condition. Finally, some moderate bone loss was noted on both the mesial and distal aspects of implant 21.

Treatment options
All of the treatment modalities listed below were theoretically an option and were presented to the patient for discussion:

- Infection control at site 11 following the CIST protocol (Mombelli and Lang 1998) with or without a tissue-regeneration procedure, aiming to achieve re-osseointegration of the coronal implant segment, with the final decision about maintaining the implant to be taken after reevaluation.
- Infection control and timely removal of implant 11, including transformation of the implant-supported crown 11 to a cantilever unit extended from implant 21 as a temporary solution, to be replaced by a new cantilever restoration later, also discussing the option of placing a new implant as part of the proposal.
- Infection control and removal of implant 11, followed by fabrication of a tooth/implant-supported three-unit fixed partial denture for sites 12 to 21.
- Infection control and removal of both implants, followed by fabrication of a tooth-supported four-unit fixed prosthesis for sites 12 to 22.
- Infection control and removal of both implants, followed by bone grafting and, upon completion of healing, placement of two new implants.
- Infection control, removal of both implants, and extraction of teeth 12 and 22, followed, if required, by bone grafting after healing and insertion of two new implants at sites 12 and 22 to support a four-unit FDP for replacement of the four maxillary incisors.
- Infection control, removal of both implants, and extraction of teeth 12 and 22, followed by fabrication of a tooth-supported six-unit fixed prosthesis for sites 13 to 23.

The advantages and inconveniences inherent in each of these treatment options were presented to the patient with a view of obtaining her informed consent. She was extremely worried and disappointed at what had happened to her recently incorporated two-unit implant-supported prosthesis. She was adamant that she could not envision wearing a removable prosthesis and asked for a durable fixed solution that would predictably meet her high esthetic expectations. According to the esthetic risk assessment table (Martin and coworkers 2006), the patient showed a high-risk profile and fell into the "complex" category of the SAC classification (Dawson and Chen 2009). Trying to maintain the severely infected implant at site 11 was considered inadequate by the authors in this specific situation, and the same considerations applied to the other implant at site 21, whose labial malposition had already given rise to pronounced mucosal recession. Teeth 12 and 22 were periodontally compromised and constituted risk factors for various reasons. A consensus was eventually reached that both implants and both lateral incisors should be removed, followed by insertion of two reduced-diameter implants at sites 12 and 22 to support a four-unit fixed partial denture. Given the prospect of a vertical bone deficiency, a restorative design with artificial gingiva was anticipated.

As expected, a major horizontal and vertical tissue deficiency was confirmed when 3 months of uneventful healing had passed following removal of both central maxillary implants and teeth 12 and 22 (Fig 2).

It was decided to perform a ridge augmentation procedure, aiming to create conditions that would allow implant placement at a future point of time. A mucoperiosteal flap was elevated and exposed a large crater-like bone defect at site 11 (Fig 3a), requiring the use of a block graft harvested from the right mandibular ramus area (Fig 3b). Since a simultaneous procedure was not considered advisable at the time, it was decided to postpone the insertion of implants at sites 12 and 22. A low-substitution bone filler (BioOss; Geistlich, Wolhusen, Switzerland) was applied mainly to the vestibular aspect of the edentulous jaw segment (Fig 3c). The grafted site was covered with a double layer of collagen membrane to protect and stabilize the applied bone filler (Fig 3d). The procedure was finalized by carefully performing incisions of the periosteum at the base of the flap to permit tension-free wound closure with interrupted sutures (Fig 3e).

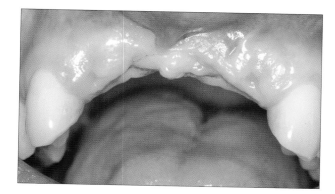

Fig 2 Labial view 3 months after removal of implants 11 and 21 and teeth 12 and 22. A major horizontal and vertical tissue deficiency was noted in the area previously occupied by the implants.

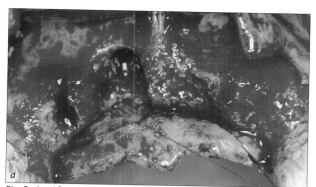

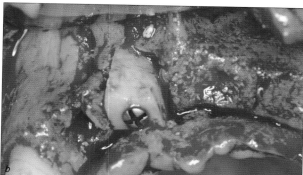

Figs 3a-b After elevation of a mucoperiosteal flap, a large crater-like bone defect became visible at the site of the removed implant 11, requiring application of a block graft harvested from the mandibular right retromolar area. A fixation screw was used to ensure positional stability of the graft.

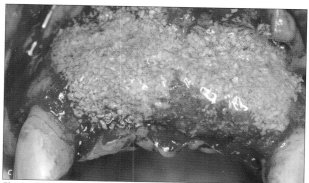

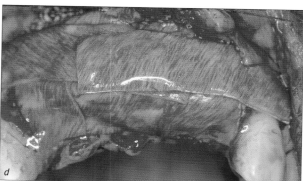

Figs 3c-d A slowly resorbing bone filler (Bio Oss; Geistlich, Wolhusen, Switzerland) was applied to the vestibular aspect, in accordance with the concept of contour augmentation, and was covered with a double layer of a bioabsorbable collagen membrane (Bio Guide; Geistlich).

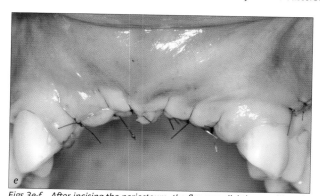

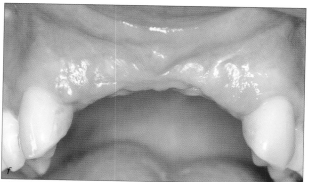

Figs 3e-f After incising the periosteum, the flap was slightly repositioned coronally and then secured with interrupted sutures. Five months after uneventful healing (right), the anterior maxillary area displayed adequate horizontal crest width, whereas the vertical deficiency persisted.

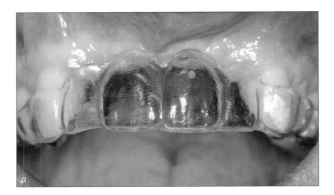

After uneventful healing and 5 months of tissue maturation, the anterior maxillary area was judged adequate for implant therapy (Fig 3f). A simple surgical guide was fabricated to provide two indispensable landmarks for correct three-dimensional implant positioning: (1) the future emergence line of the implant-supported restorations and pontics from the alveolar mucosa and (2) the future positions of the incisal edges (Fig 4a). Exposure of the area by elevation of a mucoperiosteal flap revealed both a favorable crest width and the fixation screw of the block graft to be removed before implant surgery (Fig 4b).

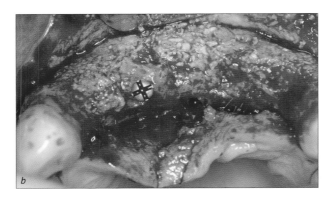

Figs 4a-b A simple surgical guide was fabricated to visualize the prospective tooth locations and their axial orientations, as well as the emergence line of the future clinical crowns from the soft tissue. Excellent crest width (indicated by the position of the fixation screw) under the elevated flap.

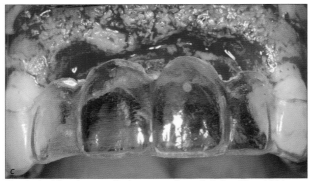

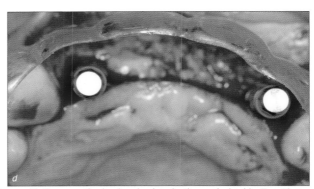

Figs 4c-d Minor bone scalloping was performed at sites 12 and 22 in accordance with the respective landmarks given by the surgical guide. Two 10-mm Narrow Neck implants were inserted under strict observance of basic implant-axis requirements (i.e. axial orientation needs to ensure accessibility of the screw located palatal to the incisal edge line).

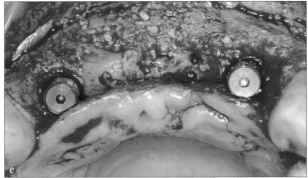

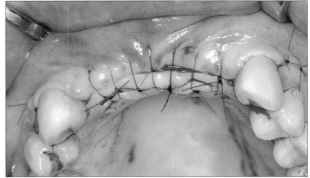

Figs 4e-f Appropriate healing caps were selected to permit both tension-free primary wound closure and easy access creation for later re-entry.

With the surgical guide in place, the distance between the bone crest and the cervical border of the stent was evaluated, a minor bone scalloping performed (Fig 4c), and an implant axis palatal to the planned incisal edge line chosen (Fig 4d). After insertion of two Narrow Neck implants (diameter 3.3 mm, length 12 mm), short healing caps were placed (Fig 4e), followed by primary wound closure with interrupted sutures (Fig 4f). Eight weeks after uneventful healing (Fig 5a), a minimally invasive access to the implants was established and excision of the low-inserting central frenulum simultaneously carried out to enhance the depth of the vestibulum (Fig 5b).

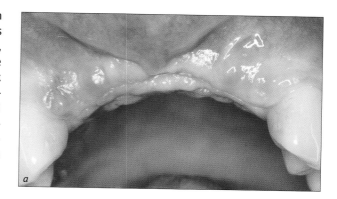

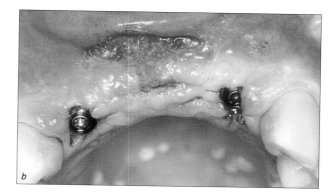

Fig 5a-b   Eight weeks after implant placement and uneventful soft-tissue healing, access to the implant shoulder was established to replace the short healing caps by longer ones. At the same time, a frenectomy was performed (right) to increase vestibular depth. Throughout the postsurgical phase, the patient was wearing a provisional removable denture.

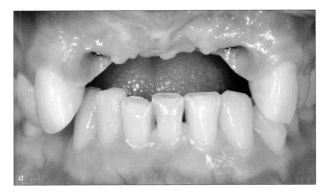

Three weeks later, at the time of inserting the provisional fixed partial denture, healthy peri-implant soft tissue was noted, although in conjunction with a vertical ridge that was clearly further apical than at the two adjacent canines (Figs 6a-b). As seen on the working cast, therefore, major changes in tooth proportion (i.e. unnatural length-to-width ratios) became apparent in the screw-retained four-unit provisional prosthesis.

In fact, the laboratory technician had tried to compensate for the missing soft-tissue height by increasing the length and volume (interproximal contact zones) of the tooth-colored clinical crowns (Figs 7a-b).

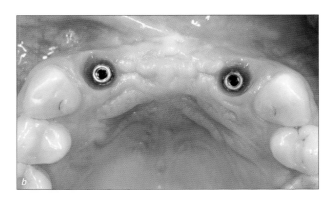

Figs 6a-b   The frontal view on the left was photographed prior to inserting an implant-supported screw-retained four-unit provisional prosthesis. Adequate soft-tissue height mesially of the canines, whereas the edentulous alveolar crest from sites 12 to 22 was located at a significantly more apical level and lacked a scalloped mucosal profile. The occlusal view, by contrast, confirmed a favorable crest width and excellent tissue thickness labial to the two Narrow Neck implants.

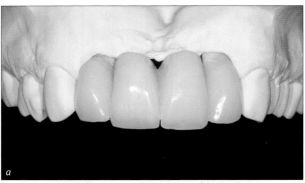
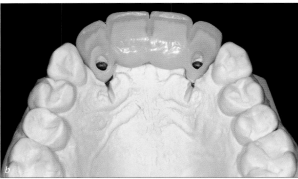

Figs 7a-b   Labial (left) and palatal (right) view of the implant-supported screw-retained four-unit provisional prosthesis on the working cast.

Once the provisional prosthesis was placed in the patient's mouth (Figs 8a-b), all the aforementioned esthetic shortcomings were confirmed. In other words, given this high smile line, the unbalanced relative tooth dimensions created visual tension through the abrupt vertical discontinuities of the mucosal line between the canines and lateral incisors. The impossibility of effectively compensating for missing pink by adding white in this smile environment was particularly striking in lateral views (Figs 8c-d).

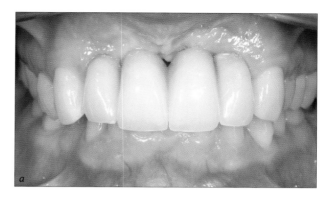

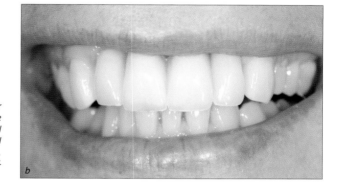

Figs 8a-b The markedly unbalanced length-to-width ratio of the four maxillary incisors due to vertical lack of soft tissue became apparent once the screw-retained four-unit provisional prosthesis was in place. Unnatural mesiocervical appearance of crowns 12 and 22. Furthermore, the clinical crowns exhibited an increased volume, notably in a coronoapical direction. Given the patient's high smile line, the aforementioned shortcomings affected the overall appearance and were therefore unacceptable.

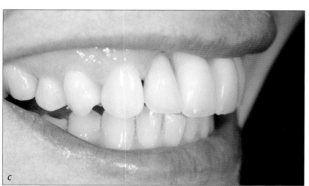

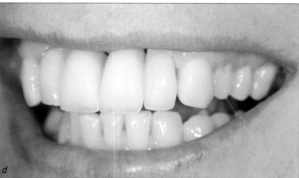

Figs 8c-d The lateral views underlined the limitations of a traditional prosthodontic design not permitting visual compensation for the consequences of vertical tissue deficiencies between the mesial aspects of crowns 12 and 22.

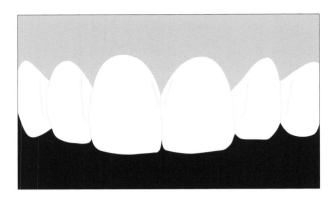

Fig 9a Schematic representation of an optimal maxillary anterior dentition, comprising both harmonious tooth proportions and a continuously scalloped soft-tissue line with complete closure of the interproximal embrasures.

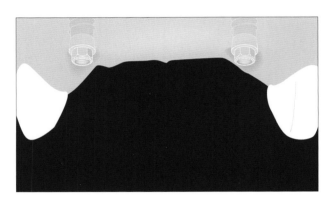

Fig 9b Schematic representation of the anterior maxilla after virtual loss of the four incisors and placement of two Narrow Neck implants at sites 12 and 22.

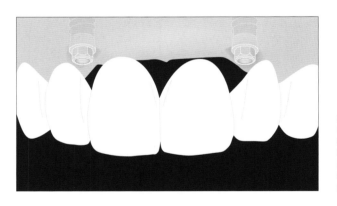

Fig 9c Schematic representation of restoring the original anatomical crowns of the four missing maxillary incisors. Unsightly black triangles resulting from the marked loss of soft-tissue height and problematic spatial relations between the implant shoulders and the optimal positions of the lateral incisors. The latter is a consequence of keeping the implants at a safe distance from the canines and of placing them in a slightly more palatal position than the original roots.

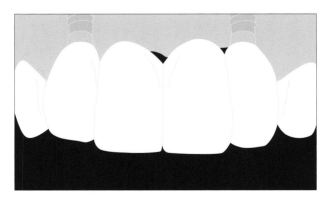

Fig 9d Schematic representation of the anterior maxilla after virtual insertion of a traditional implant-supported four-unit fixed partial denture replacing the four incisors. The clinical crowns have been enhanced in length and volume to compensate for the lack of soft-tissue height. These abnormal tooth proportions create an unnatural appearance and visual tension.

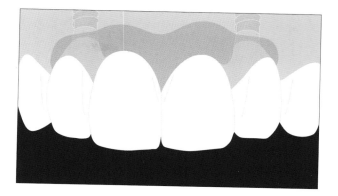

Fig 9e Schematic representation of the anterior maxilla after virtual insertion of an implant-supported four-unit fixed partial denture replacing both the four incisors and the associated soft tissue. Normal tooth proportions including harmonious soft-tissue contours are restored and succeed in giving the restoration a natural appearance.

Frequently encountered consequences of multiple tooth loss in the anterior maxilla (due to trauma, infection, or implant failure) and available treatment options are schematically represented in Figs 9a-e. The first example (Fig 9a) illustrates an intact anterior dentition showing harmonious tooth proportions, interproximal closure, and a maxillary anterior sextant whose cervical segment is characterized by a triangular gingival emergence line, with zeniths of the teeth located slightly distally of their long axis.

Following tooth loss and implant placement, a dramatic loss of tissue height associated with loss of the originally scalloped soft-tissue line may ensue (Fig 9b).

Any attempt to restore the original clinical crown shapes in the presence of a vertical tissue deficiency like that would result in massively open embrasures ("black triangles") and lack of tissue contact on the cervical aspect of the two imaginary central pontics (Fig 9c).

In situations of this type, an attempt is made to reduce the embrasure openings and to establish more extended contact zones between the cervical aspect of the pontics and the local alveolar ridge (Fig 9d). Frequently, this strategy will create visual tension by unbalanced relative tooth dimensions. In patients whose unforced smile displays any cervical portions of implant-supported restorations, the use of artificial gingiva may be considered (Fig 9e). The design principles of implant-supported fixed dental prostheses with integrated artificial gingiva have recently been described in detail by Vailati and Belser (2011) as the pink power concept. Its aim is to create the optical illusion of an intact anterior dentition even in the presence of vertical tissue deficiencies, including balanced relative tooth proportions and a harmonious, continuously scalloped soft-tissue line. The main challenge is to reconcile ideal esthetics with adequate access for hygiene instruments – i.e. to create a convex profile of the "pink" extension similar to the one considered mandatory in ovate pontics.

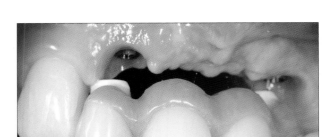
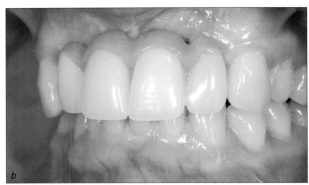

Figs 10a-b   Clinical view of inserting a screw-retained four-unit provisional prosthesis. Mesial access for Superfloss was created on crowns 12 and 22. Furthermore, the pink color of the acrylic gingival extension was far too saturated and therefore could not be perceived as "natural" gingiva.

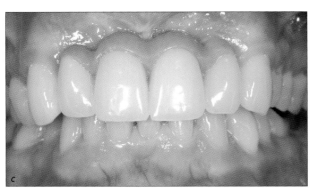
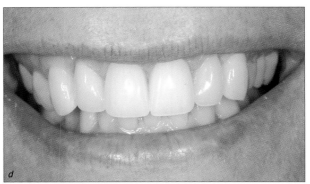

Figs 10c-d   Frontal views with the lips reflected (left) and in their normal position (right). The effect of the integrated artificial gingiva harmonized the tooth proportions and the soft-tissue line.

This can only be achieved if the edentulous ridge areas have a concave profile. Accordingly, a four-unit provisional fixed prosthesis with integrated artificial gingiva was fabricated for the present patient (Figs 10a-d). This approach is recommended to clinically test and, if required, optimize the design prior to using it as a guide for fabrication of the definitive metal-ceramic prosthesis. The patient immediately accepted the second pro-visional prosthesis, except for its shade (Fig 11). Besides the location of the apical border of the gingival extension, the most difficult feature to achieve is an optimal transition between the pink portion of the restoration and adjacent natural papillae (Figs 12a-b). In fact, the pink component has to end at the cervical zenith of an implant-supported crown adjacent to its natural neighbor (Figs 13a-b).

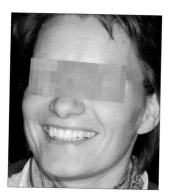

Fig 11   At normal communication distance, the relaxed smile of the patient generates a certain impression of visual harmony between the anterior maxillary dentition and the perioral region.

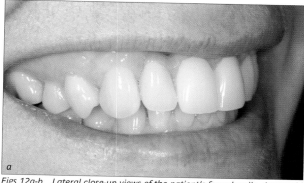

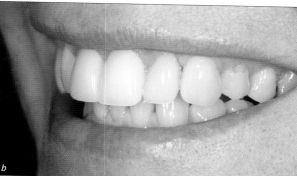

Figs 12a-b   Lateral close-up views of the patient's forced smile. Acceptable integration of the implant-supported provisional fixed prosthesis with the surrounding natural dentition, including the transitions between the implant-supported crowns 12 and 22 and the neighboring canines.

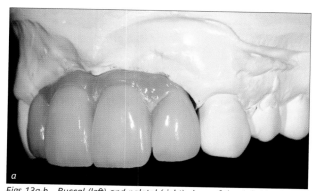

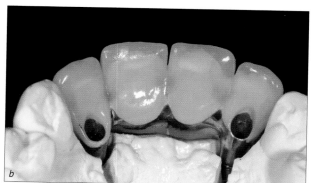

Figs 13a-b   Buccal (left) and palatal (right) views of the definitive implant-supported four-unit metal-ceramic fixed partial denture in its bisque state. A rather pale color had been selected for the artificial gingiva.

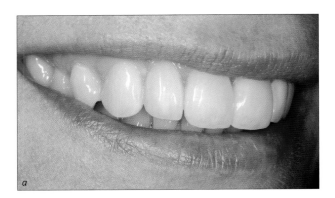

At the clinical try-in (Figs 14a-b), the clinician has to verify not only the routine parameters (interproximal contacts, marginal fit, occlusion, tooth form, color) but notably also the height of the artificial papillae, the aforementioned transition zones, the apical border of the pink component, access for Superfloss, and the convex profile of the extension. Figure 15 illustrates how the design parameters for fixed dental prostheses with integrated pink ceramics can be customized to meet individual requirements. It is recommended that final refinements should be made directly chairside during the bisque bake try-in (Figs 16a-d).

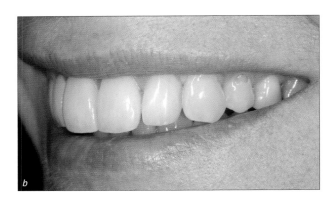

Figs 14a-b   Lateral close-up views of the patient's spontaneous smile immediately after insertion of the final screw-retained four-unit metal-ceramic prosthesis. Major features that had been approved during the provisional phase have been integrated and optimized where appropriate. A slight blanching of the soft tissue persisted mesially of the canines, indicating that some minor contour adjustments were needed prior to final delivery.

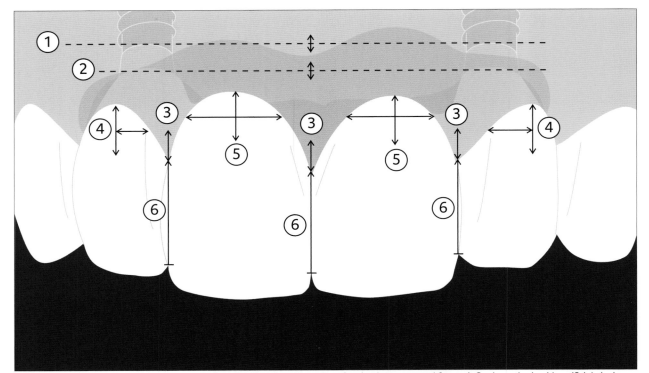

Fig 15   Schematic representation of the anterior maxilla after virtual insertion of an implant-supported four-unit fixed prosthesis with artificial gingiva replacing the four missing incisors. Variables to be considered in relation to each patient's smile line (minimal, moderate or major display of soft tissue) include (1) implant shoulder depth; (2) apical transition from pink ceramic to alveolar mucosa; (3) height of artificial papillae; (4) cervical border of pink ceramic on implant-supported crown adjacent to natural tooth; (5) cervical border of pink ceramic on pontic; and (6) apical limit of interproximal contact area.

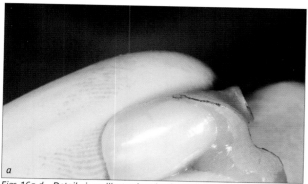
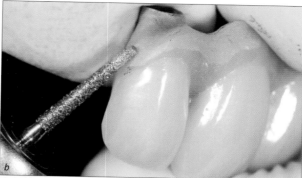

Figs 16a-d   Detail views illustrating the final contour refinements performed chairside with fine-grain diamond burs to ensure both an entirely convex profile of the cervical aspect of the prosthesis and an optimal transition between the restoration and the adjacent natural dentition.

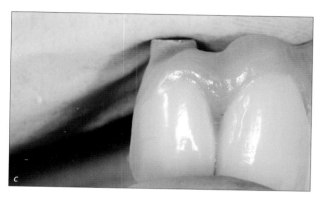
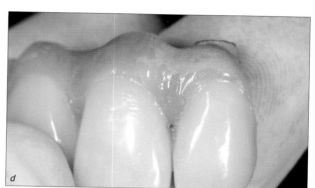

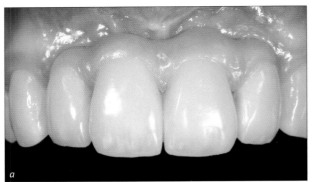 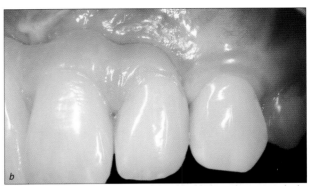

Figs 17a-b   Detail views obtained upon delivery of the final metal-ceramic prosthesis with integrated pink ceramic. An ideal balance between esthetics and accessibility was found. Favorable effect of the pale color selected for the pink segment.

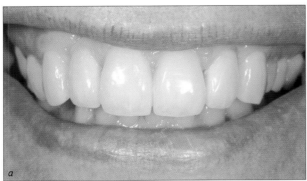 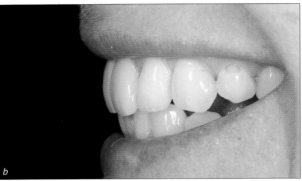

Figs 18a-b   Clinical views of the patent's natural smile. Acceptable integration of the final implant-supported prosthesis with the surrounding natural dentition was achieved, without display of the cervical pink border or the transitions from the implant-supported crowns at sites 12 and 22 to the adjacent canines.

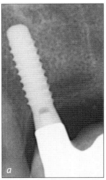 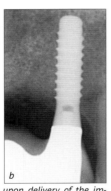

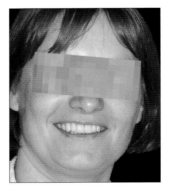

Fig 19a-b   Radiographs taken upon delivery of the implant-supported screw-retained four-unit metal-ceramic prosthesis. Acceptable marginal fit and the favorable mesiodistal peri-implant bone contours.

Fig 20   Portrait view of the patient's natural smile after treatment, confirming acceptable esthetic integration of the implant-supported four-unit fixed partial denture in the anterior maxilla.

After glazing and polishing in the dental laboratory, the final screw-retained prosthesis was delivered in the patient's mouth (Figs 17a-b and Figs 18a-b). Once this was accomplished, verification by intraoral radiographs was obtained (Figs 19a-b). The transocclusal screws were tightened to 35 Ncm and covered with Teflon tape and light-curing composite. Immediate postoperative documentation was completed by taking clinical photographs (Figs 18a-b and Fig 20) as reference for follow-up examinations.

Clinical views obtained at the 5-year follow-up intraorally with reflected lips (Figs 21a-b) and periorally of the patient's unforced smile (Figs 22a-b) confirmed stable soft-tissue conditions and esthetics. The 5-year radiographs (Figs 23a-b) also demonstrated favorable and stable bone conditions around both Narrow Neck implants supporting the four-unit prosthesis.

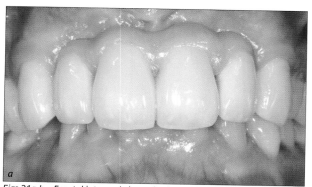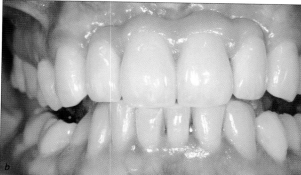

Figs 21a-b   Frontal intraoral views obtained in centric occlusion (left) and mandibular protrusion (right), documenting that major parameters of esthetics and function were unchanged after 5 years of clinical service.

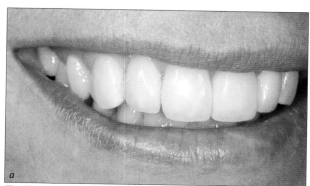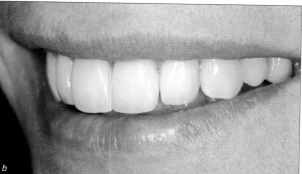

Figs 22a-b   Lateral perioral views of the patient's unforced smile, documenting that esthetic integration was fully maintained after 5 years of clinical service.

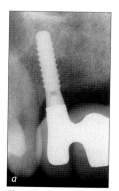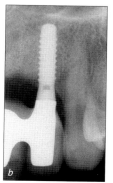

Figs 23a-b   Periapical radiographs confirming that the state of osseointegration was stable after 5 years of clinical service.

Acknowledgments

The authors wish to thank Dental Technician and Master Ceramist Alwin Schönenberger (Glattbrugg, Switzerland) for his expertise and outstanding performance once again reflected in the laboratory work that has been presented in this case study. They also acknowledge the contributions made by Dr. Francesca Vailati (Senior Lecturer at the School of Dental Medicine, University of Geneva, Switzerland) to some of the clinical photography shown.

8 <u>Conclusions</u>

J.-G. Wittneben, H. P. Weber

This volume of the ITI Treatment Guide series offers clinical recommendations for implant-supported restorations in extended edentulous areas in the esthetic zone. Such situations are usually demanding and fall into the categories of "advanced" or "complex" of the SAC Classification used by the ITI. They are commonly associated with deficiencies of the alveolar bone or soft tissues. Any replacement of multiple adjacent teeth must be preceded by a careful assessment of case-specific systemic and local parameters, including all aspects of orofacial esthetics and function. Meticulous treatment planning and risk assessment are mandatory, and the results must be matched with each clinician's individual expertise, optimizing the chances for successful short-term and long-term outcomes. In most instances, a team approach involving a surgeon, prosthodontist, and laboratory technician is required, taking advantage of the broadest possible level of knowledge and skills with ideal utilization of the available (bio)materials, technologies, and techniques.

The merits of modern technology cannot be overemphasized, particularly when it comes to diagnosis and treatment planning. One valuable technology is cone-beam computed tomography (CBCT), used in conjunction with a diagnostic template (that defines the future tooth positions based on the prosthodontic treatment plan) and an intraoral mock-up. This approach offers an opportunity to assess the surgical areas by three-dimensional visualization and yields unprecedented depth of information about existing bone deficiencies in the presurgical phase. Furthermore, implant-planning software allows the positions and angulations of dental implants to be selected properly and lets the surgeon assess whether implants can be placed simultaneously with bone grafting or whether prosthodontically optimal implant placement can only be realized after successful bone grafting. Planning software can also assist in making restorative decisions relating to abutment types and emergence profiles. On this basis, surgical guides can be fabricated for conventional or guided implant procedures, ideally integrating prosthodontic and surgical planning considerations.

Another remarkable progress in the implant-prosthetic field is the evolution of the ceramic material. Implant abutment and framework material can be custom-designed and fabricated from zirconium dioxide by CAD/CAM technology.

As in other demanding indications, staging of surgical and prosthetic procedures will enhance the predictability of a desired outcome more often than not. Provisional restorations are important to esthetically optimize the contours of the involved soft tissues and to define esthetic and functional requirements, which will ultimately be translated into the final restorations. Adjacent implants should be avoided in the esthetic zone of the maxilla, especially at lateral incisors sites. Excessive proximity between implants will result in compromised interimplant soft tissue contours. Finally, the use of pink ceramics is frequently indicated to replace missing hard or soft tissues. Prosthetic and surgical treatment plans should take into consideration that the transition from the prosthesis to the alveolar mucosa should remain concealed behind the upper lip in the patient's smile. Reconstructions of this type should be designed to offer effective access to hygiene for home maintenance.

9 <u>References</u>

Abrams H, Kopczyk RA, Kaplan AL. Incidence of anterior ridge deformities in partially edentulous patients. J Prosthet Dent. 1987 Feb; 57(2): 191-194.

Adell R, Eriksson B, Lekholm U, Brånemark PI, Jemt T. Long-term follow-up study of osseointegrated implants in the treatment of totally edentulous jaws. Int J Oral Maxillofac Implants. 1990 Winter; 5(4): 347-359.

Aglietta M, Siciliano VI, Zwahlen M, Brägger U, Pjetursson BE, Lang NP, Salvi GE. A systematic review of the survival and complication rates of implant supported fixed dental prostheses with cantilever extensions after an observation period of at least 5 years. Clin Oral Implants Res. 2009; 20(5): 441-451.

Al-Askar M, O'Neill R, Stark PC, Griffin T, Javed F, Al-Hezaimi K. Effect of single and contiguous teeth extractions on alveolar bone remodeling: a study in dogs. Clin Implant Dent Relat Res. 2011 Dec 15. [Epub ahead of print]

Araújo MG, Lindhe J. Dimensional ridge alterations following tooth extraction. An experimental study in the dog. J Clin Periodontol. 2005 Feb; 32(2): 212-218.

Araújo MG, Sukekava F, Wennström JL, Lindhe J. Ridge alterations following implant placement in fresh extraction sockets: an experimental study in the dog. J Clin Periodontol. 2005 Jun; 32(6): 645-652.

Araújo MG, Sukekava F, Wennström JL, Lindhe J. Tissue modeling following implant placement in fresh extraction sockets. Clin Oral Implants Res. 2006 Dec; 17(6): 615-624.

Araújo MG, Wennström JL, Lindhe J. Modeling of the buccal and lingual bone walls of fresh extraction sites following implant installation. Clin Oral Implants Res. 2006 Dec; 17(6): 606-614.

Baelum V, Ellegaard B. Implant survival in periodontally compromised patients. J Periodontol. 2004 Oct; 75(10): 1404-1412.

Bain CA, Moy PK. The association between the failure of dental implants and cigarette smoking. Int J Oral Maxillofac Implants. 1993; 8(6): 609-615.

Barter S, Stone P, Brägger U. A pilot study to evaluate the success and survival rate of titanium-zirconium implants in partially edentulous patients: results after 24 months of follow-up. Clin Oral Implants Res. 2012 Jul; 23(7): 873-881.

Bateli M, Att W, Strub JR. Implant neck configurations for preservation of marginal bone level: a systematic review. Int J Oral Maxillofac Implants. 2011 Mar-Apr; 26(2): 290-303.

Belser UC, Bernard JP, Buser D. Implant-supported restorations in the anterior region: prosthetic considerations. Pract Periodontics Aesthet Dent. 1996 Nov-Dec; 8(9): 875-887.

Belser UC, Buser D, Hess D, Schmid B, Bernhard JP, Lang NP: Esthetic implant restorations in partially edentulous patients: A critical appraisal. Periodontol 2000. 1998 Jun; 17: 132-150.

Belser UC, Buser D, Higginbottom F. Consensus statements and recommended clinical procedures regarding esthetics in implant dentistry. Int J Oral Maxillofac Implants. 2004; 19 Suppl: 73-74. (a)

Belser UC, Grutter L, Vailati F, Bornstein MM, Weber HP, Buser D. Outcome evaluation of early placed maxillary anterior single-tooth implants using objective esthetic criteria: a cross-sectional, retrospective study in 45 patients with a 2- to 4-year follow-up using pink and white esthetic scores. J Periodontol. 2009 Jan; 80(1): 140-151.

Belser UC, Schmid B, Higginbottom F, Buser D. Outcome analysis of implant restorations located in the anterior maxilla: a review of the recent literature. Int J Oral Maxillofac Implants. 2004: 19 Suppl: 30-42. (b)

Berglundh T, Lindhe J. Dimension of the periimplant mucosa. Biological width revisited. J Clin Periodontol. J Clin Periodontol. 1996 Oct; 23(10): 971-973.

Bernard JP, Schatz JP, Christou P, Belser U, Kiliaridis S. Long-term vertical changes of the anterior maxillary teeth adjacent to single implants in young and mature adults. J Clin Periodontol. 2004 Nov; 31(11): 1024-1028.

Bernhard N, Berner S, de Wild M, Wieland M. The binary TiZr alloy – a newly developed Ti alloy for use in dental implants. Forum Implantologicum. 2009; 5(1): 30-39.

References have been listed in strict order of the authors' names. Thus, "Miller A, Smith C ... 2009" precedes "Miller A, Young S ... 2001."

Bonewald LF. The amazing osteocyte. J Bone Miner Res. 2011 Feb; 26(2): 229-238. Review.

Bornstein MM, Balsiger R, Sendi P, von Arx T. Morphology of the nasopalatine canal and dental implant surgery: a radiographic analysis of 100 consecutive patients using limited cone-beam computed tomography. Clin Oral Implants Res. 2011 Mar; 22(3): 295-301.

Bornstein MM, Cionca N, Mombelli A. Systemic conditions and treatments as risks for implant therapy. Int J Oral Maxillofac Implants. 2009; 24 Suppl: 12-27.

Bornstein MM, Wittneben JG, Brägger U, Buser D. Early loading at 21 days of non-submerged titanium implants with a chemically modified sandblasted and acid-etched surface: 3-year results of a prospective study in the posterior mandible. J Periodontol. 2010 Jun; 81(6): 809-818.

Bosshardt DD, Schenk RK. Biologic basis of bone regeneration. In: Buser D (ed). 20 years of guided bone regeneration in implant dentistry. 2nd edition. Chicago: Quintessence Publishing; 2009.

Botticelli D, Berglundh T, Lindhe J. Hard tissue alterations following immediate implant placement in extraction sites. J Clin Periodontol. 2004 Oct; 31(10): 820-828.

Brägger U, Karoussis I, Persson R, Pjetursson B, Salvi G, Lang N. Technical and biological complications/failures with single crowns and fixed partial dentures on implants: a 10-year prospective cohort study. Clin Oral Implants Res. 2005 Jun; 16(3): 326-334.

Brägger U, Wermuth W, Török E. Heat generated during preparation of titanium implants of the ITI Dental Implant System: an in vitro study. Clin Oral Implants Res. 1995 Dec; 6(4): 254-259.

Brånemark PI, Adell R, Breine U, Hansson BO, Lindström J, Ohlsson A. Intra-osseous anchorage of dental prostheses. I. Experimental studies. Scand J Plast Reconstr Surg. 1969; 3(2): 81-100.

Brånemark PI, Zarb GA, Albrektsson T. Tissue-integrated prostheses: osseointegration in clinical dentistry. Chicago: Quintessence Publishing; 1985.

Braut V, Bornstein MM, Belser U, Buser D. Thickness of the anterior maxillary facial bone wall—a retrospective radiographic study using cone beam computed tomography. Int J Periodontics Restorative Dent. 2011 Apr; 31(2): 125-131.

Brindis MA, Block MS. Orthodontic tooth extrusion to enhance soft tissue implant esthetics. J Oral Maxillofac Surg 2009 Nov; 67 (11 Suppl): 49-59. Review

Brodala N. Flapless surgery and its effect on dental implant outcomes. Int J Oral Maxillofac Implants. 2009; 24 Suppl: 118-125. Review.

Brugnami F, Caleffi C. Prosthetically driven implant placement. How to achieve the appropriate implant site development. Keio J Med. 2005 Dec; 54(4): 172-178.

Busenlechner D, Tangl S, Arnhart C, Redl H, Schuh C, Watzek G, Gruber R. Resorption of deproteinized bovine bone mineral in a porcine calvaria augmentation model. Clin Oral Implants Res. 2012 Jan; 23(1): 95-99.

Buser D, Belser UC, Wismeijer D (eds). ITI Treatment Guide, Vol 1: Implant therapy in the esthetic zone—Single-tooth replacements. Berlin: Quintessence Publishing; 2007: 11-20. (a)

Buser D, Belser UC. Correct three-dimensional implant placement: the concept of danger and comfort zones. In: Buser D, Belser UC, Wismeijer D (eds). ITI Treatment Guide, Vol 3: Implants in extraction sockets. Berlin: Quintessence Publishing; 2008.

Buser D, Bernard JP, Hofmann B, Lussi A, Mettler D, Schenk RK. Evaluation of bone filling materials in membrane-protected defects of the mandible. A histomorphometric study in miniature pigs. Clin Oral Implants Res. 1998 9(3): 137-150. (a)

Buser D, Chen ST, Weber HP, Belser UC. Early implant placement following single-tooth extraction in the esthetic zone: biologic rationale and surgical procedures. Int J Periodontics Restorative Dent. 2008 Oct; 28(5): 441-551.

Buser D, Chen ST. Implant placement in postextraction sites. In: Buser D (ed). 20 years of guided bone regeneration in implant dentistry. 2nd edition. Chicago: Quintessence Publishing; 2009: 153-194.

Buser D, Cho JY, Yeo ABK. Surgical Manual of Implant Dentistry. Step-by-step Procedures. Berlin: Quintessence Publishing; **2007**: 47. **(b)**

Buser D, Dula K, Hirt HP, Schenk RK. Lateral ridge augmentation using autografts and barrier membranes. A clinical study in 40 partially edentulous patients. J Oral Maxillofac Surg. **1996** Apr; 54(4): 420-432.

Buser D, Halbritter S, Hart C, Bornstein MM, Grütter L, Chappuis V, Belser UC. Early implant placement with simultaneous GBR following single tooth extraction in the esthetic zone: 12-months results of a prosthetic study with 20 consecutive patients. J Periodontol. **2009** Jan; 80(1): 152-162.

Buser D, Hoffmann B, Bernard JP, Lussi A, Mettler D, Schenk RK. Evaluation of filling materials in membrane-protected bone defects. A comparative histomorphometric study in the mandible of miniature pigs. Clin Oral Implants Res. **1998** Jun; 9(3): 137-150. **(b)**

Buser D, Martin W, Belser UC. Optimizing esthetics for implant restorations in the anterior maxilla: anatomic and surgical considerations. Int J Oral Maxillofac Implants. **2004**; 19 Suppl: 43-61.

Buser D, Martin W, Belser UC. Surgical considerations with regard to single-tooth replacements in the esthetic zone: standard procedure in sites without bone deficiencies. In: Buser D, Belser UC, Wismeijer D (eds). ITI Treatment Guide, Vol 1: Implant therapy in the esthetic zone—single-tooth replacements. Berlin: Quintessence; **2007**: 26-37. **(c)**

Buser D, Mericske-Stern R, Bernard JP, Behneke A, Behneke N, Hirt HP, Belser UC, Lang NP. Long-term evaluation of non-submerged ITI implants. Part 1: 8-year life table analysis of a prospective multicenter study with 2359 implants. Clin Oral Implants Res. **1997** Jun; 8(3): 161-172.

Buser D, Wittneben J, Bornstein MM, Grutter L, Chappuis V, Belser UC. Stability of contour augmentation and esthetic outcomes of implant-supported single crowns in the esthetic zone: 3-year results of a prospective study with early implant placement postextraction. J Periodontol. **2011** Mar; 82(3): 342-349.

Cardaropoli G, Araújo M, Hayacibara R, Sukekava F, Lindhe J. Healing of extraction sockets and surgically produced augmented and non-augmented defects in the alveolar ridge. An experimental study in the dog. J Clin Periodontol. **2005** May; 32(5): 435-440.

Cardaropoli G, Araújo M, Lindhe J. Dynamics of bone tissue formation in tooth extraction sites. An experimental study in dogs. J Clin Periodontol. **2003** Sep; 30(9): 809-818.

Cardaropoli G, Lekholm U, Wennström JL. Tissue alterations at implant-supported single-tooth replacements: a 1-year prospective clinical study. Clin Oral Implants Res. **2006** Apr; 17(2): 165-171.

Carlsson GE. Dental occlusion: modern concepts and their application in implant prosthodontics. Odontology. **2009** Jan; 97(1): 8-17.

Chee WW. Provisional restorations in soft tissue management around dental implants. Periodontol 2000. **2001**; 27: 139-147. Review.

Chee WW. Treatment planning and soft-tissue management for optimal implant esthetics: a prosthodontic perspective. J Calif Dent Assoc. **2003** Jul; 31(7): 559-563.

Chen S, Buser D, Cordaro L. Surgical modifying factors. In: Dawson A, Chen S (eds). The SAC classification in implant dentistry. Berlin: Quintessence Publishing; **2009**: 18-20. **(b)**

Chen S, Dawson A. Esthetic modifiers. In: Dawson A, Chen S (eds). The SAC classification in implant dentistry. Berlin: Quintessence Publishing; **2009**: 15-17. **(a)**

Chen S, Dawson A. General modifiers. In: Dawson A, Chen S (eds). The SAC classification in implant dentistry. Berlin: Quintessence Publishing; **2009**: 12-14. **(b)**

Chen S, Beagle J, Jensen SS, Chiapasco M, Darby I. Consensus statements and recommended clinical procedures regarding surgical techniques. Int J Oral Maxillofac Implants. **2009**; 24 Suppl: 272-278. **(c)**

Chen S, Buser D. Clinical and esthetic outcomes of implants placed in postextraction sites. Int J Oral Maxillofac Implants. **2009**; 24 Suppl: 186-217. Review.

Chen S, Buser D. Implants in post-extraction sites: A literature update. In: Buser D, Belser UC, Wismeijer D (eds). ITI Treatment Guide, Vol 3: Implants in extraction sockets. Berlin: Quintessence; **2008**: 9-15.

Chen S, Darby IB, Reynolds EC and Clement JG. Immediate implant placement post-extraction without flap elevation. J Periodontol. **2009** 80(1): 163-172. **(a)**

Chen S, Darby IB, Reynolds EC. A prospective clinical study of non-submerged immediate implants: clinical outcomes and esthetic results. Clin Oral Implants Res. **2007** Oct; 18(5): 552-562.

Chen S, Wilson TG, Hämmerle CH. Immediate or early placement of implants following tooth extraction: review of biologic basis, clinical procedures, and outcomes. Int J Oral Maxillofac Implants. **2004**; 19 Suppl: 12-25.

Chiapasco M, Abati S, Romeo E, Vogel G. Clinical outcome of autogenous bone blocks or guided bone regeneration with e-PTFE membranes for the reconstruction of narrow edentulous ridges. Clin Oral Implants Res. **1999** Aug; 10(4): 278-288.

Chiapasco M, Casentini P, Zaniboni M, Corsi E, Anello T. Titanium-zirconium alloy narrow diameter implants (Straumann Roxolid) for the rehabilitation of horizontally deficient edentulous ridges: prospective study on 18 consecutive patients. Clin Oral Implants Res. **2011** Aug 18. [Epub ahead of print]

Chiapasco M, Casentini P, Zaniboni M. Bone augmentation procedures in implant dentistry. Int J Oral Maxillofac Implants. **2009**; 24 Suppl: 237-259.

Cho SC, Shetty S, Froum S, Elian N, Tarnow D. Fixed and removable provisional options for patients undergoing implant treatment. Compend Contin Educ Dent. **2007** Nov; 28(11): 604-608.

Chuang SK, Wei LJ, Douglass CW, Dodson TB. Risk factors for dental implant failure: a strategy for the analysis of clustered failure-time observations. J Dent Res. **2002** Aug: 81(8): 572-577.

Coachman C, Salama M, Garber D, Calamita M, Salama H, Cabral G. Prosthetic gingival reconstruction in fixed partial restorations. Part 1: Introduction to artificial gingiva as an alternative therapy. Int J Periodontics Restorative Dent. **2009** Oct; 29(5): 471-477.

Coachman C, Salama M, Garber D, Calamita M, Salama H, Cabral G. Prosthetic gingival reconstruction in fixed partial restorations. Part 3: laboratory procedures and maintenance. Int J Periodontics Restorative Dent **2010** Feb;30(1):19-29.

Cochran D, Schou SS, Heitz-Mayfield LJ, Bornstein MM, Salvi GE, Martin WC. Consensus statements and recommended clinical procedures regarding risk factors in implant therapy. Int J Oral Maxillofac Implants. **2009**; 24 Suppl: 86-89.

Cochran DL, Hermann JS, Schenk RK, Higginbottom FL, Buser D. A Biologic width around titanium implants. A histometric analysis of the implanto-gingival junction around unloaded and loaded nonsubmerged implants in the canine mandible. J Periodontol. **1997** Feb; 68(2): 186-198.

Cooper LF. Objective criteria: guiding and evaluating dental implant esthetics. J Esthet Restor Dent. **2008**; 20(3): 195-205.

Cordaro L, Amadé DS, Cordaro M. Clinical results of alveolar ridge augmentation with mandibular block bone grafts in partially edentulous patients prior to implant placement. Clin Oral Implants Res. **2002** Feb; 13(1): 103-111.

Cordaro L, Torsello F, Roccuzzo M. Implant loading protocols for the partially edentulous posterior mandible. Int J Oral Maxillofac Implants. **2009**; 24 Suppl: 158-168.

Darby I, Chen ST, Buser D. Ridge preservation techniques for implant therapy. Int J Oral Maxillofac Implants. **2009**; 24 Suppl: 260-271.

Dawson A. Martin W. Restorative modifiers. In: Dawson A, Chen S (eds). The SAC classification in implant dentistry. Berlin: Quintessence Publishing; **2009**: 21-24.

Dawson T, Chen ST. The SAC classification in implant dentistry. Berlin: Quintessence Publishing; **2009**.

den Hartog L, Meijer HJ, Stegenga B, Tymstra N, Vissink A, Raghoebar GM. Single implants with different neck designs in the aesthetic zone: a randomized clinical trial. Clin Oral Implants Res. **2011** Nov; 22(11): 1289-1297.

Edel A. The use of a connective tissue graft for closure over an immediate implant with an occlusive membrane. Clin Oral Implants Res. **1995** Mar; 6(1): 60-65.

Elian N, Tabourian G, Jalbout ZN, Classi A, Cho SC, Froum S, Tarnow DP. Accurate transfer of peri-implant soft tissue emergence profile from the provisional crown to the final prosthesis using an emergence profile cast. J Esthet Restor Dent. **2007**; 19(6): 306-314.

Ellegaard B, Baelum V, Karring T. Implant therapy in periodontally compromised patients. Clin Oral Implants Res. **1997** Jun; 8(3): 180-188.

Ellegaard B, Baelum V, Kølsen-Petersen J. Non-grafted sinus implants in periodontally compromised patients: a time-to-event analysis. Clin Oral Implants Res. **2006** Apr; 17(2): 156-164.

Esposito M, Grusovin MG, Willings M, Coulthard P, Worthington HV. Interventions for replacing missing teeth: different times for loading dental implants. Cochrane Database Syst Rev. **2007** Apr 18; (2): CD003878.

Evans CD, Chen ST. Esthetic outcomes of immediate implant placements. Clin Oral Implants Res. **2008** Jan; 19(1): 73-80.

Fritz ME. Implant therapy II. Ann Periodontol. **1996** Nov; 1(1): 796-815.

Froum SJ. Implant complications: scope of the problem. In: Froum SJ (ed). Dental implant complications – etiology, prevention, and treatment. Chichester, West Sussex, UK: Wiley-Blackwell Publishing; **2010**: 1-8.

Fu JH, Yeh CY, Chan HL, Tatarakis N, Leong DJ, Wang HL. Tissue biotype and its relation to the underlying bone morphology. J Periodontol. **2010** Apr; 81(4): 569-574.

Fürhauser R, Florescu D, Benesch T, Haas R, Mailath G, Watzek G. Evaluation of soft tissue around single-tooth implant crowns: the pink esthetic score. Clin Oral Implants Res. **2005** Dec; 16(6): 639-644.

Garber DA, Belser UC. Restoration-driven implant placement with restoration-generated site development. Compend Contin Educ Dent. **1995** Aug; 16(8): 796, 798-802, 804.

Gelb DA. Immediate implant surgery: three-year retrospective evaluation of 50 consecutive cases. Int J Oral Maxillofac Implants. **1993**; 8(4): 388-399.

Giglio GD. Abutment selection in implant-supported fixed prosthodontics. Int J Periodontics Restorative Dent. **1999** Jun; 19(3): 233-241.

Goodacre CJ, Bernal G, Rungcharassaeng K, Kan JY. Clinical complications with implants and implant prostheses. J Prosthet Dent. **2003** Aug; 90(2): 121-132.

Grunder U, Spielman HP, Gaberthüel T. Implant-supported single tooth replacement in the aesthetic region: a complex challenge. Pract Periodontics Aesthet Dent. **1996** Nov-Dec; 8(9): 835-842.

Grütter L, Belser UC. Implant loading protocols for the partially edentulous esthetic zone. Int J Oral Maxillofac Implants. **2009**; 24 Suppl: 169-179.

Guichet DL. Load transfer in screw- and cement-retained implant fixed partial denture design (abstract). J Prosthet Dent. **1994**; 72: 631.

Hämmerle CH, Chen ST, Wilson TG Jr. Consensus statements and recommended clinical procedures regarding the placement of implants in extraction sockets. Int J Oral Maxillofac Implants. **2004**; 19 Suppl: 26-28.

Hämmerle CH, Stone P, Jung RE, Kapos T, Brodala N. Consensus statements and recommended clinical procedures regarding computer-assisted implant dentistry. Int J Oral Maxillofac Implants. **2009**; 24 Suppl: 126-129.

Hämmerle CH, Wagner D, Brägger U, Lussi A, Karayiannis A, Joss A, Lang NP. Threshold of tactile sensitivity perceived with dental endosseous implants and natural teeth. Clin Oral Implants Res. **1995** Jun; 6(2): 83-90.

Hannink RHJ, Kelly PM, Muddle BC. Transformation toughening in zirconia-containing ceramics. J Am Ceram Soc. **2000**; 83(3): 461-487.

Harris RJ. Soft tissue ridge augmentation with an acellular dermal matrix. Int J Periodontics Restorative Dent. **2003** Feb; 23(1): 87-92.

Hebel KS, Gajjar RC. Cement-retained versus screw-retained implant restoration: achieving optimal occlusion and esthetics in implant dentistry. J Prosthet Dent. **1997** Jan; 77(1): 28-35.

Heitz-Mayfield LJ, Huynh-Ba G. History of treated periodontitis and smoking as risks for implant therapy. Int J Oral Maxillofac Implants. **2009**; 24 Suppl: 39-68.

Hermann JS, Buser D, Schenk RK, Higginbottom FL, Cochran DL. Biologic width around titanium implants. A physiologically formed and stable dimension over time. Clin Oral Implants Res. **2000** Feb; 11(1): 1-11.

Hermann JS, Cochran DL, Nummikoski PV, Buser D. Crestal bone changes around titanium implants. A radiographic evaluation of unloaded nonsubmerged and submerged implants in the canine mandible. J Periodontol. **1997** Nov; 68(11): 1117-1130.

Higginbottom F, Belser UC, Jones JD, Keith SE. Prosthetic management of implants in the esthetic zone. Int J Oral Maxillofac Implants. **2004**; 19 Suppl: 62-72.

Hirsch E, Wolf U, Heinicke F, Silva M. Dosimetry of the cone beam computed tomography Veraviewepocs 3D compared with the 3D Accuitomo in different fields of view. Dentomaxillofac Radiol. **2008** Jul; 37(5): 268-273.

Hürzeler MB, Kohal RJ, Naghshbandi J, Mota LF, Conradt J, Hutmacher D, Caffesse RG. Evaluation of a new bioresorbable barrier to facilitate guided bone regeneration around exposed implant threads. An experimental study in the monkey. Int J Oral Maxillofac Surg. **1998** Aug; 27(4): 315-320.

Januario AL, Barriviera M, Duarte WR. Soft tissue conebeam computed tomography: a novel method for the measurement of gingival tissue and the dimensions of the dentogingival unit. J Esthet Restor Dent. **2008**; 20(6): 366-373.

Januario AL, Duarte WR, Barriviera M, Mesti JC, Araújo MG, Lindhe J. Dimension of the facial bone wall in the anterior maxilla: a cone-beam computed tomography study. Clin Oral Implants Res. **2011** Oct; 22(10): 1168-1171.

Jensen SS, Aaboe M, Pinholt EM, Hjørting-Hansen E, Melsen F, Ruyter IE. Tissue reaction and material characteristics of four bone substitutes. Int J Oral Maxillofac Implants. **1996** Jan-Feb; 11(1): 55-66.

Jensen SS, Bornstein MM, Dard M, Bosshardt DD, Buser D. Comparative study of biphasic calcium phosphates with different HA/TCP ratios in mandibular bone defects. A long-term histomorphometric study in minipigs. J Biomed Mater Res B Appl Biomater. **2009** Jul; 90(1): 171-181.

Jensen SS, Broggini N, Hjørting-Hansen E, Schenk R, Buser D. Bone healing and graft resorption of autograft, anorganic bovine bone and beta-tricalcium phosphate. A histologic and histomorphometric study in the mandibles of minipigs. Clin Oral Implants Res. **2006** Jun; 17(3): 237-243.

Jensen SS, Terheyden H. Bone augmentation procedures in localized defects in the alveolar ridge: clinical results with different bone grafts and bone-substitute materials. Int J Oral Maxillofac Implants. **2009**; 24 Suppl: 218-236.

Jensen SS, Yeo A, Dard M, Hunziker E, Schenk R, Buser D. Evaluation of a novel biphasic calcium phosphate in standardized bone defects. A histologic and histomorphometric study in the mandibles of minipigs. Clin Oral Implants Res. **2007** Dec; 18(6): 752-760.

Jung RE, Holderegger C, Sailer I, Khraisat A, Suter A, Hämmerle CH. The effect of all-ceramic and porcelain-fused-to-metal restorations on marginal peri-implant soft tissue color: a randomized controlled clinical trial. Int J Periodontics Restorative Dent. **2008** Aug; 28(4): 357-365.

Jung RE, Sailer I, Hämmerle CH, Attin T, Schmidlin P. In vitro color changes of soft tissues caused by restorative materials. Int J Periodontics Restorative Dent. **2007** Jun; 27(3): 251-257.

Jung RE, Schneider D, Ganeles J, Zwahlen M, Hämmerle CH, Tahmaseb A. Computer technology applications in surgical implant dentistry: a systematic review. Int J Oral Maxillofac Implants. **2009**; 24 Suppl: 92-109.

Kan JY, Rungcharassaeng K, Fillman M, Caruso J. Tissue architecture modification for anterior implant esthetics: an interdisciplinary approach. Eur J Esthet Dent. **2009** Summer; 4(2): 104-117.

Kan JY, Rungcharassaeng K, Lozada JL. Bilaminar subepithelial connective tissue grafts for immediate implant placement and provisionalization in the esthetic zone. J Calif Dent Assoc. **2005** Nov; 33(11): 865-871.

Kan JY, Rungcharassaeng K, Sclar A, Lozada JL. Effects of the facial osseous defect morphology on gingival dynamics after immediate tooth replacement and guided bone regeneration: 1-year results. J Oral Maxillofac Surg. **2007** Jul; 65(7 Suppl 1): 13-19.

Kan JY, Rungcharassaeng K, Umezu K, Kois JC. Dimensions of peri-implant mucosa: an evaluation of maxillary anterior single implants in humans. J Periodontol. **2003** Apr; 74(4): 557-562.

Kan JY, Rungcharassaeng K. Interimplant papilla preservation in the esthetic zone: a report of six consecutive cases. Int J Periodontics Restorative Dent. **2003** Jun; 23(3): 249-259.

Kapos T, Ashy LM, Gallucci GO, Weber HP, Wismeijer D. Computer-aided design and computer-assisted manufacturing in prosthetic implant dentistry. Int J Oral Maxillofac Implants. **2009**; 24 Suppl: 110-117.

Kelly JR, Benetti P. Ceramic materials in dentistry: historical evolution and current practice. Aust Dent J. **2011** Jun; 56 Suppl 1: 84-96.

Kim Y, Oh TJ, Misch CE, Wang HL. Occlusal considerations in implant therapy: clinical guidelines with biomechanical rationale. Clin Oral Implants Res. **2005** Feb; 16(1): 26-35.

Kois JC. The restorative-periodontal interface: biological parameters. Periodontol 2000. **1996** Jun; 11: 29-38.

Kokich VO Jr, Kiyak HA, Shapiro PA. Comparing the perception of dentists and lay people to altered dental esthetics. J Esthet Dent. **1999**; 11(6): 311-324.

Kokich VO Jr, Kokich VG, Kiyak HA. Perceptions of dental professionals and laypersons to altered dental esthetics: asymmetric and symmetric situations. Am J Orthod Dentofacial Orthop. **2006** Aug; 130(2): 141-151.

Kourkouta S, Dedi KD, Paquette DW, Mol A. Interproximal tissue dimensions in relation to adjacent implants in the anterior maxilla: clinical observations and patient aesthetic evaluation. Clin Oral Implants Res. **2009** Dec(12); 20: 1375-1385.

Kreissl ME, Gerds T, Muche R, Heydecke G, Strub JR. Technical complications of implant-supported fixed partial dentures in partially edentulous cases after an average observation period of 5 years. Clin Oral Implants Res. **2007** Dec; 18(6): 720-726.

Labban N, Song F, Al-Shibani N, Windsor LJ. Effects of provisional acrylic resins on gingival fibroblast cytokine/growth factor expression. J Prosthet Dent. **2008** Nov; 100(5): 390-397.

Landsberg CJ. Socket seal surgery combined with immediate implant placement: a novel approach for single-tooth replacement. Int J Periodontics Restorative Dent. **1997** Apr; 17(2): 140-149.

Laney WR (ed). Glossary of oral and maxillofacial implants. Berlin: Quintessence Publishing, **2007**.

Lang NP, Pjetursson BE, Tan K, Brägger U, Egger M, Zwahlen M. A systematic review of the survival and complication rates of fixed partial dentures (FPDs) after an observation period of at least 5 years. II. Combined tooth-implant-supported FPDs. Clin Oral Implants Res. **2004** Dec; 15(6): 643-653.

Larsson C, Holm L, Lövgren N, Kokubo Y, Vult von Steyern P. Fracture strength of four-unit Y-TZP FPD cores designed with varying connector diameter. An in-vitro study. J Oral Rehabil. **2007** Sep; 34(9): 702-709.

Lewis S, Parel S, Faulkner R. Provisional implant-supported fixed restorations. Int J Oral Maxillofac Implants. **1995** May-Jun; 10(3): 319-325.

Lindh T, Gunne J, Tillberg A, Molin M. A meta-analysis of implants in partial edentulism. Clin Oral Implants Res. **1998** Apr; 9(2): 80-90.

Lobbezoo F, Van Der Zaag J, Naeije M. Bruxism: its multiple causes and its effects on dental implants – an updated review. J Oral Rehabil. **2006** Apr; 33(4): 293-300.

Luterbacher S, Fourmousis I, Lang NP, Brägger U. Fractured prosthetic abutments in osseointegrated implants: a technical complication to cope with. Clin Oral Implants Res. **2000** Apr; 11(2): 163-270.

Madrid C, Sanz M. What impact do systemically administrated bisphosphonates have on oral implant therapy? A systematic review. Clin Oral Implants Res. **2009** Sep; 20 Suppl 4: 96-106.

Mankoo T. Single-tooth implant restorations in the esthetic zone – contemporary concepts for optimization and maintenance of soft tissue esthetics in the replacement of failing teeth in compromised sites. Eur J Esthet Dent. 2007 Autumn; 2(3): 274-295.

Martin W, Lewis E, Nicol A. Local risk factors for implant therapy. Int J Oral Maxillofac Implants. 2009; 24 Suppl: 28-38.

Martin WC, Morton D, Buser D. Pre-operative analysis and prosthetic treatment planning in esthetic implant dentistry. In: Buser D, Belser UC, Wismeijer, eds. ITI Treatment Guide Vol 1: Implant therapy in the esthetic zone—single-tooth replacements. Berlin: Quintessence Publishing; 2007: 9-24.

Marx RE, Sawatari Y, Fortin M, Broumand V. Bisphosphonate-induced exposed bone (osteonecrosis/osteopetrosis) of the jaws: risk factors, recognition, prevention, and treatment. J Oral Maxillofac Surg. 2005 Nov; 63(11): 1567-1575.

McDermott NE, Chuang SK, Woo VV, Dodson TB. Complications of dental implants: identification, frequency, and associated risk factors. Int J Oral Maxillofac Implants. 2003 Nov-Dec; 18(6): 848-855.

Michalakis KX, Hirayama H, Garefis PD. Cement-retained versus screw-retained implant restorations: a critical review. Int J Oral Maxillofac Implants. 2003 Sep-Oct; 18(5): 719-728.

Miron RJ, Gruber R, Hedbom E, Saulacic N, Zhang Y, Sculean A, Bosshardt DD, Buser D. Impact of bone harvesting techniques on cell viability and the release of growth factors of autografts. Clin Implant Dent Relat Res. 2012 Feb 29. [Epub ahead of print]

Miron RJ, Hedbom E, Saulacic N, Zhang Y, Sculean A, Bosshardt DD, Buser D. Osteogenic potential of autogenous bone grafts harvested with four different surgical techniques. J Dent Res. 2011 Dec; 90(12): 1428-1433.

Mitrani R, Adolfi D, Tacher S. Adjacent implant-supported restorations in the esthetic zone: understanding the biology. J Esthet Restor Dent. 2005; 17(4): 211-222.

Mombelli A, Lang NP. The diagnosis and treatment of peri-implantitis. Periodontol 2000. 1998 Jun; 17: 63-76.

Moráguez OD, Belser UC. The use of polytetrafluoroethylene tape for the management of screw access channels in implant-supported prostheses. J Prosthet Dent. 2010 Mar; 103(3): 189-191.

Mortensen M, Lawson W, Montazem A. Osteonecrosis of the jaw associated with bisphosphonate use: presentation of seven cases and literature review. Laryngoscope. 2007 Jan; 117(1): 30-34.

Moy PK, Medina D, Shetty V, Aghaloo TL. Dental implant failure rates and associated risk factors. Int J Oral Maxillofac Implants. 2005 Jul-Aug; 20(4): 569-577.

Nyman S, Lang NP, Buser D, Brägger U. Bone regeneration adjacent to titanium dental implants using guided tissue regeneration. A report of 2 cases. Int J Oral Maxillofac Implants. 1990 Spring; 5(1): 9-14.

Olsson M, Lindhe J. Periodontal characteristics in individuals with varying form of the upper central incisors. J Clin Periodontol. 1991 Jan; 18(1): 78-82.

Pjetursson BE, Brägger U, Lang NP, Zwahlen M. Comparison of survival and complication rates of tooth-supported fixed dental prostheses (FDPs) and implant-supported FDPs and single crowns (SCs). Clin Oral Implants Res. 2007 Jun; 18 Suppl 3: 97-113.

Pjetursson BE, Karoussis I, Bürgin W, Brägger U, Lang NP. Patients' satisfaction following implant therapy. A 10-year prospective cohort study. Clin Oral Implants Res. 2005 Apr; 16(2): 185-193.

Pjetursson BE, Lang NP. Prosthetic treatment planning on the basis of scientific evidence. J Oral Rehabil. 2008 Jan; 35 Suppl 1: 72-79.

Priest G. Developing optimal tissue profiles implant-level provisional restorations. Dent Today. 2005 Nov; 24(11): 96-100.

Priest G. Esthetic potential of single-implant provisional restorations: selection criteria of available alternatives. J Esthet Restor Dent. 2006; 18(6): 326-338.

Quinn JB, Quinn GD, Sundar V. Fracture toughness of veneering ceramics for fused to metal (PFM) and zirconia dental restorative materials. J Res Natl Inst Stand Technol. **2010** Sep; 115(5): 343-352.

Rodríguez-Ciurana X, Vela-Nebot X, Segalà-Torres M, Calvo-Guirado JL, Cambra J, Méndez-Blanco V, Tarnow DP. The effect of interimplant distance on the height of the interimplant bone crest when using platform-switched implants. Int J Periodontics Restorative Dent. **2009** Apr; 29(2): 141-151.

Sailer I, Philipp A, Zembic A, Pjetursson BE, Hämmerle CH, Zwahlen M. A systematic review of the performance of ceramic and metal implant abutments supporting fixed implant reconstructions. Clin Oral Implants Res. **2009** Sep; 20 Suppl 4: 4-31.

Salama H, Salama M. The role of orthodontic extrusive remodeling in the enhancement of soft and hard tissue profiles prior to implant placement: a systematic approach to the management of extraction site defects. Int J Periodontics Restorative Dent. **1993** Aug; 13(4): 312-333.

Salama M, Coachman C, Garber D, Calamita M, Salama H, Cabral G. Prosthetic gingival reconstruction in the fixed partial restoration. Part 2: diagnosis and treatment planning. Int J Periodontics Restorative Dent. **2009** Dec; 29(6): 573-581.

Salama M, Ishikawa T, Salama H, Funato A, Garber D. Advantages of the root submergence technique for pontic site development in esthetic implant therapy. Int J Periodontics Restorative Dent. **2007** (Dec); 27(6): 521-527.

Salvi GE, Brägger U. Mechanical and technical risks in implant therapy. Int J Oral Maxillofac Implants. **2009**; 24 Suppl: 69-85.

Santosa RE. Provisional restoration options in implant dentistry. Aust Dent J. **2007**; 52(3): 234-242.

Schenk RK, Buser D, Hardwick WR, Dahlin C. Healing pattern of bone regeneration in membrane-protected defects: A histologic study in the canine mandible. Int J Oral Maxillofac Implants. **1994** Jan-Feb; 9(1): 13-29.

Schroeder A, Pohler O, Sutter F. Tissue reaction to an implant of a titanium hollow cylinder with a titanium surface spray layer [article in German]. SSO Schweiz Monatsschr Zahnheilkd. **1976** Jul; 86(7): 713-727.

Schroeder A, van der Zypen E, Stich H, Sutter F. The reactions of bone, connective tissue, and epithelium to endosteal implants with titanium-sprayed surfaces. J Maxillofac Surg. **1981** Feb; 9(1): 15-25.

Schulte W. Implants and the periodontium. Int Dent J. **1995** Feb; 45(1): 16-26.

Seibert JS. Reconstruction of deformed, partially edentulous ridges, using full thickness onlay grafts. Part I. Technique and wound healing. Compend Contin Educ Dent. **1983** Sep-Oct; 4(5): 437-453.

Sherif S, Susarla SM, Hwang JW, Weber HP, Wright RF. Clinician- and patient-reported long-term evaluation of screw- and cement-retained implant restorations: a 5-year prospective study. Clin Oral Investig. **2011** Dec; 15(6): 993-999.

Small PN, Tarnow DP, Cho SC. Gingival recession around wide-diameter versus standard-diameter implants: a 3- to 5-year longitudinal prospective study. Pract Proced Aesthet Dent. **2001** Mar; 13(2): 143-146.

Stafford GL. Survival rates of short-span implant-supported cantilever fixed dental prostheses. Evid Based Dent. **2010**; 11(2): 50-51.

Tarnow D, Elian N, Fletcher P, Froum S, Magner A, Cho SC, Salama M, Salama H, Garber DA. Vertical distance from the crest of bone to the height of the interproximal papilla between adjacent implants. J Periodontol. **2003** Dec; 74(12): 1785-1788.

Tarnow DP, Cho SC, Wallace SS. The effect of inter-implant distance on the height of inter-implant bone crest. J Periodontol. **2000** Apr; 71(4): 546-549.

Tarnow DP, Magner AW, Fletcher P. The effect of the distance from the contact point to the crest of bone on the presence or absence of the interproximal dental papilla. J Periodontol. **1992** Dec; 63(12): 995-996.

Taylor TD, Agar JR, Vogiatzi T. Implant prosthodontics: current perspective and future directions. Int J Oral Maxillofac Implants. **2000** Jan-Feb; 15(1): 66-75.

Taylor TD, Wiens J, Carr A. Evidence-based considerations for removable prosthodontic and dental implant occlusion: a literature review. J Prosthet Dent. **2005** Dec; 94(6): 555-560.

Theoharidou A, Petridis HP, Tzannas K, Garefis P. Abutment screw loosening in single-implant restorations: a systematic review. Int J Oral Maxillofac Implants. **2008** Jul-Aug; 23(4): 681-690.

Thoma DS, Jones AA, Dard M, Grize L, Obrecht M, Cochran DL. Tissue integration of a new titanium-zirconium dental implant: a comparative histologic and radiographic study in the canine. J Periodontol. **2011** Feb 22; 82(10): 1453-1461.

Turck D. A histologic comparison of the edentulous denture and non-denture bearing tissues. J Prosthet Dent. **1965** May-Jun; 15: 419-434.

Tymstra N, Raghoebar GM, Vissink A, Den Hartog L, Stellingsma K, Meijer HJ. Treatment outcome of two adjacent implant crowns with different implant platform designs in the aesthetic zone: a 1-year randomized clinical trial. J Clin Periodontol. **2011** Jan; 38 (1): 74-85.

Uchida H, Kobayashi K and Nagao M. Measurement in vivo of masticatory mucosal thickness with 20 MHz B-mode ultrasonic diagnostic equipment. J Dent Res. **1989** Feb; 68(2): 95-100.

Vailati F, Belser UC. Implant-supported fixed prostheses with integrated artificial gingiva for the esthetic zone: the pink power concept. Forum Implantologicum. **2011**; 7(2): 108-123.

von Arx T, Buser D. Horizontal ridge augmentation using autogenous block grafts and the guided bone regeneration technique with collagen membranes: a clinical study with 42 patients. Clin Oral Implants Res. **2006** Aug; 17(4): 359-366.

Weber HP, Cochran DL, The soft tissue response to osseointegrated dental implants. J Prosthet Dent. **1998** Jan; 79(1): 79-89.

Weber HP, Morton D, Gallucci GO, Roccuzzo M, Cordaro L, Grütter L. Consensus statements and recommended clinical procedures regarding loading protocols. Int J Oral Maxillofac Implants. **2009**; 24 Suppl: 180-183.

Welander M, Abrahamsson I, Berglundh T. The mucosal barrier at implant abutments of different materials. Clin Oral Implants Res. **2008** Jul; 19(7): 635-641.

Wilson TG Jr.. The positive relationship between excess cement and peri-implant disease: a prospective clinical endoscopic study. J Periodontol. **2009** Sep; 80(9): 1388-1392.

Wittneben JG, Buser D, Belser U, Brägger U. Peri-implant soft tissue conditioning with provisional restorations in the esthetic zone—the dynamic compression technique. Int J Periodontics Restorative Dent. **2012** (accepted for publication).

Zitzmann NU, Scharer P, Marinello CP. Factors influencing the success of GBR. Smoking, timing of implant placement, implant location, bone quality and provisional restoration. J Clin Periodontol. **1999** Oct; 26(10): 673-682.

Zuccati G, Bocchieri A. Implant site development by orthodontic extrusion of teeth with poor prognosis. J Clin Orthod. **2003** Jun; 37(6): 307-311.